Acknowledgements

The successful launching of a survey of this size and complexity depends upon the efforts of many individuals. Firstly I would like to thank all the other staff in Social Survey Division who have contributed to the project at some stage from its infancy to its completion. Secondly I would like to thank the dental organisers from the Department of Dental Health, of the University of Birmingham with whom we have collaborated throughout the project. It was they who made all the arrangements for the team of dental examiners, and carried out all the training functions, which was no mean task with a team of seventy dentists. I would also like to thank the many Local Education Authorities and schools involved for their help and co-operation.

On behalf of both survey staff and dental organisers I would like to thank the team of dentists who went through the training course and subsequently carried out the thirteen thousand dental examinations, and then returned yet again to complete the calibration test.

We would like to say a special thank you to the children who volunteered to help us in the training and calibration sessions, who as a result were each examined innumerable times. They came from Foundry Junior School, Birmingham; Chapel Fields, Langley and St Margarets Church of England Junior Schools, Solihull; and Kineton High School and Wootton Wawen Church of England Junior and Infants School, Warwickshire.

In addition we would like to thank the interviewers who recorded the dental data for the examiners and who also interviewed the mothers, but of course no survey could reach fruition without the co-operation of the people selected to take part, in this case the thirteen thousand children who underwent a dental examination for us and the three thousand mothers who answered the interview questions for us.

To all these we would like to express our thanks and appreciation of the part they all played in making the survey of children's dental health possible.

Notes to readers

Base numbers have been given in italics and where no base numbers are shown the whole age group is included. The base number for each age group can be found on the first table in the Table Section. Where a base number is less than twenty, statistics have not been given and this is shown by an asterisk. A dash in a table represents a proportion of less than 0.5% or an average of less than 0.05.

At the time of the survey the re-organisation of local authority areas and health areas had not taken place. The sample was, in any case, only large enough to withstand regional analysis on the basis of grouped economic planning regions, rather than individual economic planning regions. The results are therefore only available in terms of national figures or very broad regional figures, not in terms of the new area health authorities.

Most of the tables present a large amount of information in a relatively small space, which has resulted in a particular use of the percentage sign. Where the sign is at the head of a column then the figures sum to 100%. A percentage sign at the side of an individual figure signifies that this proportion of people had the attribute being discussed and that the complementary proportion (not shown on the table) did not. In some of the more complex tables both the side and column headings define the group of people eligible while the main heading indicates the attribute being considered. The percentage thus shows the proportion of those eligible who have the given attribute. For example, Table 7.5 (first row, first column) shows that there were 579 children aged five who had no debris and of this group 10% had some gum inflammation (90% did not). The first row, second column shows that there were 374 five year olds who had some debris of whom 51% had some inflammation (and 49% did not).

The data collected for this survey is very detailed and inevitably, if a report is to be published within a reasonable space of time, some issues have to be excluded. The author would be interested to receive any comments on aspects either not already included, or of value in more detail. No guarantee can be given that any request for further information would be included in future publications but any suggestion made before December 1975 would receive consideration.

Social Survey Division
Office of Population Censuses and Surveys
St. Catherines House
10 Kingsway
London

OFFICE OF POPULATION CENSUSES AND SURVEYS
SOCIAL SURVEY DIVISION

Children's Dental Health in England and Wales 1973

A survey carried out by Social Survey Division
of the Office of Population Censuses and Surveys
in collaboration with the Department of Dental
Health, University of Birmingham for the Department
of Health and Social Security

J E Todd

London: Her Majesty's Stationery Office 1975

ISBN 0 11 700687 4*

Contents

PART II - The home background

The dental organisers

Professor PMC James
Professor TD Foster
Dr R J Anderson
Dr JF Beal
Dr PH Gordon

from the Department of Dental Health, University of Birmingham

We would like to express our thanks to Professor GL Slack of the London Hospital Medical College Dental School for his advice at the preliminary planning stages

1 Introduction

In 1972 the Department of Health and Social Security and the Welsh Office, in collaboration with the Department of Education and Science, asked the Office of Population Censuses and Surveys to carry out a survey to provide information on the dental health of school children in England and Wales, and to investigate the factors which might influence the level of dental health. The study was to cover children of all ages from five to fifteen, and so complement the Survey of Adult Dental Health* carried out in 1968 on a sample of the general population aged 16 or more.

Information about the dental health of certain groups of school children was already available but a national survey of a random sample of children throughout the age range of compulsory education had not previously been undertaken. As with the earlier adult survey the children's survey was to consist of both a dental examination and an interview. Although for the older age groups it might well have been possible to interview the children themselves this would not have been possible with the younger children, so it was decided that the interviews should all be conducted with the mother of the child (or whoever was responsible for looking after the child).

The Office of Population Censuses and Surveys has no dental resources to call on, so the Department of Health invited the Department of Dental Health, University of Birmingham to collaborate on the study and to be responsible for the organisation of the dental examination, and dental training for the study. From the outset the Social Survey Division and the Department of Dental Health, University of Birmingham worked in close liason to ensure cohesion of design for the study as a whole. .

As the study was based on children of statutory school age the Department of Education asked for co-operation from the Local Education Authorities and the School Dental Service. Their co-operation was invaluable as it meant that the dental examinations could be carried out in the schools and that the authorities could be asked to nominate a dentist to attend the training course and then carry out the examinations required in each authority.

---

* Adult Dental Health in England and Wales in 1968 by P G Gray, J E Todd, G L Slack, J S Bulman. Carried out by the Government Social Survey (now a division of the Office of Population Censuses and Surveys) and the London Hospital Medical College Dental School, for the Department of Health and Social Security.

As the statutory school leaving age had not, at the time of the survey, been raised to sixteen, we were concerned with the age range five to fifteen. This age range covers the whole of the transition from a child having only deciduous teeth to having only permanent teeth. In order to establish the pattern of dental development through this period of rapid change a very large sample of children was required so that they could be analysed by year of age and sometimes by month.

We therefore aimed at a sample size of approximately 1000 children per year of age, ie a total sample size of about 11000. This size sample is very large by normal survey standards and we could not have achieved it without the co-operation of the education authorities, the schools and the School Dental Service.

With so many groups involved in the launching of the study it was essential that we could say at an early stage which local authorities were to be involved and what would be required of them in terms of dental manpower. First of all therefore we tried to estimate the workload required of one dental examiner.

We decided that the absolute upper limit to the number of dentists we could train was eighty (forty in each of two one-week courses). The maximum number of local authorities that could be involved was therefore eighty.

We planned that the dental examination should take about 6 minutes, and that the examiner could probably complete about 40 examinations a day. But the dentist might have to change schools in the middle of the day, or visit a school which had fewer than twenty children in the sample and so take less than half a day, so a certain amount of non-productive time had to be allowed for. We therefore estimated that the work load per dentist per unit* was one week's training, one week's field work and a single day later for final testing.

For the sample we randomly selected 80 specially constructed sampling units* of groups of schools. We then noted which authorities these units fell in, for they would be the authorities involved in the survey; altogether 69 authorities were involved. In the case of the large local authorities it was possible that more than one unit fell within their boundaries. In fact the very large authorities had 3 or 4 units. We asked all authorities which contained more than one unit if they would like to nominate more dentists for training, or whether they would prefer one dentist to spend longer on the field work. All the authorities which had two units agreed to let their nominated dentist do a double work load. Those authorities with 3 or 4 units mostly chose to send two dentists who each did double work loads.

Had the authorities not chosen to maximise the value of the training but to nominate more dentists we would have been in some difficulty as another issue had arisen which affected the distribution of resources. The Welsh Office put in a request to have information for Wales alone. On our original scheme the size of that part of the sample that would be in Wales was too small to allow separate Welsh analysis. To meet this new requirement meant increasing the

---

* See Section 1.1 for design of sample.

sample size in Wales three-fold. The effect of increasing the sample size in
Wales was that the total sample size was increased to about 13000 and instead
of selecting 80 units as a basis for the sample we had then to select 89. If
the authorities containing two units or more had nominated a dentist for each
unit we would have exceeded our maximum training capacity, but as it was, the
number of dentists to train was 71.

All except one of the local authorities were able to nominate a dentist to carry
out their work load. The authority which could not was happy that one of the
dental organisers should carry out the examinations on the authority's behalf.

The first letters asking for co-operation were sent to the local authorities by
the Department of Education and Science in June/July 1972 and the training and
the main fieldwork were planned to commence on January 15th 1973.

Although the inquiry was designed to combine both examination and interview data
there were insufficient resources to attempt to interview the mothers of all the
13000 children. We therefore chose to interview the mothers of some age groups
only. Once the examinations in school were completed the interviewers approached
all the mothers of the five year old children and all the mothers of the fourteen
year old children, thus finding out background information for the beginning and
end of school life. We chose to interview mothers of fourteen year olds rather
than fifteen year olds since by February-March, some of the fifteen year olds
had already left school, thus making the sample for that year incomplete.

In addition we interviewed some mothers of eight year olds and some mothers of
twelve year olds. The resources available for interviewing did not allow us to
include all of these mothers so we randomly selected one in two for interview.
We thus planned to interview about 1000 mothers of 5 year olds, 1000 mothers
of 14 year olds, 500 mothers of 8 year olds and 500 mothers of 12 year olds.

The dental examinations were completed by the middle of February and then the
interview was carried out with the mother at home, by one of Social Survey's
trained interviewers. The fieldwork on the interview side went on until April.
The documents used ie the dental examination chart, the criteria for dental
assessment, and the interview questionnaire are reproduced in the appendix.

A pilot trial of the whole procedure, the examinations and the interviews was
carried out during October 1972. This involved 7 examiners, 27 schools, 840
dental examinations and approximately 200 interviews.

1.1 The design of the sample

Before describing the sample design it is worth emphasizing that designing and
selecting a national sample involves some difficulties which would not be
encountered on a project carried out within one local authority. The sample
design is given so that the reader may understand the basis of the national study
but we are in no way suggesting that such a design should be used for local
studies.

One of the first decisions was that the survey should be restricted to maintained schools since the Local Education Authorities did not have the same responsibilities for other types of schools. It was also decided to exclude children in maintained special schools as their problems are likely to be much greater than those of children in ordinary schools. To include them would have greatly increased our organisational problems and would not have resulted in a large enough sample to give separate figures about their dental condition.

Once the decision had been made that the survey was to be launched with the co-operation of the local authorities, and with school dentists carrying out the examinations in schools, then some of the sampling decisions were already settled.

The best estimates of dental health would be obtained if the sample was spread over as many schools as possible since children in the same school are likely to have some similar characteristics eg environmental factors. On the other hand we had to have some kind of clustering in the sample or the costs would be prohibitive.

We needed a compromise between examining all the children in the schools selected and having as many schools to visit as children to examine. If the design were to involve selection of a random sample of children within schools then this meant visiting all the selected schools to sample from the registers. There are considerable advantages at the sampling stage, and fieldwork stage, therefore, if there can be some clustering of the schools. All schools are grouped to some extent in so far as they are within a particular education authority; but these authorities vary greatly in the population they cover and their geographical area and are rather too large to use as sampling units. We therefore decided to make up new 'units' specially for our sampling process. As long as each school went into one unit and one unit only then we could design the sample so that every child had an equal chance of being selected. In terms of sampling theory these units could be formed by grouping on any criteria. We decided to use factors which would help us in the organisation of the survey and make the units as like each other as possible. The work involved in making up special units was very great indeed and it fell on our sampling staff to carry this out.

The work was conducted in such a way that we obtained the maximum amount of information necessary for the administration of the inquiry as quickly as possible. This was so that we could inform the Department of Education and Science which local authorities contained some of our sample and which did not. They could then request co-operation from the relevant authorities.

We began by grouping all secondary maintained schools in England and Wales into what we called 'secondary units'. Each 'secondary unit' contained both boys and girls. Small denominational schools were grouped with non-denominational schools, and the size of the 'secondary units' was kept within the range of about 400 - 1000 pupils. If the 'secondary units' contained more than one school then an attempt was made to make the geographical grouping logical. None of the 'secondary units' contained schools from different education authorities.

In this way all secondary schools were grouped into some 4500 'secondary units'. The number of units in each education authority was counted and accumulated. We had estimated that we could afford to spread our sample through something like 80 of such units (this number was amended to 89 when the sampling for Wales was increased). The local authorities were ordered geographically and from a random start and thereafter at a constant interval, 89 'secondary units' were selected. This determined which authorities were involved and which were not. The practical organisation with the local authorities and the School Dental Service then began.

At this point in time we did not identify which particular 'secondary units' had been selected but merely determined which education authorities had at least one of our 'selected' units within their boundaries. This was because we still had to allot primary schools to our 'secondary units', and we did not wish any bias to creep into the grouping due to prior knowledge. In theory all primary schools had to be allotted to one and only one of the 'secondary units' giving us a final unit containing perhaps ten schools covering children of all ages. The number of primary schools is so large, (approximately 23,000), that to do this for the whole of England and Wales was an enormous task; but we had determined which education authorities were involved with a 'secondary unit' and which were not. We could therefore discard all the authorities and all their primary schools, which contained no selected 'secondary units', and this more than halved the work, and we were left with 69 education authorities to deal with. For these 69 education authorities we obtained information about the number and size of all their primary schools. We then allotted these primary schools to all the 'secondary units' whether or not they had been selected for the sample*. Only when all the primary schools had been allotted were the selected units identified.

We thus finally had 89 sampling units which were groups of schools, the 89 having been selected with equal probability. The next stage was to select children from those units. To retain an equal chance of selection for each child the sampling through the school registers was also carried out with a random start and at a constant interval.

Before the selection of children was carried out one further modification was made. Because there are a large number of primary schools many units contained ten or more schools. In addition many of the primary schools were very small and would only have yielded a handful of sample children for examination. We felt that the amount of time that would be spent by the dentist changing schools was going to be too high so we decided to reject at random one in two of the primary schools and double the number of children selected at those which remained. This retained the same chance of selection per child but concentrated the workload of the dentist. So in secondary schools children were selected at the rate of 1 in 18 and in half of the original primary schools they were selected at the rate of 1 in 9.

The original sample was designed as a self-weighting scheme but once the decision had been made to increase the sample for Wales then a weighting factor was

---

* The grouping was carried out on the basis of about equal numbers of primary schools per unit, with sensible geographical grouping where possible.

introduced. In Wales groups of schools, that is sampling units, had a three times greater chance of selection than did groups of schools in England. Thus the children in Wales had a three times greater chance of selection. This gave us a big enough sample to examine the Welsh position separately but of course in all analyses where England and Wales are grouped together the Welsh sample is down-weighted by a factor of three to restore the proper balance.

The sample covers all children in maintained schools aged 5-15 on December 31st 1972. But not all children aged 15 on December 31st 1972 were still in school. Some children aged 15 during the year would have left school before the October in which we selected the sample. It is likely that those who had left school at the first opportunity were not representative of all 15 year olds. The sample of 15 year olds still in school is likely to be better dentally than a sample of all 15 year olds and this leads to some anomalies, for since disease and treatment progress one would expect a deterioration with age. The apparent deterioration from 14 to 15 years shown by the survey results is probably never as great as it would be had the 15 year old age group been complete and is, in fact, sometimes reversed as a result of the loss of the early school leaver.

1.2 The administration

One of the major challenges in this inquiry was the administrative organisation required to launch it. The collaboration between survey organisers and dental organisers required frequent communications between Birmingham and London. At the outset this had to be viewed as a potential difficulty but in the event it worked very smoothly. Maybe this was because right at the beginning we defined exactly where the responsibilities lay for the different parts of the operation.

Of course, the major administrative headache was the large number of people and authorities who were to be involved in the inquiry. Initially the Department of Education and Science contacted the 69 local authorities and requested co-operation from the Chief Education Officer and the Chief Medical Officer and through him the Chief Dental Officer. Once co-operation in principle had been received, Social Survey Division contacted these people again to explain what would be required. At the same time a letter of explanation and a request for co-operation was sent to the head teacher of each of the schools which had come up in the sample (and that amounted to 506 schools).

We felt that the head teachers would, with justification, want to know exactly what to expect and when, so we worked out a timetable for the whole of our sample saying which day(s) or half-days we would wish to be in the school. This information was sent in the autumn of 1972 and referred to dates in the following January and February 1973. The head teachers were very co-operative indeed. Obviously there were some instances in which we had selected days on which the school could not accommodate us, but we only had to amend the arrangements for about 30-40 of the 500 or so schools.

The consequence of arranging the actual days that the dentist would visit the school so far in advance was that we also had to allocate the nominated dentist to the two training courses so that his availability agreed with the timetable. We made this allocation on the basis that all the dentists who had large workloads to carry out should attend the first training course so that they could have a week's head start on the fieldwork. Again we were very fortunate as there were only one or two instances where we in fact had to change the dentist from one course to another because of an immovable prior commitment.

On this first contact with the schools we also had to make a general arrangement about visiting the schools to carry out the sampling from the school registers. This work was carried out by Social Survey interviewers during October 1972.

We did not, at this stage, identify to the Chief Dental Officer or the nominated dentist which schools had been selected in the sample, although we did inform the Chief Education Officer in which of his schools we were sampling and later examining. The reason for witholding the information from the dentist was that we did not wish in any way to influence the programme of school inspections to be carried out in the autumn term and some schools that had just been or were about to be inspected were bound to be contained in our sample. Neither did we particularly want the nominated dentist to be chosen on the basis of the schools selected in the sample. We appreciate that in some instances this probably made the administration a bit more difficult at the local level.

When we planned the timetable for visiting schools we tried to make the journeys and changes from school to school as geographically sensible as we could. But our knowledge of the areas concerned was limited compared with local knowledge, especially in rural parts of Wales. But the administrative enormity of trying to obtain local advice when we had over 500 schools and very little time to get the survey launched made a local approach impossible. At the time of the field-work we are sure that some of the dentists suffered because of rather inefficient itineraries. If that was so we apologise but the time available and the size of the problem just did not allow us to go any further.

Early in January 1973 we notified the nominated dentists of the schools they would be going to and we wrote again to all the schools confirming the dates. We also sent the head teacher a list of the children we would wish to see. This in itself was a large administrative task since the lists involved 13000 children.

Meanwhile the dental organisers had been planning and organising the week's training course for the nominated dentists. They had been contacting the dentists independently to make arrangements for accommodation for the course and to circulate the dental examination information. The amount of organisation that was required to set up the training course and repeat it for the second set of dentists was enormous and is described in the appendix.

With the training courses and fieldwork being carried out in January and February we faced possible loss of examinations due to sickness, both of the children, and of the dentists. Two examiners were taken ill just before the training course began; the authorities concerned could not at that late stage provide replacements but two other authorities whose dentists did not have very big workloads obligingly seconded their examiners to complete the work. As far as sickness among the children was concerned the dentists made recall visits wherever possible to examine children absent at the first visit so our losses were reduced to the minimum.

At this time of year we also faced the possibility of bad weather, but fortunately January and February 1973 were unseasonably mild.

Because of these risks some people might criticise the launching of a National Dental Survey at this time of year, but there were other factors besides sickness and weather which affected our decision. Any time later in the school year we would have had serious problems with examinations in secondary schools, and an even higher proportion of fifteen year olds would have left school. When sampling from school registers one must carry out the selection process on the appropriate year's registers. To sample in the summer term when all the classes would change in the autumn would be grossly inefficient, and the schools must be allowed a reasonable time in the autumn to start the new school year and get their own organisation in hand before requesting access to the registers. After the initial selection had been done in schools some checking and further sampling processes had still to be done at Headquarters, as well as the preparation of lists of children required for examination. By this stage one has run into Christmas holidays, and the earliest it seemed feasible to launch the fieldwork was after the schools had settled back after the Christmas break. We could not, in fact, train the dentists until the children were back at school and available as subjects* so this determined our starting date of January 15th.

1.3 An outline of the dental examination

A full description of the dental criteria, training and calibration, together with copies of the documents used, will be found in the appendix.

The examination took on average 3 or 4 minutes once the examiners had become accustomed to it. Initially it took a little longer and we had made all our time-tables in terms of an examination rate of about ten children an hour.

The examination covered four main areas of interest, the effects and consequences of decay, the evidence of trauma, the condition of the soft tissues and the orthodontic condition of the child. In the time available for examination some of these areas were necessarily covered only briefly. The content of the examination is most easily described in the order in which it was executed.

The dental examination did not include any assessment by the dentist as to the reason for the loss of any missing deciduous teeth. The presence or absence of teeth was recorded in respect to the 32 possible tooth positions. Over the range where both permanent and deciduous teeth could be found the dentition was identified for those teeth present. Where the deciduous and permanent tooth were simultaneously present for the same tooth position this fact was recorded, but the detailed information about the condition of the tooth was confined to the permanent tooth.

Where there was no tooth present the dentist recorded the reason for the absence of the permanent tooth. If the dentist felt that a permanent tooth had been removed he was asked to assess, by asking the child and from his clinical

---

* See Appendix C.

experience, the reason for the loss, in terms of decay, orthodontic treatment or trauma.

For each tooth present the dentist recorded the condition of each surface in terms of any filling or decay. Surfaces recorded as filled included only those surfaces with satisfactory fillings. Surfaces which involved decay were recorded in one of three categories.

(a) decayed, but restorable

(b) decayed, involving the pulp and is unrestorable (see the dental criteria, Appendix C)

(c) filled and decayed, but restorable.

If a filled surface was also so badly decayed that it was no longer restorable by routine methods then it was recorded as unrestorable and the filling was ignored.

The information collected about the surfaces of the teeth present was summarised to obtain the following categories for each tooth position.

(i)	Tooth is sound and untreated	
(ii)	Tooth is filled otherwise sound (F or f)	
(iii)	Tooth is filled, but decayed	
(iv)	Tooth is decayed not previously treated	(D or d)
(v)	Tooth is decayed and unrestorable	
(vi)	Permanent tooth is unerupted	
(vii)	Permanent tooth is missing (Caries)	(M)
(viii)	Permanent tooth is missing (Trauma)	(T)
(ix)	Permanent tooth is missing (Orthodontic)	(O)

The dentist then examined the four upper and four lower incisors for any evidence of trauma, and recorded whether the child had a denture or not.

The dentist next examined the gums to see whether or not there was any inflammation and the extent of its seriousness. He also examined the mouth for any visual evidence of debris (plaque, materia alba, etc.) and calculus. All the soft tissue measurements were carried out in each of six segments* of the mouth.

The remainder of the examination dealt with the occlusion and position of the teeth. The dentist measured the overbite and overjet. The former was measured in terms of the fraction of lower teeth covered by upper teeth, the latter was measured to the nearest millimetre. The existence of buccal crossbite, instanding incisors and mucosal trauma were recorded and an estimate made of the occlusal classification. The mouth was examined, in six segments, for any signs of actual or potential crowding, and the existence of any orthodontic appliance was recorded. For children aged 8 or more the dentist asked the child about any experience of wearing an orthodontic appliance. The dentist then recorded his opinion as to whether orthodontic treatment was likely to be necessary. This judgement was made in terms only of the occlusion and position of the teeth. The dentists were asked to ignore the level of decay and the oral hygiene condition. Finally the dentist noted any dental anomaly which existed but was outside the main criteria for the examination.

---

* Upper 8-4, 3-3, 4-8; Lower 8-4, 3-3, 4-8

1.4 An outline of the interview

The interview was designed to obtain, from the mother, a fairly simple history of the child's dental experience. This included whether the child had ever been to the dentist, and whether he had ever had any dental treatment, and if so, whether the child had any experience of conservation or extraction. The mother was also asked about the range of dental services which the child had experienced (eg private, NHS, local authority). Details were obtained relating to any accidents which had involved the teeth, any bouts of toothache and any problems with growth and development. We also asked some questions about visiting the dentist's surgery, and how the mother felt the child reacted to such visits and what she did about it.

In a section less directly related to the dentist and dental treatment we obtained background information about early childhood in terms of feeding, the use of dummies and thumb sucking. We asked the mothers some questions about dental development in childhood and their opinions about dental hygiene and dental visits.

We also asked some questions about the kind of food that was generally eaten, the consumption of sweets and biscuits and the knowledge the mother had about fluoride.

In addition to the information related to the child selected in the sample we found out about the size of the family and his position in it. We also found out about the dental status of his mother and father, their attendance pattern and their dental expectation for their offspring. In addition we collected basic data such as the age of the parents and the occupation of the father upon which social class is based.

The interview took on average about an hour and co-operation was very high. The questionnaire is reproduced in full in the appendix.

1.5 The response

The response on this survey was very high, both at the dental examination level and at the interview level. For the sample of children involved in the interview stage we only intended to contact the mother if the child had been examined in school. So the level of response at the examination stage affected the level that could be achieved at the interview stage.

Before we could carry out the dental examinations at all we had to obtain the permission of the head teacher to carry out the survey in his school. The initial selection meant that we contacted 506 schools, whereupon we found that seven had closed without an identifiable replacement. Among the 499 remaining schools one secondary school declined to take part. We estimate that we would have sampled 42 children for examination from this school. The remaining 498 schools produced a total of 12910 children for examination. One school, although agreeing to co-operate, could not fit in a visit from us during the fieldwork period and so a further 33 possible examinations were lost. Among the 497 schools we visited some children were found to have left that school, and others were absent at all visits. Overall, including losses for all reasons we examined 95% of the original sample.

Table 1.1
Co-operation achieved

Response at Examination Stage

	Children	%
Left that school (district)	335	
Absent, all calls	236	
No reason given - probably absent	38	5
Schools withdrawn*	75	
Refusal±	11	
Other reasons (deceased medical ineligible)	7	
	}702	
Total children examined	12250	95
Original Sample	12952	100

Response at Interview Stage

	Children	%
Not dentally examined	195	6
'Mother' not interviewed: Refused	73	2
Non contact	35	1
'Mother' interviewed	3137	91
Total	3440	100

* Includes an estimated 42 children from a school that declined to take part.

± A few schools notified the parents in advance of the examination resulting in six children being withdrawn at the request of the parents: the other five children themselves declined the examination.

The success of the examination stage was due very largely to the co-operation
of the schools and conscientious efforts of the dental examiners to make re-calls
at the schools in order to examine, where possible, the children absent from school
at the time of the first visit.

The co-operation achieved from the mothers was also very high.   Among the sample
of mothers selected for interview 6% were lost because a dental examination had
not been achieved with the child and it seemed pointless to proceed with the
interview.   Losses of mothers in addition to this were very small; only 2% of
mothers declined to be interviewed and a further 1% were not contacted (mainly
because they had moved).   We thus achieved examinations and interviews with 91%
of the sample selected for both parts of the inquiry.

Part I

Dental condition

2 Dental development

The changing pattern of dentitions between the ages of five and fifteen means
that at the time of the survey examination some of the children in our sample had
no permanent teeth yet erupted whereas others had no deciduous teeth remaining.
The variations in dental development ranged widely even among children born in
the same calendar year. We found that among five to seven year olds some
children had a wholly deciduous dentition and among nine to fifteen year olds
some children had lost all their deciduous teeth but for each age group there
was a proportion of children with a mixed dentition. This proportion varied
with age from 42% of five year olds to 100% of eight year olds, decreasing to
5% of fourteen year olds.

Examining the process of the loss of the deciduous dentition is, of course,
complicated by the premature loss of some teeth extracted because of decay.
Nevertheless it is of interest to look in some detail at the teeth which would
be expected to be the first to exfoliate naturally. For this purpose we examine
the proportion of children still retaining their lower left central deciduous
incisor, grouping the children by month of birth (two months at a time).

Table 2.1

Proportion of children retaining their lower
left central deciduous incisor by month of birth

Age	Month born	Lower left central deciduous incisor present	
Five	Nov-Dec	96%	118
	Sept-Oct	87%	132
	July-Aug	84%	180
	May-June	76%	168
	Mar-Apr	64%	178
	Jan-Feb	52%	182
Six	Nov-Dec	48%	162
	Sept-Oct	34%	172
	July-Aug	23%	200
	May-June	19%	171
	Mar-Apr	11%	200
	Jan-Feb	13%	174
Seven	Nov-Dec	4%	167
	Sept-Oct	4%	170
	July-Aug	3%	200

Even among the youngest children some of the lower left central deciduous incisors were lost, (this might have been due to extraction rather than exfoliation) but the great majority, 96%, were still present. The reduction in this proportion with each two monthly increase of age suggests that normal exfoliation rather than extraction is responsible for the majority of the loss from then on. The process of exfoliation has affected the lower left central deciduous incisor to a greater extent in each group of children who are on average two months older but it is not until the children are aged seven that the proportion with the tooth still present falls to a very low level. Thus the first stages of transition from deciduous to permanent dentition can occur within a considerable range of age, indicating that dental development and chronological age are not particularly closely related.

The divergence between dental development and chronological age can also be shown by the eruption patterns of the permanent teeth.

2.1 Permanent tooth eruption by sex and age (in two-monthly groups)

We obtained detailed results of the eruption pattern of the different teeth for boys and girls separately and we divided each year of age into six two-monthly groups. This increase in the number of points we could plot made some of the base numbers rather small. We therefore calculated a three point moving average to reduce the random fluctuations in the results. The results are shown in Figure 2.1.

The rate of eruption of permanent teeth among boys and girls is generally similar but at any particular age a greater proportion of girls have the given tooth erupted. This difference is most noticeable for the lower canines where, between the ages of nine years four months and ten and a half years, these teeth have erupted for over 30% more girls than boys. The upper canines maintain this difference, reaching 25% among those aged ten years four months and ten and a half years. The upper first molars are the only teeth where the relationship between age and proportion of children having that tooth erupted is the same for both sexes.

It can be seen from the diagrams that variations of the eruption of any particular tooth with age is considerable for both boys and girls. This is best illustrated by the lower second premolars. Eruption of this tooth has occurred for some children aged seven whilst for others it is still not present by the age of fifteen, although it has erupted for over 90% of girls aged thirteen and boys aged fourteen. The tooth showing the least variation of eruption with age is the lower central incisor. In this case the tooth was already present among the five year olds (10% of both sexes at five years four months) and had erupted for nearly all girls (97%) by the age of seven years four months and nearly all boys (99%) by the age of seven years ten months.

Thus the diagrams show that both sexes experience the same large variations in the age at which particular teeth erupt but for boys the whole process tends to occur later than for girls, this time lag being as much as a year for the lower canines.

Figure 2.1   Permanent tooth eruption patterns by sex and age in two-month
intervals

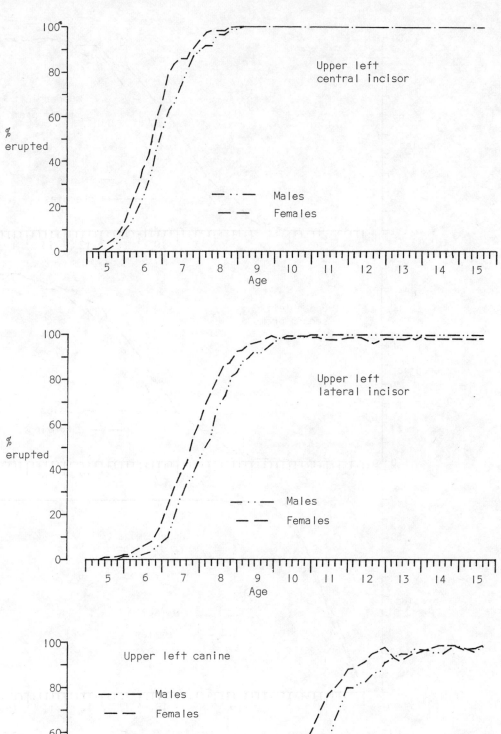

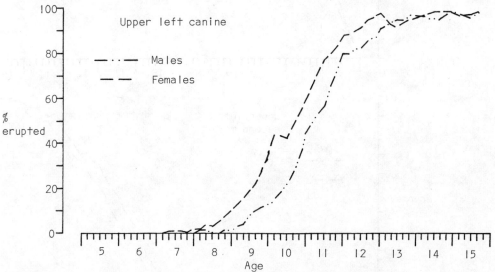

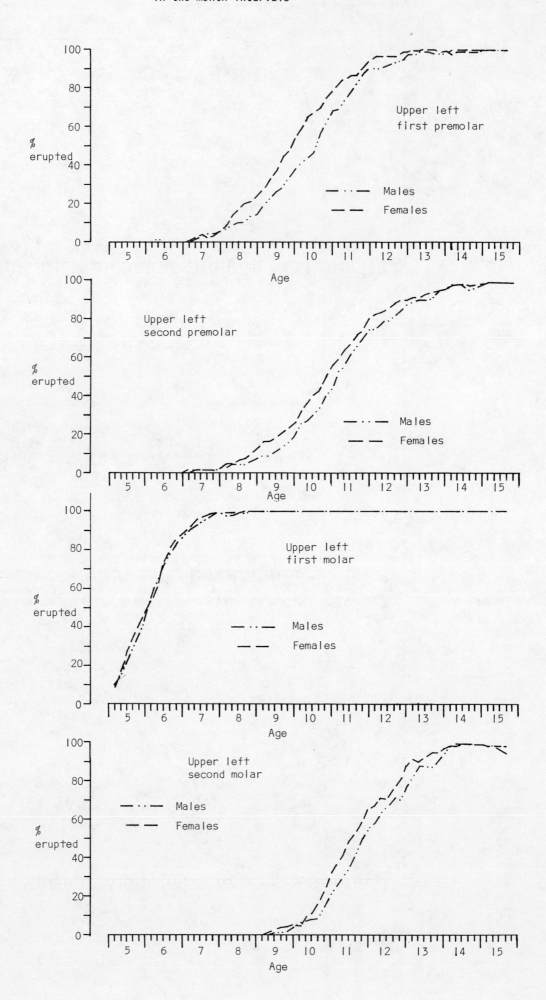

Figure 2.1 (contd) Permanent tooth eruption patterns by sex and age
in two-month intervals

18

Figure 2.1 (contd)   Permanent tooth eruption patterns by sex and age
                     in two-month intervals

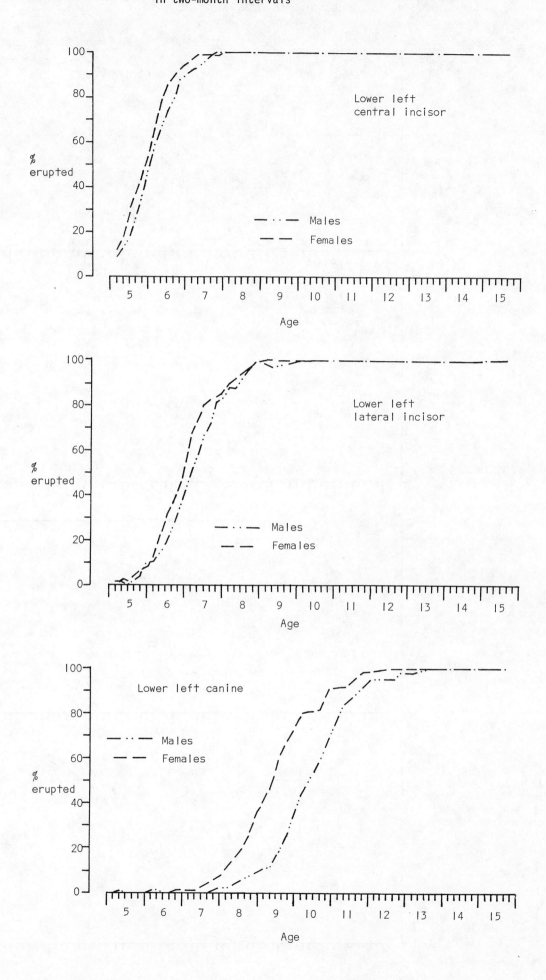

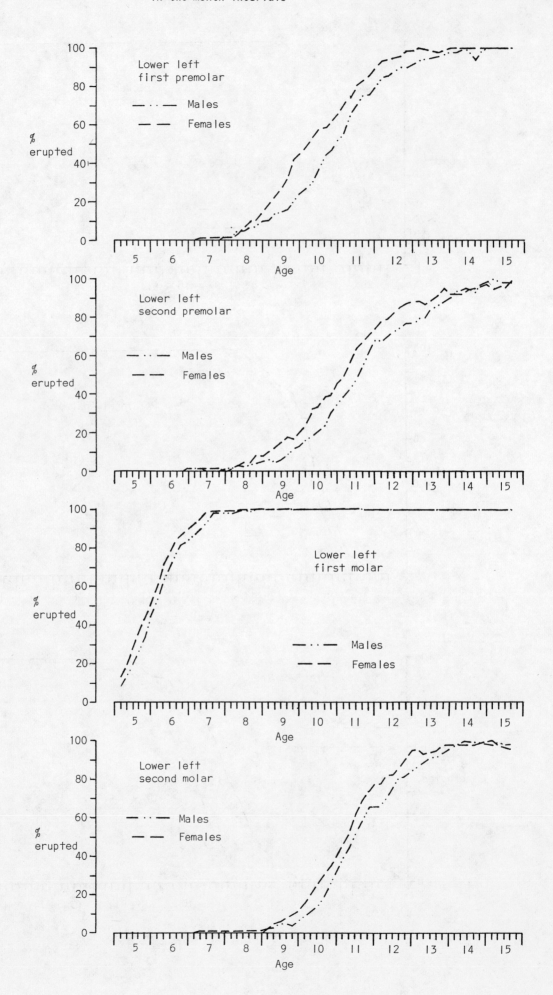

Figure 2.1 (contd) Permanent tooth eruption patterns by sex and age
in two-month intervals

2.2 Dental development and total decay experience

Any measurement of dental development and total decay experience is complicated
by the natural pattern of tooth development. Normally in childhood, twenty
deciduous teeth erupt and during their lifetime these teeth may or may not
become decayed; and the decay may or may not be treated, either by conservation
or extraction. Whatever the dental history of the deciduous teeth they will, in
due course, naturally drop out, if they have not already been extracted for decay
reasons. Once the teeth are gone it is not possible to say with certainty
whether there had been any decay or not, and as soon as the permanent teeth start
to erupt it is easy to concentrate entirely on these and forget the deciduous
antecedents. In the absolute sense, however, the decay experience of an
individual is the sum of what happens to fifty-two teeth.

Assessing the likely decay experience of missing permanent teeth is not nearly
such a formidable task since permanent teeth are not naturally shed, and in the
age group 5-15 years the numbers of missing permanent teeth are relatively small.
The dental examiners were therefore asked to assess whether missing permanent
teeth were absent due to decay, orthodontic extraction, through damage from an
accident, or as yet unerupted. In doing this they used their dental knowledge
and experience, and they asked the child when they felt this would clarify the
position.

As far as the deciduous dentition was concerned the dental examiners were asked
not to make any assessment as to the decay experience of missing deciduous teeth.
This was because the survey covered children of widely varying ages and with a team
of 70 dentists carrying out approximately 13000 examinations we needed the
criteria for examination to be well defined and universally applicable.

The dental examination as carried out thus includes only known decay experience,
that is permanent teeth classified as filled, decayed or missing, or deciduous
teeth classified as filled or decayed.

Wherever the survey results deal with disease experience the reader's attention
is drawn to the fact that the survey only measured known disease experience.

This is not to say that an estimate of total disease cannot be made. Such
estimates are, in fact, discussed in detail in Chapter 4. It must be
understood however that these estimates are derived from certain specific
assumptions, and then applied to the data after it has been collected, not
by the dentist at the time of collection.

Because of the difficulties in assessing total disease for deciduous teeth there
are many advantages in analysing the two dentitions separately. In some
circumstances however, such as when one is determining the total current need
for treatment, it would seem more relevant to look at the mouth regardless of
dentition. Another factor worth taking into account is the likely use of the
results in comparison with other studies. Such comparisons are impossible if the
presentation is fundamentally different.

For these reasons the detailed tables giving distributions of the number of
children with varying numbers of teeth in varying conditions have been produced

for the dentitions together and separately. We hope that this will result in the most flexible presentation allowing the biggest range of comparisons. One hazard of presenting results in such detail is that, due to rounding, some of the figures do not add exactly. For example the average number of teeth with known disease experience can be viewed in all its component parts and for separate dentitions. In some instances the reader may find that the component parts do not exactly add to the overall figure, since they have each been separately rounded.

3   Dental decay and treatment

3.1 Active decay

The average number of teeth that need treatment provides an overall picture of
the situation but it is of interest also to look at the extent of current
treatment need among children. At the time of the examination 63% of five year
olds had some active decay. In no age group except the fifteen year olds* did
this proportion fall below 60% and it was as high as 78% among the eight year
olds. Among the younger children the current decay was, of course, mainly in
the deciduous dentition but even among five year olds we found a few children
with erupted permanent first molars which were already decayed.

Table 3.1

Proportion of children with some active decay

Age	Proportion of children with some active decay		
	Deciduous teeth	Permanent teeth	Either dentition
Five	63%	3%	63%
Six	68%	12%	69%
Seven	68%	27%	73%
Eight	72%	40%	78%
Nine	66%	42%	76%
Ten	51%	46%	69%
Eleven	32%	53%	66%
Twelve	15%	54%	61%
Thirteen	7%	58%	61%
Fourteen	2%	61%	62%
Fifteen	1%	57%	57%

Active decay involving permanent teeth was found among as many as 40%
of eight year olds; for twelve year olds 54% had some active decay involving
permanent teeth and the proportion was as high as 61% among the fourteen year
olds.   With this proportion of children involved with active decay at the
time of the survey it is of considerable interest to examine the proportion
of children with a large number of teeth actively decayed when we examined
them.

---

* This was probably due to the fact that the fifteen year old group excluded
early school leavers, see Section 1.1.

The determination of what is 'a large number' is again complicated by the different stages of dental development and, so, for illustration we present two levels, those of five or more and ten or more teeth involved with active decay at the time of the examination.

Nearly a quarter of children in the age range 5-8 had five or more actively decayed teeth (of either dentition) when we examined them. Among the five and six year olds this was mainly due to decay in the deciduous dentition, but from then on the permanent dentition was making its contribution. As the deciduous dentition is lost the permanent dentition is itself contributing more towards extensive decay, and in combination the proportion of children with five or more teeth actively decayed remained above 10%. Throughout the age range there was a small group of children (1-3%) who had as many as ten decayed teeth at the time of examination.

Table 3.2
Proportion of children with extensive active decay

Age	Proportion of children with active decay in					
	Deciduous teeth		Permanent teeth		Either dentition	
	5 or more teeth	10 or more teeth	5 or more teeth	10 or more teeth	5 or more teeth	10 or more teeth
Five	23%	5%	-	-	23%	5%
Six	22%	3%	-	-	23%	3%
Seven	19%	1%	-	-	27%	3%
Eight	11%	-	1%	-	23%	3%
Nine	8%	-	-	-	18%	2%
Ten	4%	-	2%	-	14%	1%
Eleven	1%	-	6%	-	13%	-
Twelve	-	-	8%	1%	10%	1%
Thirteen	-	-	10%	1%	11%	1%
Fourteen	-	-	12%	2%	14%	2%
Fifteen	-	-	10%	2%	10%	2%

At the age of eleven the proportion of children with five or more actively decayed teeth was 6% and this rose with age until among the fourteen year olds we found 12% of children with 5 or more currently decayed permanent teeth (the lower figure for 15 year olds is probably due to the loss from the sample of the early school leavers).

3.2 Filled teeth
Since decay is so widespread the form of treatment received for decay is of paramount importance in terms of retaining a functional dentition. First we show the amount of restorative treatment that was evident among the children we examined.

Among five year olds a quarter of children had some filled* teeth when we examined them. At this age the fillings were in deciduous teeth only (although we have

---

* Filled otherwise sound. See Section 1.3.

Table 3.3

Proportion of children with some filled* teeth

Age	Proportion of children with some filled* teeth		
	Deciduous teeth	Permanent teeth	Either dentition
Five	26%	-	26%
Six	38%	5%	39%
Seven	42%	17%	47%
Eight	45%	37%	57%
Nine	44%	50%	64%
Ten	33%	61%	67%
Eleven	21%	66%	70%
Twelve	10%	75%	76%
Thirteen	4%	77%	77%
Fourteen	1%	81%	81%
Fifteen	1%	88%	88%

* *Filled otherwise sound.*

seen that in fact in this age group some permanent first molars were decayed). Among the six year olds two out of five children had some filled teeth and by this age some of the fillings were in the permanent dentition. Among seven year olds 17% had some filled permanent teeth and nearly half the children had some filled teeth. Among eight year olds over a third had some filled permanent teeth and over a half had some filled teeth in either dentition. The proportion of children with some filled teeth increased with age reaching three-quarters of twelve year olds and over 80% of fourteen year olds (the high proportion for fifteen year olds probably reflects the loss from that group of the early school leavers). We look next at the proportion of children who have (for their age) a fairly large number of filled teeth. By the age of twelve nearly a quarter of children had five or more filled teeth. Among the thirteen year olds 8% had as many as ten or more filled teeth, among fourteen year olds 13% had ten or more filled teeth.

Table 3.4

Proportion of children with extensive numbers of filled* teeth

Age	Proportion of children with				
	Deciduous teeth	Permanent teeth		Either dentition	
	5 or more filled* teeth	5 or more filled* teeth	10 or more filled* teeth	5 or more filled* teeth	10 or more filled* teeth
Five	3%	-	-	3%	-
Six	5%	-	-	7%	-
Seven	6%	-	-	11%	-
Eight	7%	-	-	16%	2%
Nine	6%	1%	-	18%	1%
Ten	3%	2%	-	19%	2%
Eleven	1%	11%	1%	22%	2%
Twelve	-	19%	3%	23%	3%
Thirteen	-	35%	8%	35%	8%
Fourteen	-	46%	13%	47%	13%
Fifteen	-	61%	19%	60%	19%

* *Filled otherwise sound.*

3.3 Extracted teeth

Treatment by extraction can only be shown with respect to permanent teeth as the dental examination did not include any assessment of why deciduous teeth had been lost*. From the age of seven onwards we found that some children had had some permanent teeth extracted.

Table 3.5

Proportion of children with some extracted permanent teeth

Age	Proportion of children with	
	One (or more) permanent teeth extracted for decay	Four (or more) permanent teeth extracted for decay
Five	-	-
Six	-	-
Seven	1%	-
Eight	4%	-
Nine	8%	1%
Ten	13%	3%
Eleven	18%	4%
Twelve	23%	6%
Thirteen	28%	6%
Fourteen	31%	9%
Fifteen	33%	9%

By the age of ten, one in ten children had lost at least one permanent tooth by extraction. By the age of fourteen about 30% had lost at least one permanent tooth by extraction, in fact by the age of fourteen nearly one child in ten had four or more permanent teeth extracted for decay reasons.

3.4 Dental condition of individual deciduous teeth

The summary information about the whole mouth (eg total disease experience, DMF + df) is the resultant of many varying components. The situation is complicated not only by the two dentitions but also by the variation in ages at which the different deciduous teeth naturally exfoliate and the permanent teeth erupt. The effect of dental disease in children of different ages is somewhat simplified by examining the progress (or deterioration) of particular teeth. In this chapter we confine ourselves to the deciduous dentition. Figure 3.1 shows diagrammatically the contribution being made to dental health by different teeth at different ages. The diagrams show the proportion of teeth that are decayed and the proportion that have been filled. In addition the proportion that are sound are shown and also the proportion of permanent teeth that have erupted at each age to replace the deciduous dentition. Only the left side of the mouth has been used to illustrate the situation as the disease and treatment pattern was symmetrical. Tables 63-73 in the Table Section give the full results for all teeth.

---

* See Section 4.2 for estimate of total disease experience of deciduous teeth.

As far as deciduous incisors were concerned only the tail end of their lifespan came into the survey age range. The difference between the proportion of deciduous incisor teeth still present and the permanent teeth erupted was very small, indicating that most of deciduous incisor tooth loss was due to natural exfoliation with fairly rapid eruption of the permanent incisors. The vast majority of deciduous incisors present at the examination were sound although at the age of five 14% of upper 'a's were decayed as were 7% of upper 'b's. The deciduous incisors did not have any fillings.

The deciduous canines 'c' contributed for a much longer time to the dental health of the children in the sample. The vase majority of these teeth were disease free.

Most of the disease found in the deciduous canines was untreated although a small number of the teeth had been filled. The loss of the deciduous canine and its replacement by a permanent tooth occurred at very different ages in different children. The first losses occurred at seven and eight years old with permanent tooth eruption among some eight year olds. At the other extreme some deciduous canines were still retained at thirteen, fourteen and fifteen. Despite the long range there were relatively few children for whom neither deciduous nor permanent tooth was present at examination. There was nothing to suggest that this was not the natural state of affairs.

The deciduous first molars ('d') made a somewhat shorter contribution towards the lifespan of the deciduous dentition than did the deciduous canines, but they made a much greater contribution to disease experience. By the age of seven 30% of children had a decayed or filled deciduous first molar present. Of the diseased teeth present fewer than half were filled at any age. The lower first molar experienced more disease than the upper equivalent. The difference between the proportion of lower first deciduous molars present, and the proportion of erupted permanent teeth is much larger than was shown with the canines and probably indicates the level of extraction of deciduous molars for caries reasons.

The deciduous second molar ('e') contributed more than any other tooth towards disease in the primary dentition. Among the diseased teeth still present nearly a half of second molars were filled. Again there was a considerable disparity between missing deciduous 'e's and erupting permanent teeth. For example some lower second molars were missing in children aged five although no permanent teeth erupted in that position until the age of eight. This early loss of deciduous second molars for decay reasons occurred much more frequently in the lower jaw than in the upper.

From the diagrams it can be seen that over the range of age 5-15 it is the deciduous molars which make a marked contribution to disease and treatment in deciduous teeth, the incisors are very quickly lost and the canines are not so prone to decay.

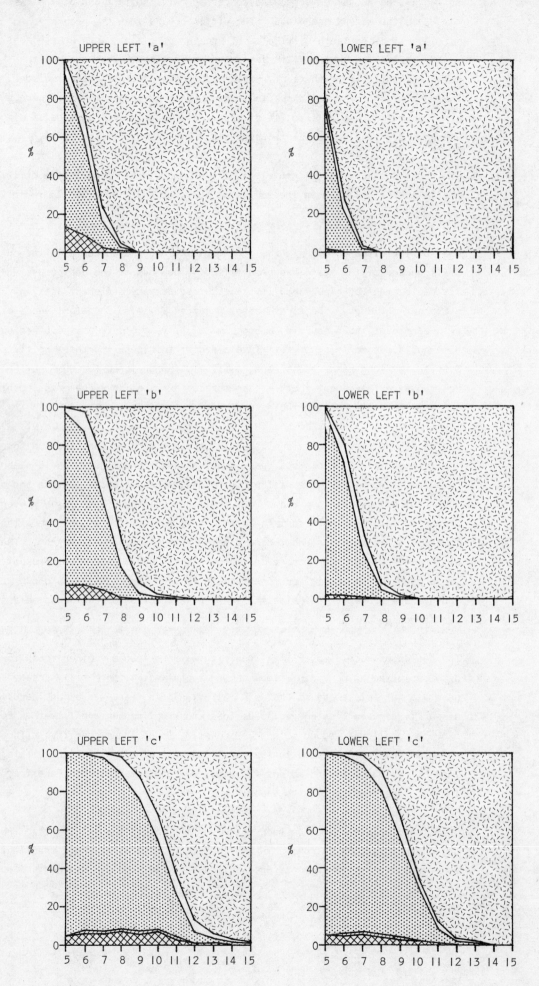

Figure 3.1 Deciduous incisors and canines

Figure 3.1 (contd) Deciduous first molars

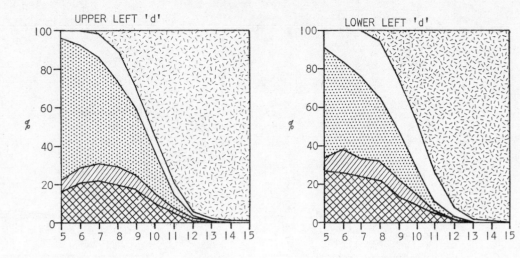

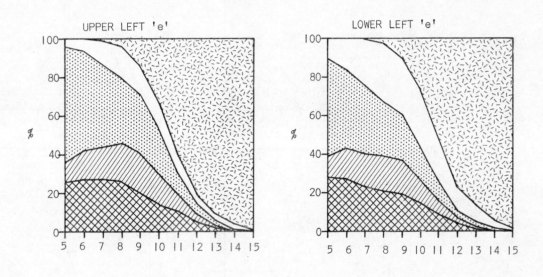

KEY

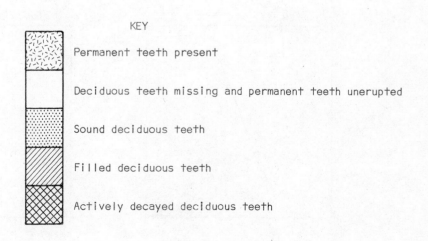

Permanent teeth present

Deciduous teeth missing and permanent teeth unerupted

Sound deciduous teeth

Filled deciduous teeth

Actively decayed deciduous teeth

Figure 3.2   Decay and treatment experience of individual permanent teeth

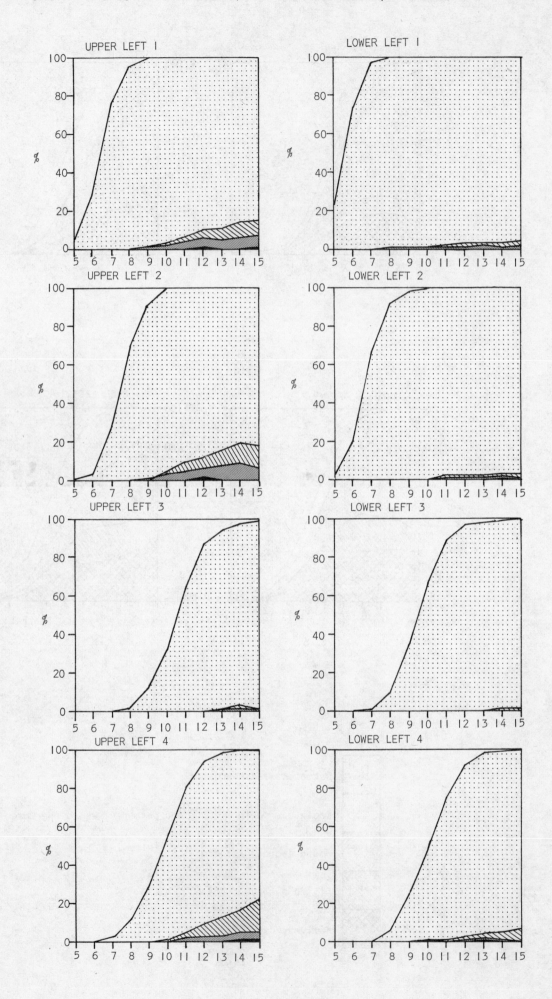

Figure 3.2 (contd)   Decay and treatment experience of individual permanent
                     teeth

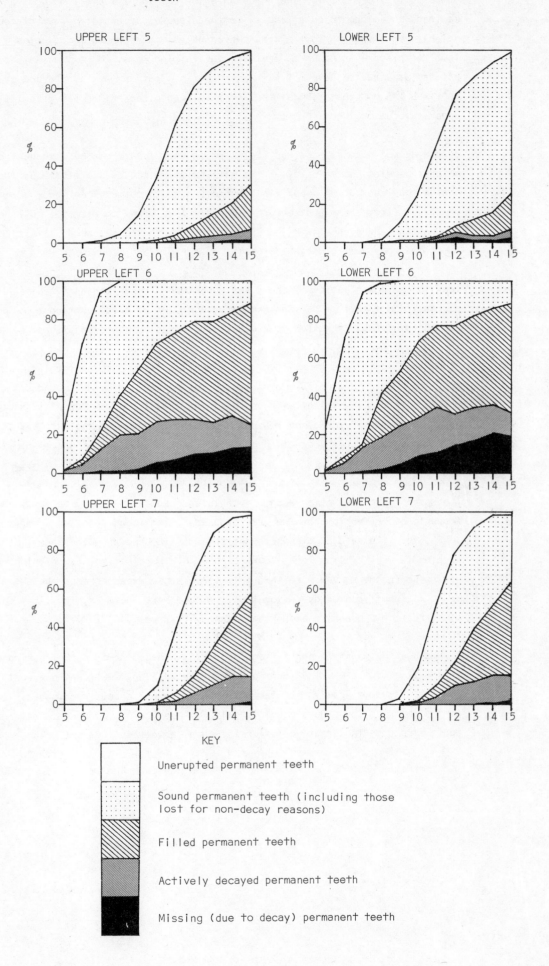

KEY

Unerupted permanent teeth

Sound permanent teeth (including those
lost for non-decay reasons)

Filled permanent teeth

Actively decayed permanent teeth

Missing (due to decay) permanent teeth

3.5 Dental condition of individual permanent teeth

Compared to the posterior teeth the anterior permanent teeth (incisors and canines) do not contribute largely to the disease pattern of permanent teeth in children aged five to fifteen. Nevertheless there was a fairly high level of disease in upper central and lateral incisors. More than half of the disease appeared to have met with restorative treatment but by the age of fourteen 14% of upper central incisors had been diseased, as had been 19% of upper lateral incisors.

By the age of nine disease was beginning to show itself on the permanent pre-molars. Again, the majority of the decayed teeth had been filled. By the age of fourteen 20% of upper first premolars had disease experience; however, the lower first premolars were considerably less prone to disease. Differences between the upper and lower jaw did not occur with the second premolars where among fourteen year olds, 20% of both had decay experience.

The biggest contribution to the disease pattern of the permanent teeth came, of course, from the first permanent molar. Over 20% of first permanent molars were present among the five year olds. There was evidence of disease very early in its lifespan, and by the age of nine a half of first molars had become diseased. In the age range five to fifteen the first permanent molar is the only tooth which appreciably contributes towards the 'missing' component of the 'DMF + df' classification. In the lower jaw as many as 20% of first molars had been extracted for decay reasons among the fourteen year olds. Throughout the age groups studied more than a half of the first molars found to be diseased had been filled.

The second permanent molar erupts much later than the first. The tooth is first found to be present among nine year olds and first found diseased among ten year olds. The rate of disease experienced by the second molar once it has erupted is very similar to that experienced by the first molar. Within the age range in the survey more than half the disease experience of the second molar had been treated by restoration. There were, however, the first signs of extractions occurring among the teenage children.

Although a few fourteen and fifteen year olds had got some of their third molars at the time of the examination the proportion was very small and not worth showing diagrammatically. So far they had not experienced any disease. Looking at the contribution made to dental health by the various permanent teeth one is again struck by the great variation in dental development of children.

4 Total decay experience

4.1 Known decay experience

The average number of teeth with known disease experience can be separated by the kind of treatment they have received, that is whether they have been filled, extracted (if a permanent tooth), or whether the decay is as yet untreated.

Figure 4.1 shows diagrammatically the inter-relation of disease and treatment, part (a) shows both dentitions together and parts(b) and (c) show the dentitions seperately.

Among five year olds it is only deciduous teeth which contribute to disease experience, but from the age of six onwards the permanent teeth make a continually larger contribution to disease until, among the fourteen year olds only permanent teeth contribute to the average number of teeth with disease experience. The total amount of active decay (D + d) increases between the ages of five and eight years (from 2.6 teeth for five year olds to 2.8 teeth for eight year olds) and then decreases with age to 1.9 teeth for fourteen year olds and 1.6 teeth for fifteen year olds.

The five year olds have, on average, 0.7 filled teeth (F + f) and this figure increases with age to 6.0 for the fifteen year olds. From the age of ten onwards the average number of filled teeth exceeds the average number of teeth with active decay. The average number of missing permanent teeth rises steadily from 0.1 at eight years old to 0.8 for fifteen year olds.

From Figure 4.1 (a) one can see that deciduous teeth have proportionately far less restorative treatment than do the permanent teeth. For the former, the average number filled never exceeds the average number with active decay, whereas for the latter the average number filled is greater than the average number decayed for those children aged eight years and above.

Figure 4.1 (a) is complicated by the mixed dentitions and so we give, in addition, diagrams representing the two dentitions separately. Figure 4.1 (b) shows that the five year olds have an average of 2.6 deciduous teeth with active decay; this figure decreases with age due to the natural loss of deciduous teeth. The number of filled deciduous teeth reaches a maximum of 1.2 teeth at eight years old.

Figure 4.1 (a)   Average number of DMF and df teeth by age

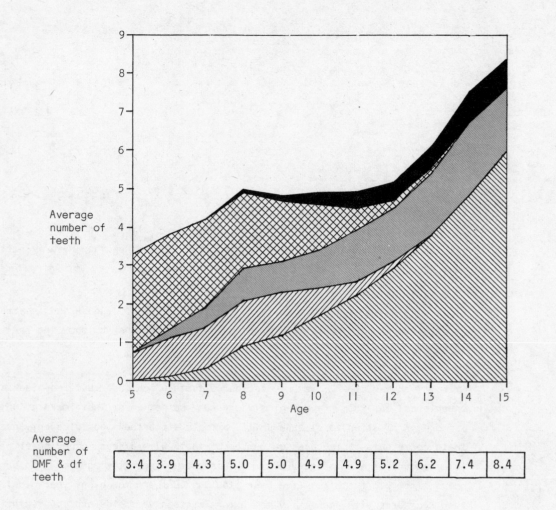

3.4	3.9	4.3	5.0	5.0	4.9	4.9	5.2	6.2	7.4	8.4

Average number of DMF & df teeth

(b)   Average number of deciduous teeth which have decay experience by age

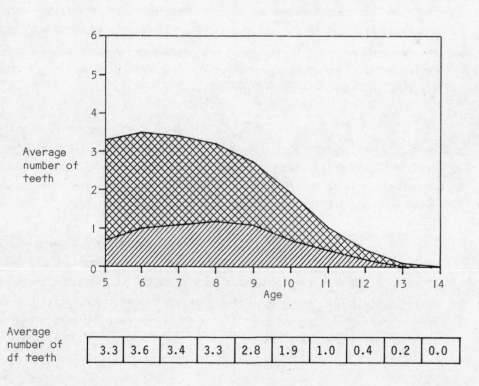

Average number of df teeth

3.3	3.6	3.4	3.3	2.8	1.9	1.0	0.4	0.2	0.0

(c)   Average number of permanent teeth
which have decay experience by age

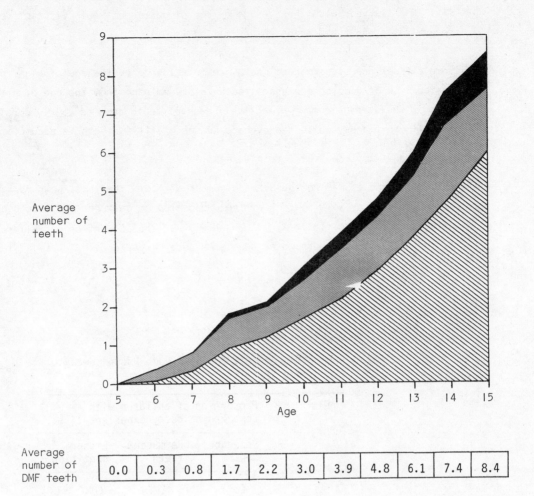

| Average number of DMF teeth | 0.0 | 0.3 | 0.8 | 1.7 | 2.2 | 3.0 | 3.9 | 4.8 | 6.1 | 7.4 | 8.4 |

KEY

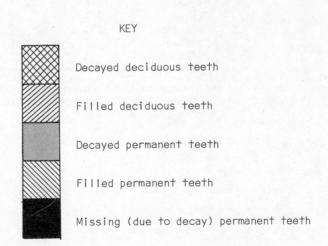

Decayed deciduous teeth

Filled deciduous teeth

Decayed permanent teeth

Filled permanent teeth

Missing (due to decay) permanent teeth

Figure 4.1 (c) shows that decay in permanent teeth begins before the age of
six. For six year olds the average number of permanent teeth with active
decay is 0.2 and the average number filled is 0.1.

Some extractions of permanent teeth are in evidence by the age of eight but the
restoration of decayed permanent teeth is predominant from the age of about
nine. The average number of actively decayed teeth remains fairly constant at
the different ages, while the average number of filled teeth is accumulated
with age.

In addition to examining the average number of teeth that are known to have
experienced decay we also look at the proportion of children who have been
affected by disease (Table 4.1). We show first the proportion of children at the
different ages who are known to have some decay experience.

Table 4.1

Proportion of children with some known* decay
experience

Age	Proportion of children with some known* decay experience		
	Deciduous teeth	Permanent teeth	Either dentition
	(df)	(DMF)	(DMF + df)
Five	71%	3%	71%
Six	79%	16%	80%
Seven	83%	39%	86%
Eight	85%	65%	91%
Nine	81%	74%	93%
Ten	63%	85%	93%
Eleven	43%	90%	95%
Twelve	21%	93%	95%
Thirteen	10%	95%	95%
Fourteen	3%	96%	96%
Fifteen	1%	97%	97%

* Deciduous teeth absent at examination are
  unaccounted for in terms of disease and are
  therefore excluded.

Even among the youngest children seven out of ten had evidence of decay
experience. At this age (five) most of the decay was of course on deciduous
teeth, but even at that stage 3% of children had some decay experience on
permanent teeth. The proportion of children with decayed (treated or untreated)
permanent teeth rose very sharply with age, so that at the age of eight two
thirds of children were involved. The proportion continued to increase with
age reaching 90% of children with decay experience on permanent teeth at the
age of eleven. Even this was not the ceiling, by the age of fourteen fewer
than 5% of children had no evidence of decay on their permanent teeth.

We were also interested to know how many children have extensive decay
experience. The definition of 'extensive' depends very largely on age. We

have selected different levels to highlight the position at different ages.
The full distributions appear in the Table Section so that the reader can,
if he wishes, use his own definition of 'extensive'.

Table 4.2

Proportion of children with extensive known* decay experience

| Age | Proportion of children with known* decay experience in | | | | |
| | Deciduous teeth | | Permanent teeth | | |
	5 or more teeth	10 or more teeth	5 or more teeth	10 or more teeth	15 or more teeth
Five	31%	6%	-	-	-
Six	34%	3%	-	-	-
Seven	34%	1%	1%	-	-
Eight	27%	-	2%	-	-
Nine	22%	-	4%	-	-
Ten	12%	-	11%	-	-
Eleven	4%	-	28%	2%	-
Twelve	-	-	43%	9%	1%
Thirteen	-	-	59%	17%	3%
Fourteen	-	-	72%	27%	7%
Fifteen	-	-	80%	36%	9%

*Deciduous teeth absent at examination are unaccounted for in terms of
disease and are therefore excluded.*

When considering the deciduous dentition these figures must of course be a
minimum estimate since any missing deciduous teeth that were decayed are
excluded. The problems of estimating total decay experience for deciduous
teeth have already been discussed in Section 2.2 and the reader will find in
Section 4.2 a discussion of the estimating procedure we have used and the
results obtained.

As far as Table 4.2 is concerned we know that at least 6% of five year olds had
ten or more teeth involved with decay.

For the permanent teeth we first of all examined the proportion of children
who had five or more permanent teeth with decay experience. This level was
used so as to exclude those whose total disease experience on permanent teeth
involved only the first permanent molars. This level of decay experience was
very low until the age of eight (2%), it then increased to 4% for nine year
olds, and 11% for ten year olds. By the age of eleven over a quarter of
children had 5 or more permanent teeth involved with decay. By this age 2% of
children had 10 or more teeth decayed. At twelve 9% of children had 10 or more
teeth involved and at thirteen years old the proportion was 17%. By this age
3% of children had, in fact, 15 or more teeth decayed and the proportion of
children with this high level of involvement increased to 7% at fourteen and
9% at fifteen.

We have discussed earlier the proportion of children who were known from the
survey to have some active decay. If for each age group, we compare this
proportion to the proportion of children who had some decay experience, we

Table 4.3

Proportion of children with some known decay experience compared to the proportion with current treatment need

| Age | Proportion of children with | | | | | |
| | Deciduous teeth | | Permanent teeth | | Either dentition | |
	Some known decay experience	Some active decay	Some known decay experience	Some active decay	Some known decay experience	Some active decay
Five	71%	63%	3%	3%	71%	63%
Six	79%	68%	16%	12%	80%	69%
Seven	83%	68%	39%	27%	86%	73%
Eight	85%	72%	65%	40%	91%	78%
Nine	81%	66%	74%	42%	93%	76%
Ten	63%	51%	85%	46%	93%	69%
Eleven	43%	32%	90%	53%	95%	66%
Twelve	21%	15%	93%	54%	95%	61%
Thirteen	10%	7%	95%	58%	95%	61%
Fourteen	3%	2%	96%	61%	96%	62%
Fifteen	1%	1%	97%	57%	97%	57%

can see what proportion of children were, at the time of the survey, dentally fit through dental treatment. Among the children in their first year at school (the five year olds) 71% were known to have (had) decay and 63% had some active decay, so 8% of five year olds had evidence of past decay but no current decay and were therefore dentally fit as the result of dental treatment. When we look at the last full age group in school (14 year olds) we find that 4% had no decay experience, 34% were free from decay at the time of the examination as a result of treatment and 62% were currently in need of treatment. Thus the proportion of children found to be dentally fit through dental treatment ranged through the age groups as follows:- 8%, 11%, 13%, 13%, 17%, 24%, 29%, 34%, 34%, 34%, 40%, proportions which compare somewhat unfavourably with those referring to the presence of active decay.

With decay being so widespread the future prognosis for children who experience no restorative treatment is fairly bleak. We compare in Table 4.4 the proportion of children who are known to have some decay experience and the proportion who have some filled teeth, the difference between these two figures being the proportion of children who have no apparent experience of restorative dentistry but have experienced decay.

For example among five year olds 71% are known to have (had) decay and 26% have some filled teeth, thus 45% of five year olds are known to have had decay but have no filled teeth. The proportion of children known to have had decay but who had no filled teeth at the time of examination was for the different ages:- 45%, 41%, 39%, 34%, 29%, 26%, 25%, 19%, 18%, 15%, 9%. Among fourteen year olds, the last full age group in school at the time of the survey, 15% had some decay experience but no evidence of restorative treatment.

Table 4.4

Proportion of children with some known decay experience compared to the proportion with some filled* teeth

Age	Proportion of children with					
	Deciduous teeth		Permanent teeth		Either dentition	
	Some known decay experience	Some filled* teeth	Some known decay experience	Some filled* teeth	Some known decay experience	Some filled* teeth
Five	71%	26%	3%	-	71%	26%
Six	79%	38%	16%	5%	80%	39%
Seven	83%	42%	39%	17%	86%	47%
Eight	85%	45%	65%	37%	91%	57%
Nine	81%	44%	74%	50%	93%	64%
Ten	63%	33%	85%	61%	93%	67%
Eleven	43%	21%	90%	66%	95%	70%
Twelve	21%	10%	93%	75%	95%	76%
Thirteen	10%	4%	95%	77%	95%	77%
Fourteen	3%	1%	96%	81%	96%	81%
Fifteen	1%	1%	97%	88%	97%	88%

Filled otherwise sound.

4.2 Estimated total decay experience of deciduous teeth among five year olds

In Chapter 2 we discussed the problems of estimating total decay experience and how this was really a problem confined to the deciduous dentition, arising from the fact that deciduous teeth naturally exfoliate and once they are gone it is not possible to say with certainty whether they were decayed or not before they were lost.

In terms of changing dentitions the age range of our sample was very wide, 5-15 years, thus embracing the total period of mixed dentitions. However, we decided at the planning stage that the examination criteria needed to be designed so that they were applicable to all children. We therefore asked the dental examiners not to make any estimate of the state of health of missing deciduous teeth. If a study is confined to one age group, especially if that age group is the five year olds, then it is much more feasible to estimate the condition of the missing deciduous teeth at the time of the examination since dental knowledge and experience indicates what is likely to be a natural situation and what is likely to be the result of dentist intervention.

Because the five year olds are the youngest and, therefore, the least likely age group to have extensive loss through natural exfoliation we have studied them in detail and have made several estimates to show the effect of various different assumptions on the estimated total disease experience of their deciduous teeth.

Estimate I:-   Assume all missing deciduous teeth in five year olds were extracted for decay reasons, or were diseased before they exfoliated.

Estimate II:-   Assume all missing deciduous teeth (except lower central incisors) in five year olds were extracted for decay reasons or were diseased before they exfoliated.

Assume missing lower central incisors had exfoliated without being diseased unless any of the lower anterior teeth (canine to canine) were present and diseased, or either canine was missing; in which case assume the missing lower central incisors had been decayed

Estimate III:-   Assume all missing deciduous teeth (except incisors) in five year olds were extracted for decay reasons or were diseased before they exfoliated.

Assume missing upper incisors (central or lateral) had exfoliated without being diseased unless 3 or 4 of the upper incisors were currently absent without any eruption of the permanent dentition.

Assume missing lower incisors (central or lateral) had exfoliated without being diseased unless any of the lower anterior teeth (canine to canine) were present and diseased, or either canine was missing, in which case assume the missing lower incisors had been decayed.

Estimate IV:-   Assume all missing deciduous teeth (except incisors) in five year olds were extracted for decay reasons or were diseased before exfoliation.

Assume missing incisors were naturally exfoliated with no disease experience.

Estimate V
(known decay
experience):-   The survey measured the amount of disease present at the time of examination and thereby provides the minimum estimate of total disease experience. The exclusion of the missing deciduous teeth is equivalent to assuming that all missing deciduous teeth in five year olds were not decayed before they were lost.

The estimate most likely to be closest to the true figure of total decay experience is Estimate III, where all missing canines and molars are presumed decayed and missing incisors are presumed decayed only if there is evidence of disease in that part of the mouth. The detailed definition was arrived at after close scrutiny of the dental charts of the five year olds.

Table 4.5 shows the range of variation of estimated total disease according to the assumptions made. The survey examination found on average, 3.3 decayed or filled deciduous teeth. This rose to 3.9 if one assumed that all missing incisors were not decayed but any other missing deciduous teeth were decayed. If one assumed that evidence of decay in the proximity of missing incisors indicated that they had been diseased then the average rose to 4.0 teeth per child. The assumption that all deciduous missing teeth except lower central incisors were lost through decay, including lower centrals only if there was evidence of decay in the other lower incisors or canines caused the average to rise to 4.2. If one assumed, rather unrealistically, that all missing deciduous teeth were decayed before being lost then the average number of teeth estimated as having experienced decay in five year olds is 4.6.

Table 4.5
Estimated total deciduous decay experience in five year olds

	Five year olds		
	No deciduous teeth with decay experience	Ten (or more) deciduous teeth with decay experience	Average number of deciduous teeth with decay experience
Estimate I	21%	15%	4.6
Estimate II	26%	13%	4.2
Estimate III	28%	11%	4.0
Estimate IV	28%	10%	3.9
Estimate V	29%	6%	3.3

If Estimate III is the best of our estimates then 28% of five year olds have had no decay on their deciduous teeth, and 11% have had ten or more teeth involved with decay. The assumptions about decay in deciduous incisors make relatively little difference to the proportion of children estimated as decay free since it is unlikely that incisor decay exists in the absence of deciduous molar decay. The proportion of children with ten or more teeth estimated as having had decay experience is 11% for Estimate III. This is considerably higher than the proportion of children known to have ten or more teeth involved. This is as one would expect since all our Estimates I-IV assume that canine and molar absences are due to decay whereas Estimate V (known decay) excludes any such assumption.

A few of the five year olds in our sample had some decayed permanent teeth (first molars). We therefore calculated the total decay experience for five year olds for either dentition and found that the amount of decay in the permanent dentition was, in fact, so small that it did not affect the average number of teeth decayed, the proportion of children with no decay or the proportion of children with ten or more teeth decayed.

4.3 Estimated total deciduous decay experience among children aged six and over

The total estimated deciduous decay for the five year olds was obtained by estimating the condition of each missing deciduous tooth for each child according to the definitions given. It is not possible to continue such a method of estimation among the older children since too high a proportion of deciduous teeth have been shed.

Once we have arrived at a detailed estimate for the five year olds we can use this information to make some assumptions about the likely decay level among the six year olds as a group. This permits us to estimate the proportion of each of the twenty deciduous teeth likely to have experienced decay among six year olds, and this can be expressed as the average number of decayed deciduous

teeth per child. Firstly a decision has to be made as to which teeth were
likely to have been extracted for caries, and which are likely to have been
affected by natural exfoliation. The former are all included as decayed, the
latter are assessed, on a group basis, according to the decay experience of
that tooth type among five year olds. The estimates thus obtained for the six
year olds can then be used in the same way to estimate the total disease
experience of deciduous teeth in seven year olds and so on.

In this way an estimate can be made, year by year, of the likely total decay
experience of deciduous teeth (both present and absent). The calculations made
in order to arrive at these estimates were intricate and very time consuming
since disease experience was estimated individually for each tooth type, for
all the ages from six to fourteen. The workload was reduced by taking
advantage of the symmetry of caries and calculating for the left side of the
mouth only and doubling the result. Even so the process involved ten separate
estimates for each of nine different age groups.

Any estimate of total disease experience of deciduous teeth carried out re-
trospectively must be based on a series of assumptions. Other people might
well choose to make different assumptions from the ones we finally chose. In
order to explain the basis of our estimate we reproduce a worked example for
one tooth type and one age group in the appendix.

Using our preferred estimate for the total decay experience of five year olds
(Estimate III) and assuming that by a certain age natural exfoliation must be
a major cause of loss, we arrived at the estimates given in Table 4.6.

Table 4.6
Estimated total decay experience of
deciduous teeth

Age	Estimated average number of deciduous teeth with decay experience
Five	4.0
Six	4.9
Seven	5.6
Eight	6.3
Nine	6.4

The estimate was of decay experience during the tooth's lifetime, using the
state of the younger children to estimate the previous experience of the older
children. One would therefore expect the accumulation of decay experience to
reach a maximum and remain at that level. This was in fact the case and the
maximum level reached was an average of 6.4 and this was first reached among
the nine year olds. We therefore conclude that an average one third of deciduous
teeth suffer from decay during their lifetime.

Of course, some deciduous teeth contribute much more towards decay experience
than others. For example the teeth estimated to be most prone to decay were

the lower 'e's of which three-quarters were estimated as being decayed at some
time.   The next most decay prone teeth were the upper 'e's and lower 'd's of
which two-thirds suffered decay at some stage.   Among the upper 'd's one half
were decayed in their lifetime.   Not more than 20% of the deciduous canines
and the upper central incisors had been decayed.   Fewer than one in ten of the
upper lateral incisors and the lower incisors ever experienced decay.   The
deciduous molars thus played a far larger part in the decay experience of the
deciduous dentition than did the deciduous canines and incisors.

5 Accidental damage

As part of the examination the dentists were asked to inspect each child's incisors to see if there was any evidence of accidental damage. They were asked to record the extent of the damage ranging from a fracture of the enamel not involving the dentine to the provision of a temporary crown or the extraction of the tooth.

It was anticipated that more damage would be found among boys than girls since boys are more likely to be involved in rougher games and body sports. Below we show the proportion of children, for boys and girls separately, whom we found to have suffered damage to their incisors. Among the five and six year olds some of this damage involved deciduous teeth, but from then on it was the permanent incisors that were involved.

Table 5.1

Proportion of children found to have some damage to incisors in either dentition by sex

Age	Proportion of children with some damage to incisors*		
	Male	Female	All
Five	8%	7%	8%
Six	5%	3%	4%
Seven	4%	3%	3%
Eight	9%	4%	7%
Nine	14%	10%	12%
Ten	14%	8%	11%
Eleven	21%	9%	15%
Twelve	22%	12%	18%
Thirteen	21%	12%	16%
Fourteen	20%	12%	16%
Fifteen	15%	11%	13%

Deciduous or permanent incisors

By the age of nine more than one in ten children had suffered some damage to their incisors. Among girls this figure remained at about one in ten, but for boys one in five had damaged his incisors by the age of eleven. This level among boys was constant thereafter except for a drop among fifteen year olds. (The fifteen year old group has lost the early school leavers and is not therefore representative of the whole of that age group).

Table 5.2

Accidental damage to incisors

a) All incisors

Type of damage	Rate of damage per thousand incisors for children aged										
	5+	6+	7+	8+	9+	10+	11+	12+	13+	14+	15+
Discolouration	5.1	2.8	0.9	-	0.4	0.5	0.5	2.4	0.5	0.7	0.9
Fracture (enamel only)	4.3	1.5	2.4	6.1	10.2	11.4	14.8	15.2	11.9	12.7	12.0
Fracture (enamel and dentine)	2.4	1.4	1.4	4.4	6.5	6.5	7.6	8.6	5.7	9.2	7.5
Fracture (involving pulp)	-	-	0.2	0.5	0.8	0.6	1.0	1.0	1.2	2.6	0.9
Displacement	0.3	-	-	-	0.3	0.1	-	0.1	-	-	-
Temporary crown	-	-	-	0.1	-	-	-	-	0.4	0.3	0.7
(Semi) Permanent restoration	-	-	-	0.1	0.1	0.3	1.6	2.0	1.5	2.0	1.4
Tooth missing due to trauma	1.3	0.5	0.1	0.2	0.6	-	0.9	1.3	1.6	1.1	1.1

(b) Upper central incisors

Type of damage	Rate of damage per thousand upper central incisors for children aged										
	5+	6+	7+	8+	9+	10+	11+	12+	13+	14+	15+
Discolouration	18.9	9.3	2.2	-	0.9	1.8	2.0	6.3	1.1	2.2	2.9
Fracture (enamel only)	10.0	2.8	5.7	20.6	29.2	33.0	41.1	42.4	37.7	38.5	30.9
Fracture (enamel and dentine)	8.4	4.2	4.0	8.7	17.7	20.6	21.8	23.0	20.2	21.7	21.6
Fracture (involving pulp)	-	-	0.4	-	2.7	1.8	4.1	2.1	4.4	3.8	3.6
Displacement	1.1	-	-	-	1.3	-	-	0.5	-	-	-
Temporary crown	-	-	-	0.5	-	-	-	-	1.6	0.5	2.2
(Semi) Permanent restoration	-	-	-	0.5	0.4	1.4	5.6	5.8	4.9	5.4	3.6
Tooth missing due to trauma	4.7	1.4	0.4	0.9	1.3	-	3.5	4.7	5.5	3.8	2.9

In the majority of cases where a child had damaged his incisors one tooth only was involved, but for about a third of children who had suffered damage two or more incisors were involved. We also examined the results to see if there was any regional variation in the proportion of children damaging their teeth but there was not.

The damage that the dentist recorded included discolouration, fracture, displacement, protective restoration and extraction. Table 5.2 shows the rate at which these conditions were found per thousand incisors. Even among the incisors the risks for damage were not equal, the upper central incisors being more at risk than other incisors. We therefore show the rate of damage per thousand upper central incisors separately.

Fractures of the enamel (the least severe damage recorded) accounted for most of the damage found, fractured enamel being found on 40 out of every thousand upper central incisors examined in children aged eleven or more. Fractures involving both enamel and dentine were found on about 20 out of every thousand upper central incisors over the same age range. The more serious kinds of damage were much less common. Among children aged nine or more, between 2 and 4 upper central incisors per thousand had fractures which involved the pulp. A central upper incisor had been lost through trauma at the rate of about 5 per thousand central incisors in twelve and thirteen year olds. Temporary crowns, or semi-permanent or permanent restorations to upper central incisors occurred slightly more often than the loss of such a tooth. About 6 upper central incisors per thousand had been treated in these ways among eleven year olds and over.

Although important in terms of the demand for specialist treatment for the more serious damage, the reduction in overall dental health caused by accidental damage is small compared to the ravages of decay.

6 Dentures

In overall terms the number of children who are provided with dentures is very small. For this survey the dentists examined nearly thirteen thousand children and fewer than fifty were found to have had some denture provision. As might be expected the rate of denture provision was highest amongst the oldest children.

Table 6.1
Proportion of children with dentures

Age	Proportion of children with dentures per thousand children
Five	-
Six	-
Seven	1 per thousand
Eight	-
Nine	-
Ten	2 per thousand
Eleven	6 per thousand
Twelve	7 per thousand
Thirteen	10 per thousand
Fourteen	9 per thousand
Fifteen	13 per thousand

We scutinised the dental examination chart for the children who had dentures and there were in all (unweighted) 46 children involved. One in two of the children with dentures had suffered accidental damage to the teeth, one in ten of the children had a developmental or congenital reason for the denture provision, and the remaining two in five apparently needed the denture because of extraction due to decay. All the dentures seen were upper partial dentures except for one case where the child had a lower partial denture only, and one case where the child had a full upper clearance.

It is encouraging to find that only a small number of children have been provided with dentures, although unfortunately this also means that the group is too small to carry out any more detailed analysis.

7 The condition of the gums

Although the more advanced gum conditions are much rarer in children than in adults, none the less, the initial signs of gum trouble are already apparent at an early age.

For the survey examination, the dentist looked at six segments of the mouth in turn, and for each, recorded the worst condition found in that area of the mouth. There were three different conditions which he assessed: whether there was any inflammation of the gums; the presence of any debris; and whether or not there was any calculus. In Table 7.1 we present the proportions of children who were found to have some of each of the three conditions and the proportion with any of the conditions present.

Table 7.1

Gum condition in children of different ages

Age	Proportion of children with			
	Some inflammation	Some debris	Some calculus	Some inflammation calculus, or debris
Five	26%	39%	5%	47%
Six	35%	48%	5%	58%
Seven	50%	62%	9%	72%
Eight	56%	67%	15%	78%
Nine	56%	67%	17%	78%
Ten	56%	65%	21%	76%
Eleven	59%	65%	26%	80%
Twelve	57%	64%	28%	78%
Thirteen	55%	59%	31%	75%
Fourteen	54%	56%	33%	74%
Fifteen	51%	51%	34%	71%

At the age of five just over a quarter (26%) of children were found to have some gum inflammation (not associated with the process of exfoliation and eruption of teeth). This condition was found to include a half of seven year olds and 59% of those aged eleven. The proportions were not so high in the teenage children but gum inflammation was nevertheless present in over half of those examined.

The presence of debris showed a similar pattern with age. Almost a half (48%) of six year olds and over two-thirds of those aged eight and nine were

found to have some debris present.   Again the proportions were not so high
in the teenage children but even so involved over a half of those examined.
Although a considerable proportion of the older children were found to have some
calculus present, its prevalence, especially among the younger children, was
small compared to the proportions found to have some inflammation and debris.
If we regard each of the three conditions to be a contra-indication to good oral
hygiene, then the proportion of children in any age group that had no such contra-
indications is remarkably small.   Almost half (47%) of children aged five were
found to have some involvement.   This proportion increased to over three-quarters
of those aged 8-14; therefore of children aged eight or more, fewer than one in
four was found to have a good state of oral hygiene.

We examined the results to see whether gum condition varied between boys and girls
of the same age.   In Figures 7.1, 7.2, and 7.3 we show diagrammatically how the
sexes varied in terms of the presence of each of the three conditions age for age.

Between the ages of five to seven, there was virtually no difference in gum
condition between boys and girls.   However, from the age of eight onwards, a
higher proportion of boys than girls had gum inflammation and debris.
Although not quite such a dramatic difference, the pattern is similar with regard
to calculus - a higher proportion of boys than girls having some present.

We looked to see if any particular area in the mouth was contributing more than
others towards the gum conditions found.   Tables 7.2, 7.3, and 7.4 give the
proportions of children in each age group who were found to have evidence of the
conditions in each of the six segments of the mouth.

For the measurement of gum inflammation, the dentist was not only asked to record
in which segments it was found, but a measurement of the severity as well.   Only
in the anterior sections of the mouth (upper and lower middle) did the proportions
of children having severe inflammation rise above 1% (3% of children aged 12-14
were found to have inflammation of a severe nature in the anterior segments).
Table 7.2 presents the proportions in each age group who were found to have any
gum inflammation in the six segments.   It was in the anterior segments (upper and

Table 7.2

Gum inflammation by mouth segment in children of different ages

Age	Proportion of children with some gum inflammation in					
	Upper left segment	Upper middle segment	Upper right segment	Lower right segment	Lower middle segment	Lower left segment
Five	11%	10%	8%	6%	8%	5%
Six	14%	12%	12%	6%	19%	7%
Seven	16%	19%	12%	9%	35%	8%
Eight	19%	28%	16%	9%	42%	8%
Nine	21%	32%	18%	8%	37%	8%
Ten	21%	36%	17%	10%	38%	9%
Eleven	25%	38%	21%	10%	41%	9%
Twelve	25%	38%	22%	10%	37%	9%
Thirteen	25%	37%	20%	10%	38%	12%
Fourteen	27%	35%	22%	11%	38%	11%
Fifteen	23%	30%	19%	9%	36%	12%

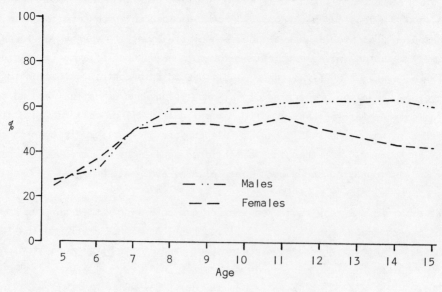

Figure 7.1   Proportion of children with some gum inflammation

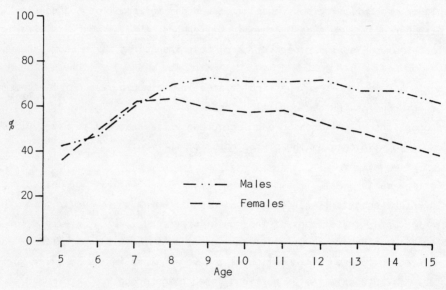

Figure 7.2   Proportion of children with some debris

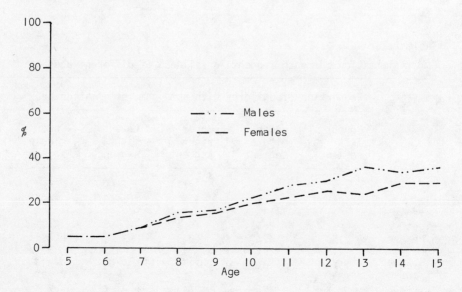

Figure 7.3   Proportion of children with some calculus

lower middle) that the greatest proportion of children were found to have inflammation. Over a third of children aged nine or more were found to have gum inflammation in the anterior segments. About a quarter of children aged eleven or more were found to have inflammation in the upper posterior segments (upper left and right) while only one in ten were found to have any present in the lower posterior segments (lower left and right). It would appear then that the anterior segments of the mouth contribute the greatest to gum inflammation in children and that generally, it is found more often in the upper jaw than in the lower.

Table 7.3 presents the proportions in each age group who were found to have any debris for each of the mouth segments separately. The dentist was asked to record whether any debris found was recent or long-standing, but for the purpose of the table, no distinction is made, as again, it was only on the anterior segments that the proportion of children having long-standing debris was above 2% (4% of children aged 10-14 were found to have long-standing debris). As in the case of gum inflammation, it is in the anterior segments (upper and lower middle) that debris was most prevalent. Over a third of children aged 8-14 had debris present in the upper middle segment and a half of children aged 8-10 were found to have some present in the lower middle segment. Also, as in the case of gum inflammation, it was the upper posterior segments which had a higher prevalence of debris than the lower posterior segments. About a third of children aged 8-14 had debris present in the upper left and right segments while only a fifth were found to have it present in the lower left and right segments.

Table 7.3

Debris by mouth segment in children of different ages

Age	Proportion of children with some debris in					
	Upper left segment	Upper middle segment	Upper right segment	Lower right segment	Lower middle segment	Lower left segment
Five	22%	17%	19%	13%	19%	14%
Six	24%	19%	23%	15%	29%	15%
Seven	29%	26%	26%	18%	46%	17%
Eight	35%	36%	30%	18%	51%	17%
Nine	34%	41%	31%	19%	50%	17%
Ten	32%	40%	29%	18%	50%	18%
Eleven	33%	42%	32%	20%	48%	20%
Twelve	35%	42%	31%	20%	47%	19%
Thirteen	34%	39%	29%	20%	42%	20%
Fourteen	33%	37%	32%	21%	39%	20%
Fifteen	29%	30%	26%	19%	34%	19%

In the measurement of calculus, the dentist was only asked to record whether or not any was present in each segment. By far the greatest contribution to the prevalence of calculus was made by the lower middle segment (Table 7.4). The proportion of children found to have calculus in this area of the mouth ranged from 4% of those aged five to 31% of those aged fifteen. The upper middle and both lower posterior (left and right) segments were virtually free from calculus. It was only in the older age groups that the upper posterior segments were found to have an appreciable level of calculus (10% of children aged 15 were found to have calculus in the upper left segment and 7% in the upper right segment).

Table 7.4

Calculus by mouth segment in children of different ages

Age	Proportion of children with some calculus in					
	Upper left segment	Upper middle segment	Upper right segment	Lower right segment	Lower middle segment	Lower left segment
Five	-	-	-	-	4%	-
Six	1%	-	1%	-	5%	-
Seven	1%	-	-	-	8%	-
Eight	2%	-	2%	1%	13%	-
Nine	2%	-	1%	1%	16%	-
Ten	3%	-	2%	1%	20%	1%
Eleven	5%	-	3%	1%	22%	2%
Twelve	6%	1%	5%	2%	25%	1%
Thirteen	7%	1%	5%	2%	28%	2%
Fourteen	8%	1%	7%	2%	30%	2%
Fifteen	10%	2%	7%	3%	31%	2%

Debris and inflammation were both fairly common even among the youngest children whereas calculus was not so evident, especially among the youngest children. We looked in more detail at the two more common conditions to see whether children without any debris were more or less likely to have inflammation than those children who did have debris. The results are shown in Table 7.5 and demonstrate very large differences indeed.

Table 7.5

Proportion of children with some gum inflammation by debris

Age	Proportion with some gum inflammation among children who have			
	No debris		Some debris	
Five	10%	579	51%	374
Six	16%	556	55%	524
Seven	24%	438	66%	699
Eight	27%	363	70%	728
Nine	28%	372	70%	757
Ten	23%	377	73%	714
Eleven	32%	343	74%	642
Twelve	29%	349	73%	608
Thirteen	26%	375	75%	540
Fourteen	26%	402	76%	521
Fifteen	26%	341	76%	355

Among the five year olds who were free from debris, only one in ten had some inflammation, while among those who had some debris, a half had some inflammation as well. The large difference between the presence of gum inflammation according to whether or not the examiner recorded the presence of debris existed for all ages.   For the teenage children, a quarter of those with no debris had gum inflammation compared with three-quarters of those children who had debris.   There was thus a strong association between the presence of debris and the presence of gum inflammation.

8 Orthodontics

The dental examination included a wide range of indicators for various aspects
of the orthodontic assessment of the child. Firstly we look at the most common
developmental problem, that is crowding.

8.1 Crowding

One of the most common anomalies of dental development is the overcrowding of
teeth in the jaw, forcing the teeth out of alignment. The survey dental
examination included an assessment of crowding, the criteria* for which included
potential crowding as well as actual crowding; for example if the space into
which two premolars had to erupt was only big enough for one such tooth then the
dentist counted this as (potential) crowding. For this assessment the mouth was
divided into six segments, upper left molars and premolars, upper canines and
incisors, upper right molars and premolars, and three similar segments in the
lower jaw. Each segment was assessed separately and initially we look at the
proportion of children who had some crowding in at least one segment (Table 8.1).
Among the five year olds the assessment of crowding, including potential crowding,
was of course the most difficult, but among the six year olds 40% were estimated
as having a crowding problem. Between the ages of seven and ten 60% or more of
children had some crowding and although the proportions were less among the older
children, they were never less than half of the children.

Table 8.1
Proportion of children with crowding

Age	Proportion with some crowding in		
	One or more segments	Two or more segments	Three or more segments
Five	18%	5%	1%
Six	40%	14%	3%
Seven	60%	30%	9%
Eight	65%	39%	14%
Nine	63%	37%	14%
Ten	62%	35%	14%
Eleven	58%	33%	13%
Twelve	55%	28%	10%
Thirteen	52%	24%	8%
Fourteen	50%	25%	8%
Fifteen	53%	25%	7%

* See appendix for examination criteria.

Table 8.1 also shows the proportion of children who had two or more, and three or more segments of the mouth that were crowded. In the middle age groups over a third of children had crowding in at least two segments, and even among the oldest children a quarter had at least two segments that were crowded. A smaller proportion of children had three or more crowded segments of the mouth, but even so in the eight to eleven age range, 14% of children examined had at least three segments of the mouth that were crowded.

Table 8.2 shows which segments of the mouth were most at risk for crowding. The middle segments involving the canines and incisors, both upper and lower, were the locations most frequently involved with crowding. Over a quarter of the oldest children had crowded upper anterior teeth and nearly a third had crowded lower anterior teeth, and by the age of fourteen and fifteen any orthodontic treatment that is likely to be undertaken has usually already been completed.

Table 8.2

Proportion of children with crowding in different locations

Age	Proportion of children with some crowding in					
	Upper left segment	Upper middle segment	Upper right segment	Lower right segment	Lower middle segment	Lower left segment
Five	1%	7%	–	–	14%	–
Six	3%	14%	4%	4%	31%	2%
Seven	9%	34%	8%	7%	40%	7%
Eight	15%	41%	13%	12%	35%	10%
Nine	13%	40%	12%	11%	34%	12%
Ten	12%	37%	13%	13%	33%	12%
Eleven	12%	36%	9%	12%	34%	13%
Twelve	8%	32%	8%	11%	30%	10%
Thirteen	6%	29%	5%	8%	31%	8%
Fourteen	7%	27%	6%	8%	31%	9%
Fifteen	3%	31%	5%	7%	33%	7%

8.2 Other orthodontic assessments

As well as assessing crowding the orthodontic part of the dental examination included an assessment of the child's occlusion, overbite and overjet, crossbite, whether any incisors were instanding and whether there was any mucosal trauma. The results of these different assessments are presented in the following sub-sections.

(a) Occlusion

The detailed description of the criteria used can be found in the appendix and a table showing the full distribution of the antero-posterior relationship of the dental arches will be found in the Table Section (Table 82). Class I of the classification denoted those with a normal or ideal arch relationship. Table 8.3 shows the proportion of children so classified. Except for the five and six year olds, among whom the deciduous dentition was still playing a major role the results show that a third or more of children did not have an ideal arch relationship.

Table 8.3

Proportion of children with class 1 occlusion

Age	Proportion with class 1 occlusion
Five	73%
Six	73%
Seven	65%
Eight	61%
Nine	64%
Ten	64%
Eleven	62%
Twelve	64%
Thirteen	65%
Fourteen	67%
Fifteen	68%

(b) Overbite and overjet

Another factor of relevance to the orthodontist is the extent to which upper teeth overlap lower teeth (overbite) and the extent to which upper teeth are horizontally in front of the lower teeth (overjet). Again the detailed results can be found in the Table Section (Tables 82 and 83). Overbite and overjet are in some ways rather difficult factors to assess for children of different ages. In the younger children a higher proportion of the measurements could not be made at all because the teeth concerned were not present. The measurements that could be made were also rather smaller in the younger age groups, reflecting that some were taken on deciduous teeth, and that others were taken on permanent teeth that were not yet fully erupted.

The assessment for overbite was carried out in terms of the proportion of the lower incisors covered by the upper incisors when in a state of natural occlusion. From the age of eight onwards the most frequent condition was that over a third and up to two-thirds of the lower incisors were covered by upper incisors. The second most common level of tooth overlap was up to one-third. Between them these two categories accounted for approximately three-quarters of children aged eight or more. In Table 8.4 we show the extremes of overbite, that is anterior open bite, zero overbite and over two-thirds overlap.

Table 8.4

Proportion of children with extremes of overbite

Age	Proportion of children with		
	Anterior open bite	Zero overbite	Over two-thirds overbite
Five	11%	10%	17%
Six	18%	9%	11%
Seven	10%	7%	12%
Eight	6%	4%	17%
Nine	3%	2%	17%
Ten	3%	2%	18%
Eleven	2%	2%	19%
Twelve	2%	2%	16%
Thirteen	2%	3%	16%
Fourteen	2%	4%	15%
Fifteen	2%	3%	14%

In many cases among the younger children the anterior open bite and zero overbite would appear to be connected with the deciduous dentition and the development of the permanent dentition. From the age of nine onwards however there is little variability in the prevalence of either open bite or zero overbite. The proportion of children with over two-thirds of the lower incisors covered by the upper incisors remains fairly constant through all age groups, and is a much more frequent occurrence (three children out of twenty) than anterior open bite (or zero overbite).

Overjet was measured on both of the central incisors in terms of the millimetre horizontal distance from the front edge of the upper incisors to the front edge of the opposing lower incisors, when the jaws were in a state of natural occlusion. The number of cases where no measurement could be made was again highest among the young children who were currently involved with the shedding of deciduous incisors. The majority of children had an overjet measurement in the range 1-4 mm. This was so for about two-thirds of the children aged five to seven and about three-quarters of children aged eight to fifteen. In Table 8.5 we show the proportions of children with the more extreme measurements of overjet, that is zero or negative, 5-6 mm and 7 or more mm.

Table 8.5

Proportion of children with extremes of overjet
(upper left central incisor)

Age	Proportion with overjet measurement of		
	Zero or negative	5-6 mm	7 mm or more
Five	7%	5%	2%
Six	4%	6%	1%
Seven	4%	9%	4%
Eight	4%	11%	7%
Nine	2%	12%	6%
Ten	3%	12%	5%
Eleven	3%	15%	6%
Twelve	3%	11%	7%
Thirteen	3%	11%	3%
Fourteen	4%	11%	4%
Fifteen	3%	11%	3%

The proportion of children with an overjet of 7mm or more was highest among the eight to twelve year olds and then declined. It is not possible from the survey data to tell whether this decline was brought about by the provision of orthodontic treatment.

(c) Mucosal trauma

Very few children had any signs of mucosal trauma, the highest proportion being 4% among the seven to ten year olds. Most of the trauma that was present occurred palatally in the upper jaw (Table Section, Table 84).

(d) Incisors that are instanding or edge to edge

Among the younger children (five to seven) a greater proportion of children had incisors that were instanding or met edge to edge when the back teeth were in occlusion, than was the case with the teenagers. About 13% of the young children had some such problems, compared with 9% or 10% of the teenagers (Table Section, Table 84).

(e) Buccal crossbite

The proportion of children who had any problem with buccal crossbite or cusp to cusp occlusion was lowest (2%) among the five year olds and highest (14-16%) among the seven to ten year olds. The proportion declined very slightly among the older children (Table Section, Table 84)

8.3 Orthodontic conditions in combination

Having examined the prevalence of various orthodontic conditions in the previous two sections we next investigate the extent to which the major conditions were interrelated. Since crowding was one of the major developmental anomalies we consider the prevalence of other orthodontic conditions in the presence or absence of crowding.

Table 8.6 shows that anterior open bite or zero overbite were no more likely to be found among children with crowding than among children with no crowding. A large overbite (over two-thirds overlap), on the other hand, was more often found among children aged seven to eleven if they had crowded teeth.

Table 8.6

The proportion of children with small and large overbite, by crowding

Age	Proportion with anterior open bite or zero overbite				Proportion with over two-thirds overbite			
	No crowding		Some crowding		No crowding		Some crowding	
Five	21%	782	24%	170	16%	782	21%	170
Six	25%	649	29%	432	12%	649	11%	432
Seven	16%	458	17%	679	10%	458	14%	679
Eight	12%	382	9%	709	12%	382	19%	709
Nine	7%	414	4%	715	12%	414	19%	715
Ten	5%	415	4%	677	15%	415	20%	677
Eleven	4%	410	4%	576	15%	410	22%	576
Twelve	4%	432	4%	525	14%	432	18%	525
Thirteen	6%	442	4%	473	14%	442	18%	473
Fourteen	5%	460	6%	463	13%	460	17%	463
Fifteen	6%	329	4%	367	11%	329	16%	367

Table 8.7 shows that there was no systematic association between negative and zero overjet and crowding, or with overjet of 5 millimetres or more with crowding. Although for one or two of the age groups the differences are significantly different the lack of systematic variation suggests no general association of the two conditions.

Table 8.7

The proportion of children with small and large overjet, by crowding

Age	Proportion with negative or zero overjet				Proportion with 5mm or more overjet			
	No crowding		Some crowding		No crowding		Some crowding	
Five	7%	782	5%	170	6%	782	11%	170
Six	5%	649	3%	432	6%	649	9%	432
Seven	5%	458	4%	679	11%	458	14%	679
Eight	3%	382	5%	709	15%	382	18%	709
Nine	2%	414	3%	715	18%	414	18%	715
Ten	1%	415	4%	677	17%	415	17%	677
Eleven	3%	410	3%	576	19%	410	22%	576
Twelve	2%	432	3%	525	15%	432	20%	525
Thirteen	2%	442	3%	473	13%	442	16%	473
Fourteen	3%	460	4%	463	13%	460	18%	463
Fifteen	5%	329	3%	367	11%	329	17%	367

Table 8.8 shows the proportion of children who had some instanding or edge to edge incisors according to whether or not the child had any crowding. Among children aged five to seven, for whom the deciduous teeth and early development of permanent incisors would have been involved there was no significant difference between the prevalence of these incisor problems and whether or not the child had crowded teeth. From the age of eight to fourteen there were approximately proportionally twice as many children with some instanding or edge to edge incisors among the children with crowded teeth.

Table 8.8

The proportion of children with incisor problems, by crowding

Age	Proportion with some instanding or edge to edge incisors			
	No crowding		Some crowding	
Five	13%	782	12%	170
Six	17%	649	11%	432
Seven	16%	458	15%	679
Eight	7%	382	14%	709
Nine	7%	414	14%	715
Ten	4%	415	15%	677
Eleven	6%	410	12%	576
Twelve	6%	432	13%	525
Thirteen	7%	442	12%	473
Fourteen	5%	460	15%	463
Fifteen	8%	329	11%	367

Table 8.9

The proportion of children with
class 1 occlusion, by crowding

Age	Proportion with class 1 occlusion	
	No crowding	Some crowding
Five	75% 782	65% 170
Six	77% 649	67% 432
Seven	74% 458	59% 679
Eight	71% 382	56% 709
Nine	71% 414	60% 715
Ten	72% 415	59% 677
Eleven	71% 410	56% 576
Twelve	71% 432	58% 525
Thirteen	71% 442	59% 473
Fourteen	75% 460	58% 463
Fifteen	75% 329	62% 367

Approximately three-quarters of the children with no crowding were classified
as having class I occlusion (Table 8.9). The comparable proportion among the
children with crowding was always lower, (in the range 56% to 67%). Although
there was obviously an association between crowding and occlusion it is
interesting to note that nearly a quarter of children with no crowding did not
have a normal arch relationship while well over half of those who had crowding
did. The association between crowding and occlusion although present was by no
means overwhelming.

For the last comparison of orthodontic conditions we examine whether or not
extreme overjet and overbite conditions are associated or not. Table 8.10 shows
that negative (or zero) overjet hardly ever exists in combination with an over

Table 8.10

Proportion of children with small or large overjet, by small
or large overbite

Age	Proportion with negative or zero overjet among children with		Proportion with 5mm or more overjet among children with	
	Anterior open bite or zero overbite	Over two-thirds overbite	Anterior open bite or zero overbite	Over two-thirds overbite
Five	18% 207	1% 158	12% 207	6% 158
Six	9% 287	3% 124	11% 287	5% 124
Seven	10% 192	3% 142	14% 192	15% 142
Eight	15% 110	2% 184	19% 110	21% 184
Nine	8% 59	- 186	18% 59	19% 186
Ten	23% 50	2% 199	26% 50	26% 199
Eleven	32% 39	2% 188	27% 39	34% 188
Twelve	13% 40	- 152	26% 40	26% 152
Thirteen	19% 44	- 149	16% 44	22% 149
Fourteen	22% 53	2% 139	14% 53	19% 139
Fifteen	32% 34	- 95	12% 34	18% 95

two-thirds overbite. The prevalence of large overjet (5mm or more) was not associated with overbite. A similar proportion of children had a large overjet whether their overbite was large or small.

8.4 Orthodontic treatment received

The previous sections have shown the orthodontic situation as it was found to be at the time of the dental examination. Dental intervention in the form of orthodontic treatment may of course in some cases have remedied or partly remedied an orthodontic problem before the time of the survey. Treatment is not the only method by which orthodontic problems may have been remedied since growth and development of the jaw also play a part. In terms of orthodontic treatment we obtained information about two forms, orthodontic extractions and orthodontic appliance therapy.

In order to alleviate crowding and improve on the positioning of teeth a dentist may need to extract some permanent teeth. It is likely that the teeth extracted for this purpose are not diseased and we therefore asked the survey dental examiners to differentiate between permanent teeth extracted for caries and permanent teeth extracted for orthodontic reasons. In making this classification he used his dental knowledge and experience and also asked the child about his dental history. Table 8.11 shows that orthodontic extraction did not occur before the age of nine. It then increased with age until one in five children had lost some teeth for orthodontic reasons. It is interesting to compare this with the proportion of children losing teeth for decay reasons. Extraction for decay reasons begins sooner than does orthodontic extraction and reaches the level of one in three children having experienced extraction of permanent teeth for decay reasons by the age of fourteen or fifteen.

Table 8.11

Proportion of children who have had orthodontic extractions compared with the proportion who have had decay extractions

Age	Proportion who have had	
	Orthodontic extractions	Decay extractions
Five	–	–
Six	–	–
Seven	–	1%
Eight	–	4%
Nine	1%	8%
Ten	2%	13%
Eleven	7%	18%
Twelve	13%	23%
Thirteen	17%	28%
Fourteen	22%	31%
Fifteen	21%	33%

The extraction of teeth may in itself be enough to correct crowding. In some cases however the child needs further treatment which involves the wearing of a brace or appliance to remedy crowding or non-alignment of the teeth. During the dental examination the dentist asked all children aged eight or more whether they had ever had to wear a brace (see Table 8.12).

Table 8.12
Proportion of children who had had
appliance therapy

Age	Proportion who	
	Had a brace at the examination	Had had a brace
Five	-	-
Six	-	-
Seven	-	-
Eight	-	1%
Nine	-	1%
Ten	1%	2%
Eleven	3%	4%
Twelve	5%	7%
Thirteen	4%	10%
Fourteen	2%	13%
Fifteen	1%	16%

On the assumption that the two groups did not overlap, about 15% of teenagers had had appliance therapy.

We have seen that the number of children with some crowding at the time of the survey decreased after the age of eight. We were interested to know whether or not this decrease could be attributed to a natural growth in the jaw or to an increased proportion of children receiving orthodontic treatment. Table 8.13 gives the proportion of children in each age group who were found to have some crowding at the time of the examination; and also the proportion of those children who had had orthodontic extractions in the past, but at present had no crowding. If we presume that these extractions were to relieve crowding then the sum of the two percentages provides an estimate of the total crowding experience of children.

If we disregard dentist intervention and growth of the jaw, we would expect the proportion of children with crowding to reach a maximum level at a certain age and remain there for children above this age. If, however, we were to consider that the situation should improve due to jaw growth we would expect this level to drop after reaching its maximum.

In Table 8.13 we see that the proportion of children with some crowding experience reaches a maximum of 65% among the eight year olds and then drops gradually to just over 60% for the teenagers. The difference between the proportion of eight year olds with crowding experience and that of the thirteen year olds is a significant one, but the downward trend is not very large. It is difficult to say whether or not this apparent improvement is due to jaw growth as extractions for other than orthodontic reasons could have helped to ease crowding during this

Table 8.13

Estimated total crowding experience

Age	Proportion of children with		
	Some present crowding (a)	No present crowding but previous orthodontic extractions (b)	Estimated total crowding experience (a+b)
Five	18%	–	18%
Six	40%	–	40%
Seven	60%	–	60%
Eight	65%	–	65%
Nine	63%	1%	64%
Ten	62%	1%	63%
Eleven	58%	4%	62%
Twelve	55%	6%	61%
Thirteen	52%	8%	60%
Fourteen	50%	11%	61%
Fifteen	53%	9%	62%

period. It would seem from the results however, that orthodontic treatment by extraction makes a bigger contribution to the alleviation of crowding than does growth or other dental treatment.

8.5 Estimated need for orthodontic treatment

The dentists were asked to estimate, in their opinion, whether the children they examined needed or would need orthodontic treatment. They were asked to make this assessment ignoring whether the mouth was well cared for or not, and whether it was likely that the child would stay the full course of treatment, but only taking account of those factors which indicated whether the dental development of the child needed orthodontic attention. The dentists also estimated whether or not they thought the treatment required would be likely to involve an appliance.

Table 8.14

Proportion of children in need of orthodontic treatment

Age	Proportion who need	
	Some orthodontic treatment	Appliance therapy
Five	17%	8%
Six	28%	15%
Seven	48%	31%
Eight	57%	40%
Nine	55%	38%
Ten	50%	35%
Eleven	46%	34%
Twelve	37%	28%
Thirteen	30%	22%
Fourteen	28%	19%
Fifteen	27%	20%

It is of course, rather difficult to predict future orthodontic need among the very young children but the dental examiners were estimating that about half of the seven year olds would need some attention. This proportion did not fall below a half until the age of eleven, thereafter the proportion declined until it reached approximately a quarter among the fifteen year olds. Even among the oldest age group one in four children were estimated to be in need of orthodontic attention.

In addition to saying whether the child would need orthodontic attention the dentists were asked to say whether they thought this would involve appliance therapy. Most of the children estimated as potentially in need of orthodontic treatment were said to be in need of appliance therapy, although at all ages there were some children who were said to be in need of orthodontic extraction only. The proportion of children said to be in need of appliance therapy was greatest among the eight year olds (40%), thereafter the proportion declined to about a fifth of the teenage children.

Among the eight, nine and ten year olds the survey dentist estimated that a half or more of the children needed orthodontic treatment. We examine, in the following tables how the level of orthodontic treatment need varied with the different orthodontic conditions found. Table 8.15 shows the proportion of children needing orthodontic treatment according to whether or not the dentist found any crowding.

Table 8.15

Proportion of children needing orthodontic treatment by crowding

Age	Proportion needing orthodontic treatment among children who have			
	No crowding		Some crowding	
Five	10%	782	47%	170
Six	10%	649	54%	432
Seven	15%	458	69%	679
Eight	21%	382	76%	709
Nine	22%	414	74%	715
Ten	18%	415	70%	677
Eleven	15%	410	67%	576
Twelve	13%	432	57%	525
Thirteen	10%	442	49%	473
Fourteen	8%	460	50%	463
Fifteen	6%	329	46%	367

The need for orthodontic treatment was highest among eight and nine year olds who had crowding, of whom three quarters needed treatment. At each age the proportion needing orthodontic treatment was much higher among those with crowding than those without. Notwithstanding the fact that crowding obviously played a major role in the assessment of treatment need, as many as one in five children with no crowding, at the age of peak need, required orthodontic treatment for other reasons. Not all of the crowding recorded in terms of the criteria laid down for the dental examination was deemed by the dental examiner to need orthodontic treatment. A quarter of eight and nine year olds, and a half of the teenagers with crowding were said not to need orthodontic treatment. Thus although there was a strong association between crowding and orthodontic treatment need the relationship was by no means one to one.

Table 8.16

Proportion of children needing orthodontic treatment by overbite and crowding

| Age | Proportion needing orthodontic treatment among children with | | | |
| | Anterior open bite or zero overbite | | Over two-thirds overbite | |
	No crowding	Some crowding	No crowding	Some crowding
Five	16% 166	59% 41	15% 122	38% 36
Six	14% 161	57% 126	10% 75	65% 49
Seven	18% 75	76% 117	13% 48	70% 95
Eight	46% 45	82% 65	24% 48	78% 136
Nine	52% 29	70% 29	27% 52	81% 134
Ten	73% 22	82% 28	26% 63	75% 136
Eleven	* 18	85% 21	19% 63	79% 124
Twelve	* 19	52% 22	26% 60	63% 92
Thirteen	28% 26	* 18	16% 62	54% 87
Fourteen	25% 24	67% 30	7% 60	53% 79
Fifteen	16% 21	* 13	14% 37	48% 58

In Table 8.16 we examine whether the proportion of children who were classified as needing orthodontic treatment varied for extremes of overbite if these were or were not also associated with crowding. The proportion needing treatment who had anterior open bite or zero overbite but no crowding rose to a peak of 73% of ten year olds. The proportion needing treatment among the teenagers was about a quarter, which perhaps suggests that by that age the worst cases, or at least those which can benefit from treatment, are more likely to have already been dealt with. For children with both anterior open bite (or zero overbite) and crowding the proportion needing treatment was significantly higher than for those with the overbite condition without any crowding.

When we looked at large overbite (over two-thirds overlap) the results showed that the treatment need for children was much lower among those without the additional problem of crowding, and that anterior open bite and zero overbite without crowding was much more likely to be assessed as in need of treatment than was over two-thirds overbite without associated crowding. There was a trend for children with extreme overbite in combination with crowding to be more likely to need orthodontic treatment than the total group of children with crowding (compare Table 8.16 with 8.15), but these differences were not large enough to be statistically significant.

There were too few children with very small overjets to analyse the relationship between crowding and orthodontic treatment need, but we could look at large overjets, that is children with an overjet of 5mm or more (see Table 8.17). Among children aged seven who had a large overjet but no crowding 67% were said to be in need of orthodontic treatment, until the age of ten the proportion

remained above half and thereafter decreased to about a quarter of fourteen year
olds. For those children who had some crowding as well as a large overjet the
proportions said to be in need of orthodontic treatment were much higher reaching
a peak of 89% of the eight year olds. As with the investigation of overbite the
children with a combination of large overjet and crowding were more likely to be
said to need orthodontic treatment than the total group of children with crowding.

Table 8.17

Proportion of children needing
orthodontic treatment, by large
overjet and crowding

Age	Proportion needing orthodontic treatment among children with overjet of 5mm or more who have			
	No crowding		Some crowding	
Five	39%	51	*	18
Six	37%	39	66%	41
Seven	67%	50	82%	98
Eight	63%	58	89%	127
Nine	55%	76	85%	128
Ten	49%	69	80%	118
Eleven	35%	80	77%	128
Twelve	45%	66	72%	105
Thirteen	23%	59	55%	74
Fourteen	24%	62	70%	85
Fifteen	15%	36	62%	63

In Table 8.18 we examine the need for orthodontic treatment of children with a
non-normal occlusion, and compare the proportions for children who also have
crowding with those for children who have not. As we have already seen for
previous combinations the proportions of children needing orthodontic treatment

Table 8.18

Proportion of children needing orthodontic
treatment by crowding and occlusion

Age	Proportion needing orthodontic treatment among children with			
	No crowding and class 2 or 3 occlusion		Some crowding and class 2 or 3 occlusion	
Five	59%	187	62%	58
Six	30%	148	73%	136
Seven	48%	113	83%	271
Eight	55%	108	85%	305
Nine	58%	117	82%	282
Ten	49%	111	86%	274
Eleven	41%	119	79%	249
Twelve	40%	121	70%	218
Thirteen	26%	125	60%	189
Fourteen	20%	116	61%	190
Fifteen	16%	79	61%	138

are much higher when a particular orthodontic anomaly is found in conjunction
with crowding. Non-normal occlusion is no exception and the highest proportion
of children needing orthodontic treatment was found among those ten year olds who
had both a class 2 or 3 occlusion and crowding, the proportion being 86%.
This dropped with age but was still over 60% among the teenagers. For those
children who had no crowding over half of eight and nine year olds needed
orthodontic treatment but this proportion decreased rapidly with age so that
only one in five of the fourteen and fifteen year olds were said to need treatment.

Table 8.19 shows the relationship between need for orthodontic treatment, crowding
and instanding or edge to edge incisors. The deciduous dentition and newly
erupting permanent teeth once again obscure the situation for the five and six
year olds. Among the seven and eight year olds who had no crowding but did have
some instanding or edge to edge incisors one quarter were said to need treatment
whereas 80% of seven year olds and over 90% of eight year olds who had some
crowding as well were said to be in need of treatment.

Table 8.19

Proportion of children needing orthodontic treatment by
crowding and instanding or edge to edge incisors

Age	Proportion needing orthodontic treatment among children with			
	No crowding but some instanding or edge to edge incisors		Some crowding and some instanding or edge to edge incisors	
Five	13%	104	59%	20
Six	17%	109	59%	47
Seven	23%	46	80%	102
Eight	25%	28	91%	99
Nine	59%	27	86%	103
Ten	*	16	88%	100
Eleven	50%	23	78%	71
Twelve	38%	24	62%	66
Thirteen	36%	30	76%	57
Fourteen	30%	22	66%	69
Fifteen	26%	26	56%	40

It can be seen from Tables 8.15 to 8.19 that children are more likely to need
orthodontic treatment if they have a second orthodontic anomaly with crowding
than if they just have crowded teeth.

9   Overall dental condition

In previous chapters we have presented information about decay, gum trouble and the orthodontic position, for children, but the topics have each been discussed separately. In this chapter we look at some of the interrelationships between these three aspects of dental health.

9.1 Gum condition and current decay

The dental examination recorded the gum condition as it was at the time of the examination, and so the measurements reflect the present situation only and can give us no indication of whether the oral hygiene position has changed over time. It seemed therefore more reasonable to compare the current gum situation with the current decay situation rather than with any estimate of total decay experience. In this way we are really comparing whether lack of dental care, as manifested in our measurements of oral hygiene, is associated at all with lack of care as indicated by the presence of current decay. Tables 9.I to 9.4 show the proportion of children who had some decay according to whether or not they had any gum contra-indications and also for each of the measurements (gum inflammation, debris, and calculus) separately.

Table 9.I shows that for every age group the proportion of children who had some decay was greater among those who had some gum trouble than among those who did not. For all except two of the age groups the differences were significant. The

Table 9.1

Proportion of children with decay by overall gum condition

Age	Proportion with some decay of children who had			
	No inflammation, debris or calculus		Some inflammation, debris or calculus	
Five	56%	508	72%	444
Six	62%	453	74%	627
Seven	64%	315	76%	822
Eight	76%	246	79%	845
Nine	73%	251	76%	878
Ten	62%	265	72%	826
Eleven	59%	193	68%	792
Twelve	54%	209	63%	747
Thirteen	47%	228	65%	686
Fourteen	53%	237	65%	686
Fifteen	49%	199	60%	497

two age groups which did not show significant differences were the eight and nine year olds where the prevalence of current decay is at its highest. With nine of the eleven age groups showing a significant difference there is little doubt that there is an association between decay and oral hygiene, but it is worth drawing attention to the fact that the prevalence of current decay is very high in the absence of any gum trouble and therefore any action which resolved whatever was responsible for this association of decay and gum trouble as measured by the survey would only make a marginal impact on the level of current decay.

In Table 9.2 we examine the relationship of gum inflammation and decay and with this particular oral hygiene indicator all age groups except the eight year olds and the fifteen year olds had a significantly higher proportion of children with current decay among the group who had some inflammation. There is no doubt that gum inflammation has some association with decay, although this may be through lack of care of gums and teeth rather than any direct relationship.

Table 9.2

Proportion of children with decay by gum inflammation

Age	Proportion with some decay of children who had			
	No gum inflammation		Some gum inflammation	
Five	58%	701	78%	251
Six	64%	703	77%	377
Seven	69%	568	76%	568
Eight	77%	480	79%	611
Nine	72%	498	78%	631
Ten	65%	480	73%	612
Eleven	62%	402	69%	583
Twelve	55%	412	66%	544
Thirteen	53%	410	67%	505
Fourteen	54%	420	68%	503
Fifteen	54%	339	60%	357

Table 9.3 shows similar information about the presence of debris and its relationship with current decay. The results were very like those concerning inflammation. For all age groups (except the nine year olds) a significantly greater proportion of children with debris present had some decay compared with those who had no debris. As mentioned earlier however, the prevalence of current decay was high even without the presence of any adverse gum condition.

Table 9.4 shows the situation with respect to decay taking account of whether or not the child had any calculus. The results for calculus were entirely different from those for gum inflammation and debris. In only two age groups was there any significant difference between the proportions of children with current decay (eight year olds and twelve year olds) and in both these cases there was a higher proportion of children with decay among those who did not have any calculus. There was, overall, no evidence among children of any association between this particular condition and decay.

Table 9.3

Proportion of children with decay,
by debris

Age	Proportion with some decay of children with			
	No debris		Some debris	
Five	58%	579	73%	374
Six	63%	556	75%	524
Seven	65%	438	77%	699
Eight	73%	363	80%	728
Nine	73%	372	77%	757
Ten	60%	377	74%	714
Eleven	56%	343	71%	642
Twelve	53%	349	66%	608
Thirteen	48%	375	70%	540
Fourteen	54%	402	68%	521
Fifteen	50%	341	64%	355

Table 9.4

Proportion of children with decay,
by calculus

Age	Proportion with some decay of children with			
	No calculus		Some calculus	
Five	63%	908	65%	44
Six	69%	1025	62%	55
Seven	73%	1037	71%	100
Eight	79%	928	72%	163
Nine	77%	941	71%	188
Ten	69%	860	71%	232
Eleven	67%	734	63%	252
Twelve	64%	687	55%	269
Thirteen	60%	631	63%	284
Fourteen	63%	622	59%	301
Fifteen	57%	462	58%	234

Thus the overall relationship between gum condition and current decay which was shown in Table 9.1 was due to gum inflammation and debris both of which individually showed an association with decay, calculus playing no part at all.

9.2 Crowding and decay and gum trouble

In this section we examine the most common of the problems which occur during dental development, that is crowding, and test whether the children with crowded teeth are more or less likely than those without crowding to have decayed teeth or gum trouble. Table 9.5 shows the results with respect to current decay. For each age group a significantly higher proportion of the children with crowding had some decay. As with the relationship between decay and gum trouble discussed earlier the association is by no means complete. A high proportion of the children with no crowding had some decay at the time of the examination, but for those with crowding the proportion was always higher.

Table 9.5

Proportion of children with decay,
by crowding

Age	Proportion with some decay of children with			
	No crowding		Some crowding	
Five	62%	782	70%	170
Six	66%	649	73%	432
Seven	67%	458	76%	679
Eight	74%	382	80%	709
Nine	71%	414	79%	715
Ten	63%	415	74%	677
Eleven	61%	410	69%	576
Twelve	56%	432	65%	525
Thirteen	56%	442	65%	473
Fourteen	57%	460	66%	463
Fifteen	47%	329	61%	367

Table 9.6 shows whether, overall, there was any association between gum trouble
and crowding. The results show that for every age group there was a higher
proportion of children with some gum trouble among the children who were
classified as having some crowding than among those who were free from crowding.
In addition to looking at the overal position with respect to the gums we
investigate whether the gum indicators (inflammation, debris and calculus), each
contributed to the association or whether some factors were of more importance
than others.

Table 9.6

Proportion of children with some
overall gum trouble, by crowding

Age	Proportion with some inflammation, calculus or debris among children who had			
	No crowding		Some crowding	
Five	43%	782	65%	170
Six	54%	649	65%	432
Seven	64%	458	78%	679
Eight	74%	382	80%	709
Nine	74%	414	80%	715
Ten	70%	415	79%	677
Eleven	73%	410	86%	576
Twelve	73%	432	83%	525
Thirteen	72%	442	78%	473
Fourteen	78%	460	80%	463
Fifteen	67%	329	75%	367

Table 9.7 shows the relationship between crowding and gum inflammation. Again
there was a positive relationship. For each age group there was a higher
proportion of children with gum inflammation among the children with some
crowding.

Table 9.7

Proportion of children with gum inflammation, by crowding

Age	Proportion with some inflammation of children who had			
	No crowding		Some crowding	
Five	23%	782	41%	170
Six	29%	649	44%	432
Seven	40%	458	57%	679
Eight	50%	382	60%	709
Nine	50%	414	59%	715
Ten	51%	415	59%	677
Eleven	50%	410	66%	576
Twelve	50%	432	63%	525
Thirteen	51%	442	59%	473
Fourteen	47%	460	62%	463
Fifteen	44%	329	58%	367

As far as debris was concerned there was, in general, an association with crowding but although for each age group the proportion of children with debris was higher among the children with crowding the differences were not significant for the eight, thirteen and fifteen year olds. However with all the other age groups demonstrating significant differences it is likely that the association does occur for debris and crowding. The results are given in Table 9.8.

Table 9.8

Proportion of children with debris by crowding

Age	Proportion with some debris of children who had			
	No crowding		Some crowding	
Five	36%	782	56%	170
Six	43%	649	57%	432
Seven	53%	458	68%	679
Eight	64%	382	68%	709
Nine	63%	414	70%	715
Ten	59%	415	69%	677
Eleven	57%	410	71%	576
Twelve	58%	432	68%	525
Thirteen	56%	442	62%	473
Fourteen	49%	460	64%	463
Fifteen	48%	329	54%	367

In the earlier part of the chapter we found that although decay was associated with gum inflammation and debris there was no evidence of association with calculus. The results in Table 9.9 show us that similarly there is no marked association between calculus and crowding. For three of the eleven age groups there was a significant difference but for the other eight there was not. We have thus seen that there is some association between decay, gum trouble and crowding.

Table 9.9

Proportion of children with some
calculus, by crowding

Age	Proportion with some calculus of children who had			
	No crowding		Some crowding	
Five	4%	782	9%	170
Six	5%	649	5%	432
Seven	8%	458	9%	679
Eight	13%	382	14%	709
Nine	15%	414	18%	715
Ten	19%	415	23%	677
Eleven	23%	410	28%	576
Twelve	25%	432	31%	525
Thirteen	26%	442	36%	473
Fourteen	31%	460	35%	463
Fifteen	30%	329	37%	367

The association between decay and gum trouble probably reflects the existence of a
third factor, dental care, which may be causative in both cases.   The association
between decay and crowding may also reflect dental care, but in this case it is
more likely that crowding causes problems in dental care which in turn affect decay.

9.3 Other conditions

The dentists were asked to record any other conditions which were apparent during
the examination.   They recorded ulceration of soft tissues for one percent of
children of each age group.   They found abscesses to be more common among the
younger children, involving 6% of five year olds but only 3% of ten year olds.   In
the middle ranges of age, seven to twelve, about one in twenty (5%) of children
had developmental anomalies involving the enamel or dentine, about the same
proportion of children had anomalies involving the teeth themselves.   Only one or
two percent of children in each age group were recorded as having any anomaly
involving the development of the face and jaws.   Acquired anomalies were only
found in one percent of children beyond the age of eight (Table Section, Table 85).

9.4 Current overall dental need

Finally we draw together the information relating to decay, gum trouble and
orthodontic need in order to assess what proportion of children needed the
attention of a dentist or hygienist at the time of the examination.   In this
assessment we use the dental examiner's estimate of orthodontic need as the
best summary of the total orthodontic position.

Any estimate of overall dental need is of course based on the criteria laid
down for the survey examination and must always be interpreted within that
framework.   The survey criteria for measuring decay will, if anything lead to
an underestimate of decay since early signs of decay were ignored.   The fact
that the estimate might be an underestimate is of little consequence in
this particular analysis since we found that from the age of six onwards nine
out of ten children examined could benefit from dental attention.

Table 9.10

Proportion of children needing some dental attention at the time of the examination

Age	Proportion of children with some decay or gum trouble or orthodontic need	
Five	79%	952
Six	87%	1080
Seven	94%	1137
Eight	97%	1091
Nine	96%	1129
Ten	95%	1092
Eleven	95%	986
Twelve	94%	956
Thirteen	90%	915
Fourteen	90%	923
Fifteen	88%	696

With the level of potential current dental need as indicated by Table 9.10 the problem facing the dental profession is obviously one of priorities.

Part II

The home background

10 Mother's dental experience, knowledge and attitudes

Nearly 13000 children of all ages from five to fifteen had a full dental examination for the survey; this was too large a sample to be able to interview all the mothers and so the interview part of the inquiry was confined to mothers of children of certain ages (five, eight, twelve and fourteen). In this way we concentrated our interviewing resources at certain points so that a fairly detailed analysis could be undertaken relating dental health to home environment, while also obtaining information about the extent to which disease, treatment and dental attitudes varied for children at different stages of their dental development. Most of the results involving the interview are presented for all these four age groups separately, although some special topics are discussed in relation to one age group only. The four age groups have not been combined for any analysis since they do not form a homogeneous or naturally recongnisable group by such amalgamation. The base numbers for the interview groups are different from those for the examination since although all of the mothers of five year olds and fourteen year olds were approached for interview a few were not able to take part. For the eight year olds and twelve year olds we only approached a random sample of one in two of the mothers whose children had been examined, and here again in a few cases the mothers were not in fact interviewed. For eight year olds and twelve year olds the interview base numbers are therefore slightly less than half the size of the group dentally examined. Mothers were not approached for interview if for any reason the child had not been dentally examined, so wherever we were successful in obtaining interview data we also have dental information for that child.*

10.1 Mother's dental status and attendance pattern

In surveys conducted on adult dental health an individual's dental status and dental attendance pattern have both been shown to be highly associated with attitudes towards dentistry and the type of dental treatment received. Since most of the day to day responsibility for bringing up children lies with the mother we begin the analysis by looking at the mother's own dental situation as a first indicator of the child's dental environment.

A considerable proportion of the mothers we interviewed had already lost all their natural teeth, this was so for 10% of the mothers of five year olds and increased

---

* See Chapter 1

through the age groups to 27% of the mothers of fourteen year olds (see Table
10.1), so at the time of the survey quite a proportion of the children did not
currently have a maternal example of how to look after their natural teeth.

Table 10.1

Mother's dental status and attendance pattern

Mother's dental status and attendance pattern	Children aged			
	5+	8+	12+	14+
	%	%	%	%
Regular	44	43	37	33
Occasional	12	12	13	11
Irregular	34	26	29	29
Edentulous	10	19	21	27
	100	100	100	100
Base	922	532	451	886

Between a quarter and a third of the mothers were irregular attenders, that is they
only went to the dentist when they were having trouble with their teeth. About
one in nine said they attended for an occasional check-up. The proportion of
mothers who said they went to the dentist for a regular check-up ranged from 44%
of the mothers of five year olds to 33% of the mothers of fourteen year olds.
Among the mothers of the older children the results showed a gradual movement away
from regular dental attendance towards less regular dental habits and a greater
likelihood of total tooth loss.

In Table 10.2 we examine the variation in the proportion of mothers who had already
lost all their natural teeth according to their social class, and the region in
which they lived. Among the highest social class group (I, II and III non-manual)
the proportion of edentulous mothers ranged from 4% to 15% over the four age groups.

Table 10.2

Proportion of mothers who are edentulous by characteristics of mother

Characteristics of mother	Proportion of mothers who are edentulous of children aged							
	5+		8+		12+		14+	
Social class I, II & III non-manual	4%	283	11%	177	14%	165	15%	284
III manual	12%	441	21%	227	23%	174	31%	396
IV and V	13%	158	22%	108	29%	92	39%	176
Region The North	16%	312	25%	173	31%	140	36%	294
Midlands and East Anglia	10%	195	26%	109	25%	88	32%	197
Wales and the South West	8%	151	17%	80	19%	77	31%	143
London and the South East	4%	264	8%	170	12%	146	12%	252

Among the lowest social class group (IV and V) the proportion of edentulous mothers
ranged from 13% among the mothers of five year olds to 39% among the mothers of
fourteen year olds. There was thus a more than twofold difference between the
prevalence of total tooth loss for the highest and lowest social class group mothers.

The variation in total tooth loss among the mothers was as great for different regions as it was between different social class groups. In the North 16% of the mothers of five year olds had already lost all their natural teeth; this proportion rising to 36% of mothers of fourteen year olds. This contrasts with the position in London and the South East where only 4% of the mothers of five year olds and only 12% of the mothers of fourteen year olds were edentulous. If the total tooth loss of the mother is related in any way to her attitudes towards the dental health and dental care of her child then we can expect the impact to be felt differentially by different social classes and different regions.

Table 10.3 shows the variations in regular dental attendance for mothers of different social classes and different regions. This table presents the complementary picture to that of total tooth loss, highlighting the locations of greatest dental awareness and interest. Among the social classes I, II and III non-manual the majority of mothers said they were regular dental attenders. The proportion was as high as 71% among the mothers of five year olds, decreasing over the age groups to 55% among the mothers of fourteen year olds. Among social classes IV and V just over a quarter of the mothers of five year olds said they were regular attenders, and this decreased to just under a fifth among the mothers of twelve and fourteen year olds.

Table 10.3

Proportion of mothers who are regular attenders by characteristics of mother

Characteristics of mother		Proportion of mothers who are regular attenders of children aged							
		5+		8+		12+		14+	
Social class	I, II & III non-manual	71%	283	65%	177	56%	165	55%	284
	III manual	35%	441	37%	227	29%	174	24%	396
	IV and V	27%	158	27%	108	17%	92	19%	176
Region	The North	39%	312	39%	173	28%	140	25%	294
	Midlands and East Anglia	39%	195	33%	109	26%	88	25%	197
	Wales and the South West	48%	151	48%	80	37%	77	36%	143
	London and the South East	51%	264	51%	170	51%	146	45%	252

As one might anticipate from Table 10.2 there was a regional difference in the proportion of mothers who were regular dental attenders, London and the South East having the best record in all age groups. Not only did this region always have the highest proportion of mothers who were regular dental attenders, but it did not suffer a significant drop in this proportion among the mothers of the older children. A significantly smaller proportion of mothers of fourteen year olds (compared with mothers of five year olds) were regular dental attenders in all the other regions.

The relationships between the mother's dental status, attendance pattern, social class and region alone indicate the potential complexities of the child's dental environment, before any analysis has been made of the mother's attitudes towards the dental situation of children in general or of her child in particular. In the

following sections we look at the mother's views of dental issues affecting
children in general, relating these to her own circumstances, and later discuss
her wishes and expectations for her own child.

10.2 Mother's knowledge about dental development

If children do not get the dental attention they need at the time that they need
it this may be because some mothers put a low priority on dental health or it may
be that some mothers do not know enough about dental development among children.
In this section we examine the level of knowledge among mothers and in later
sections we examine what priorities they attach to dental health.

The transition from deciduous teeth to permanent teeth take place over a period
of years.   We have seen in earlier chapters that some of the five year olds already
had a mixed dentition at the time of the survey while a few of the fourteen year olds
also still had a mixed dentition.   In addition to the fact that the process takes
place over a long time, the rate of change being very different for different
children, the normal pattern of the eruption of permanent teeth does not follow a
simple pattern of the replacement of deciduous teeth.   As we shall see later it
is unknown to many mothers that the first permanent molars erupt directly behind
the last deciduous molar and come through at the age of about six.   In this way the
child is provided with enough teeth to chew with throughout the period of transition
from deciduous to permanent teeth.   Since no deciduous teeth are sheed in order for
the first permanent molars to erupt it is not so surprising if some mothers think
that these are the last of the deciduous teeth coming through.   To establish whether
or not mothers did know about this part of dental development we asked them to
estimate the age at which children usually get their first permanent front teeth,
and their first permanent back teeth.   The results are shown in Table 10.4   We did
not specify in the question whether we meant mothers to estimate the age at which
the tooth first comes through the gum (which was the definition used in the dental
examination) or whether we meant when it was fully erupted, so there may have been
some variation between mothers in their interpretation.   Neither did we give the
mothers any instruction as to how to define age, so again there may have been some
variation since it is not always clear when someone refers to a particular age, say
seven, whether they include six and three-quarters or not, and whether they include
seven and three-quarters or not.   (The survey definition of the age of the child
was the age (in years) on December 31st 1972.)

We compared the answers given by the mothers with the dental information obtained
from the dental examination. The first permanent front teeth to erupt are the
lower central incisors and we took the left one as an indicator; 23% of five year
olds had the tooth present, 73% of six year olds had the tooth present, and 97% of
seven year olds had the tooth present. Thus virtually all children had their
first permanent front tooth through the gum by the age of eight. The proportion
of mothers who thought the first permanent front tooth would be through by the
age of eight can be obtained by summing the proportions up to and including age
seven, that is 81% of the mothers of five year olds, 87% of the mothers of eight
year olds, 76% of the mothers of twelve year olds, and 72% of the mothers of
fourteen year olds. Considering the possible variations in the interpretation of

Table 10.4

Mother's estimate of age at which permanent teeth first erupt

About what age do mothers think children usually get their first permanent front teeth?	Children aged			
	5+	8+	12+	14+
	%	%	%	%
Less than five	1	3	4	3
Five	11 ⎱81	11 ⎱87	8 ⎱76	8 ⎱72
Six	33	36	25	24
Seven	36	37	39	37
Eight	14	10	16	18
Nine and over	5	3	8	10
	100	100	100	100

About what age do mothers think children usually get their first permanent back teeth?				
	%	%	%	%
Less than five	3	4	3	3
Five	3 ⎱23	2 ⎱27	2 ⎱21	1 ⎱15
Six	7	8	6	4
Seven	10	13	10	7
Eight	22	18	17	21
Nine	18	18	19	21
Ten	19	21	21	21
Eleven	7	7	8	9
Twelve	7	6	9	8
Thirteen and over	4	3	5	5
	100	100	100	100
Base	922	532	451	886

age and eruption, we feel the estimates that the mothers made about front teeth are quite close to reality.

As far as the first permanent back teeth were concerned the position was rather different. The first permanent molars (sixes) are the earliest permanent back teeth to erupt and for comparative purposes we used the lower left six to compare the mothers' estimates with the dental examination information. Lower left sixes were already found to be present for almost a quarter (23%) of our youngest age group, the five year olds; among the six year olds 70% of the children had a lower left six and among the seven year olds 94% had one. We thus had a similar age cut-off point as with the front permanent tooth, since virtually all children had the lower left six by the age of eight (in fact most of them had it by the age of seven). The proportion of mothers who thought that the first permanent back tooth would be through before the age of eight bore little resemblance to the survey dental findings being 23%, 27%, 21% and 15% for the four groups of mothers. The misunderstanding about the presence of permanent back teeth in children aged six and seven was not due to a shift of merely a year or two in the estimate, but rather a shift of four years or more with 20% of mothers estimating ten years old as the age, and a further 10% suggesting that the first permanent back tooth erupted even later than that.

The difference between the mother's accuracy in estimates for front teeth and back teeth probably reflects the differences in the circumstances of eruption; firstly the fact that the front teeth are visible and secondly in the case of the front teeth the permanent incisors replace deciduous ones which therefore have to be shed, a process which is hardly likely to be allowed to pass unnoticed.

We did not ask the mothers what age they thought the last of the deciduous teeth erupted and so we have no positive evidence for all mothers as to whether they believed that the first permanent back tooth was a deciduous tooth. We could however obtain a certain amount of evidence on this point from other information in the interview. We asked mothers whether her child had ever had any teeth extracted, and if so whether these extractions had involved deciduous teeth only or not. Among the twelve year olds there were 102 children who had had some first permanent molars extracted but 45% of their mothers said that these children had only ever had milk teeth taken out.

We have already seen in Section 10.1 that there was considerable variation in the dental attendance pattern of the mothers, and that these differences were associated with social class and region. In Table 10.5 we examine whether the characteristics of the mother were associated with her knowledge of the eruption age of the first permanent back tooth. For this analysis we also included the number of children in the family on the grounds that this might reflect the mother's experience.

Table 10.5

Proportion of mothers who say first back permanent tooth erupts before the age of eight by characteristics of mother

Characteristics of mother		Proportion of mothers who say first back permanent tooth erupts before the age of eight, of children aged							
		5+		8+		12+		14+	
Dental attendance pattern	Regular	22%	407	24%	230	21%	165	13%	288
	Occasional	28%	101	16%	58	18%	52	14%	86
	Irregular	20%	309	35%	140	18%	127	19%	252
	Edentulous	20%	93	26%	98	22%	96	15%	241
Social class	I, II & III non-manual	24%	283	22%	177	24%	165	13%	284
	III manual	19%	441	25%	227	17%	174	17%	396
	IV and V	27%	158	35%	108	21%	92	16%	176
Region	The North	20%	312	27%	173	19%	140	13%	294
	Midlands and East Anglia	26%	195	29%	109	15%	88	22%	197
	Wales and the South West	22%	151	17%	80	25%	77	16%	143
	London and the South East	22%	264	28%	170	24%	146	14%	252
Number of children in the family	One	16%	86	30%	26	26%	29	18%	61
	Two	23%	386	30%	185	20%	130	15%	243
	Three	24%	226	24%	187	17%	128	16%	237
	Four	21%	131	17%	70	17%	73	14%	162
	Five or more	16%	94	32%	65	30%	92	18%	183

No particular group of mothers was especially well informed. Only rarely did as many as one third of mothers in any group estimate eruption to take place before the age of eight. Mothers in the top social class group, mothers who were regular dental attenders and mothers who had had several children were not noticeably more aware of this aspect of dental development than anyone else. Neither was there any systematic variation with region. The groups with the highest proportion of mothers saying eruption occurred before the age of eight were the lowest social class group and the irregular dental attenders among the mothers of eight year olds. This suggests that these mothers may gain the knowledge from a dentist but only when the state of the child's teeth necessitates urgent dental treatment, a situation much more likely to occur with these mothers than with those who are themselves regular dental attenders. It is perhaps less important for the dentally aware mothers to have this knowledge anyway in that the child's need for treatment will be regularly reviewed by the dentist and will not get out of control.

10.3 Mother's knowledge about decay

Another barrier to the delivery of adequate dental care might arise if mothers were under any misapprehension as to how early in a child's life dental decay could occur. To obtain some evidence on this point we asked mothers to estimate the youngest age at which they thought children's teeth might decay.

Table 10.6

Mother's estimate of youngest age at which decay could occur

What do mothers think is the youngest age at which children's teeth can decay?	Children aged			
	5+	8+	12+	14+
	%	%	%	%
Under two	23 ⎤ 54	23 ⎤ 51	23 ⎤ 51	21 ⎤ 47
Two	31 ⎦	28 ⎦	28 ⎦	26 ⎦
Three	26	25	22	23
Four	12	13	13	14
Five	5	4	9	8
Six and over	3	7	4	8
	100	100	100	100
Base	922	532	451	886

Table 10.6 shows that about half of the mothers believed that children's teeth could decay before the age of three, three-quarters said that children's teeth could decay before the age of four, and about nine out of ten believed that decay could occur before the age of five. There was thus general acknowledgement by the mothers that decay is a problem which may develop before children start school, many of them recognising that the problem may arise much sooner than that.

We were also interested to find out what mothers thought caused decay, and what might be done to help prevent it. We gave no guidance (in terms of ranges of possible answers) for these questions but recorded verbatim the spontaneous replies that the mothers gave. Each mother gave as many reasons as she wished and all of the causes and remedies she suggested were coded. The coding frame drawn up to accommodate the answers gives the range of ideas that were expressed and shows that two factors dominated the rest. These were firstly 'eating sweets and sweet things' (88%, 86%, 81%, 79% for the four groups of mothers respectively) and secondly 'not taking care of the teeth, and not cleaning them properly' (44%, 40%, 39%, 38% respectively). Table 10.7 gives the suggested reasons for decay in detail. An unbalanced diet and lack of calcium were mentioned by quite a number of mothers but beyond that the causes suggested were each mentioned by fewer than one in ten of mothers.

Table 10.7

Mother's suggestions as to the causes of decay

What do mothers think causes teeth to decay?	Children aged			
	5+	8+	12+	14+
Sweets and sweet things	88%	86%	81%	79%
Lack of care, and cleaning	44%	40%	39%	38%
Unbalanced diet	18%	18%	20%	19%
Lack of calcium	14%	17%	21%	20%
Mother's health in pregnancy	8%	8%	11%	11%
Heredity	6%	7%	8%	7%
Makeup of teeth	6%	6%	6%	6%
Dummies and dinky feeders	6%	6%	6%	6%
Eating soft, sloppy food	6%	6%	7%	8%
Child's health	5%	3%	8%	6%
Base	922	532	451	886

With such an overwhelming acceptance among mothers (8 out of 10) that eating sweets and sweet things causes decay it was of considerable interest to turn to the question of what mothers thought might help to prevent decay. As with the causes of decay there were two dominant suggestions as to how to help prevent decay. In fact these suggestions for prevention were closely related to the two causes, but the priorities were reversed. Two-thirds of mothers said regular tooth cleaning could help to prevent decay, under a half suggested avoiding sweets and cloying things to eat (see Table 10.8). Thus although the great majority of mothers recognised that the eating of sweet things contributed towards decay under half were prepared to suggest that restricting the intake of these foods would prevent decay, many more preferred to suggest cleaning the teeth as a preventive measure. The mothers thus exhibited a considerable reluctance towards changing eating habits for the sake of dental health. Their apparent belief in the efficacy of tooth brushing provides an attractive alternative that is simpler to effect and easier to enforce than a fundamental change of diet. A more detailed discussion of tooth brushing will be found in Chapter 14.

Beyond the two main suggestions for preventing decay a considerable number of mothers recommended a good balanced diet, regular dental check-ups and eating hard crunchy food. Relatively few mothers mentioned preventive methods such as water fluoridation, fluoride tablets or toothpaste or any form of preventive dental treatment.

Table 10.8

Mother's suggestions as to what might help prevent decay

What do mothers think can be done to help prevent decay?	Children aged			
	5+	8+	12+	14+
Regular tooth cleaning	73%	72%	68%	65%
Avoid sweet (cloying) food	47%	50%	45%	37%
Have a good balanced diet	28%	26%	31%	30%
Regular dental check-ups	23%	19%	24%	23%
Eat hard, crunchy food	21%	22%	23%	21%
Fluoride tablets, or toothpaste	6%	4%	3%	3%
Add fluoride to water	5%	5%	5%	6%
Have calcium in the diet	5%	4%	4%	4%
Preventive dental treatment	3%	3%	3%	2%
Base	922	532	451	886

10.4 Mother's knowledge about fluoride

A national survey such as this is not designed to provide information on the
effect of water fluoridation on children's teeth. A broad-based national sample
cannot add to the evidence since so few of the sampled children lived in areas
with fluoridated water and in fact none of the sampled schools were in areas
with a water supply that naturally had the required level of fluoride. There
are of course specially designed inquiries which have taken place in order to
measure the effect of water fluoridation on dental health, and these are the
sources of data for evidence on this issue.* Thus although we were not in a
position to measure the relationship between fluoride and decay, we were able
to investigate the mothers' general attutudes towards fluoride and so it was in
this way that we pursued the fluoride question.

Nearly all mothers, nine out of ten, said they had heard of fluoride, and we
asked all those who said they had heard of it what effect they thought fluoride
had on teeth. The answers they gave were recorded verbatim and then later
classified. About a quarter of mothers said that fluoride helps to preserve
teeth and prevent decay and a third were more specific stating that fluoride
strengthens or hardens the enamel. Over a quarter of the mothers who said they
had heard of fluoride said they did not know what effect fluoride had on teeth.
The high level of 'don't knows' may have resulted to some extent from people
thinking we wanted them to be more specific in their answers than was in fact
required. The proportion who said they did not know was fairly high even among
the regular attenders and the top social class group.

We asked all the mothers who had heard of fluoride whether they knew of any other
ways of getting fluoride apart from in the water supply. Between a quarter and
a third of mothers of the different age groups said they did not know of any
other way. Between two-thirds and three-quarters said that you could get fluoride
in toothpaste, about one in ten mentioned fluoride tablets, two or three per
hundred mentioned preventive dental treatment involving fluoride.

---

* Ministry of Health, Scottish Office and Ministry of Housing and Local Government
  1962. The conduct of the fluoridation studies in the United Kingdom and the
  results achieved after five years. (Reports on Public Health and Medical Subjects
  no.105) London, HMSO.

  Department of Health and Social Security et al., 1969. The fluoridation studies
  in the United Kingdom and the results achieved after eleven years. (Reports on
  Public Health and Medical Subjects no.122) London, HMSO.

Since toothpaste is widely advertised and fluoride tablets are not, we investigated
how the proportion of mothers who mentioned toothpaste and the proportion who
mentioned tablets varied according to the mother's characteristics. Since this
is merely a small illustrative analysis we confine the presentation to mothers
of five year olds (see Table 10.9).

Table 10.9

Proportion of mothers of five year olds who mentioned toothpaste and tablets as a
source of fluoride by characteristics of mother

Characteristics of mother		Proportion of mothers of five year olds who			
		Mentioned fluoride toothpaste		Mentioned fluoride tablets	
Dental attendance pattern	Regular	72%	407	21%	407
	Occasional	68%	101	9%	101
	Irregular	73%	309	6%	309
	Edentulous	54%	93	3%	93
Social class	I, II & III non-manual	74%	283	21%	283
	III manual	72%	441	10%	441
	IV and V	63%	158	9%	158
Region	The North	75%	312	12%	312
	Midlands and East Anglia	67%	195	11%	195
	Wales and the South West	75%	151	12%	151
	London and the South East	66%	264	17%	264

As might be expected fluoride tablets were most frequently mentioned by mothers
who were regular attenders or from social class I, II or III non-manual, 21%
from each of these groups mentioned the tablets whereas only 6% of irregular
attenders and 10% of mothers from social class III manual mentioned them.
However, in mentioning fluoride toothpaste all four groups showed the same high
frequency of about 73%. There were no marked differences between the regions.
These figures indicate that only the dentally aware know of fluoride tablets
whereas fluoride toothpaste, which is extensively advertised, comes to the
attention of a much wider population.

10.5 When should mothers first take children to the dentist?

Since mothers seemed to have few illusions as to how soon decay can start in
children and that sweets and sweet things are of fundamental importance in terms
of decay, we were interested to know when they thought children should first be
taken to the dentist. There were two main points of view expressed, one of which
was that the appropriate time was when the child had some dental trouble, the
other view point was that a certain age was the time to start. We grouped the ages
or time of life into three categories, very young (three years old or younger)
before school (about four years old) and when starting school (about five years
old). Table 10.10 shows the distribution of the answers given. About one in
six of the mothers took the view that no action was necessary until some form of
dental trouble occurred. About a half of the mothers thought it was best to
start taking a child to the dentist when he or she was still very young (three
years old or less). In all, about two thirds of mothers thought it was best to
start taking children to the dentist before they reach school age.

Table 10.10

Mother's views as to when first to take children to the dentist

When do mothers think children should first be taken to the dentist?	Children aged			
	5+	8+	12+	14+
	%	%	%	%
When has toothache (trouble)	16	16	16	15
Very young (three years or less)	60	56	54	50
Before school (four years old)	11	14	14	13
When starts school (five years)	9	9	10	15
Other answers	4	5	6	7
	100	100	100	100
Base	922	532	451	886

The attitude that the first time a child should be taken to the dentist is when he has some dental trouble might be expected to be related to the mother's own dental attendance pattern. In Table 10.11 we show, for various characteristics of the mother, which mothers were most likely to subscribe to this view. It was no surprise to find that very few (6% or less) of mothers who were regular attenders thought the first visit should be left until it was essential, while about a quarter of those mothers who were already edentulous or themselves only went to the dentist when they had trouble gave this as the criterion for a child's first visit.

Table 10.11

Proportion who say start taking children to dentist when they have toothache (or trouble) by characteristics of mother

Characteristics of mother		Proportion of mothers who say start taking children to dentist when they have toothache (or trouble) for children aged							
		5+		8+		12+		14+	
Dental attendance pattern	Regular	6%	407	6%	230	4%	165	3%	288
	Occasional	13%	101	17%	58	12%	52	14%	86
	Irregular	28%	309	24%	140	26%	127	20%	252
	Edentulous	24%	93	27%	98	25%	96	22%	241
Social class	I, II & III non-manual	9%	283	10%	177	9%	165	7%	284
	III manual	18%	441	16%	227	21%	174	17%	396
	IV and V	22%	158	23%	108	20%	92	22%	176
Region	The North	18%	312	20%	173	21%	140	19%	294
	Midlands and East Anglia	20%	195	20%	109	23%	88	15%	197
	Wales and the South West	12%	151	14%	80	13%	77	12%	143
	London and the South East	14%	264	11%	170	10%	146	13%	252

The encouraging result is the inverse of the previous statements, that is, that three-quarters of the mothers who themselves would only go the dentist when they have trouble did not give this as the criterion for when they would first take a child.

Having looked at one view of when to first take a child to the dentist, we also examine the other end of the spectrum, that is the proportion of mothers who said it was best to take a child at three or less. Overall just over a half of mothers said this and Table 10.12 shows how this proportion varied with the mother's characteristics.

Table 10.12

Proportion who say start taking children to dentist at age three or earlier by characteristics of mother

Characteristics of mother		Proportion of mothers who say start taking children to dentist at age three or earlier, of children aged							
		5+		8+		12+		14+	
Dental attendance pattern	Regular	78%	407	70%	230	76%	165	69%	288
	Occasional	54%	101	49%	58	38%	52	52%	86
	Irregular	42%	309	44%	140	39%	127	40%	252
	Edentulous	45%	93	43%	98	49%	96	38%	241
Social class	I, II & III non-manual	75%	283	67%	177	66%	165	64%	284
	III manual	54%	441	52%	227	52%	174	43%	396
	IV and V	49%	158	50%	108	38%	92	42%	176
Region	The North	55%	312	54%	173	51%	140	40%	294
	Midlands and East Anglia	52%	195	44%	109	41%	88	49%	197
	Wales and the South West	70%	151	65%	80	59%	77	55%	143
	London and the South East	64%	264	62%	170	63%	146	59%	252

Among mothers who were regular dental attenders between three-quarters and two-thirds thought three years old or younger was the age at which a child should first be taken to the dentist, while less than a half of mothers who either only went to the dentist with trouble or were edentulous subscribed to this view. Mothers in the top social class group were more likely to say that children should have an early introduction to dentistry and this attitude was also found to be more prevalent among mothers from Wales and the South West and London and the South East than elsewhere.

We asked all the mothers who thought children should be taken to the dentist before they had any specific trouble why they thought this was important. There were two main reasons given, some mothers giving both reasons. About two thirds of the mothers who advised starting dental visits before the child had toothache said the purpose of such visits was to get the child familiar with the dental surgery and chair, and the dentist, and into the habit of visiting the surgery without associating it with pain. About four out of nine mothers who advised visiting the dentist prior to the child having toothache said that it was best to keep a check on the decay situation so that any necessary steps could be taken before the situation became too serious.

It is interesting that among those mothers who recommended starting dental visits before dental emergencies arise the most frequently mentioned reason for doing so was educational, rather than the expectation of the need for treatment at that age. Thus although nearly all mothers believed that children can have decayed

teeth before the age of five, those who thought it best to start taking the child
before trouble was imminent gave reasons for doing so which implied that they
did not expect this to be the case with their children.

10.6 Do children find going to the dentist unpleasant?

We asked all the mothers what they thought children find most unpleasant about
going to the dentist, if anything. Fewer than a quarter of mothers said that they
did not think that children found anything unpleasant about it. Earlier in the
interview we had asked the mothers whether they themselves found going to the
dentist unpleasant, and we were particularly interested to see whether their
attitudes towards how children felt were associated at all with their own
personal feelings on the matter. The results are given in Table 10.13, and show
conclusively that the mothers' views about how children feel are very much
related to their own views; for example among the mothers of five year olds 34%
of those mothers who themselves found nothing unpleasant about going to the
dentist said that they thought children found nothing unpleasant about it,
whereas among mothers who themselves find it unpleasant only 18% said they thought
children do not find it so. Similar differences occurred for the four groups.

Table 10.13

Proportion of mothers who think children find nothing unpleasant about going to the
dentist, according to mother's own views

		Proportion of mothers who think children find nothing unpleasant about going to the dentist, for children aged							
		5+		8+		12+		14+	
	All mothers	21%	922	26%	532	16%	451	18%	886
Mother finds dental visit	Not unpleasant	34%	143	49%	102	33%	81	30%	184
	Unpleasant	18%	774	20%	430	12%	369	14%	697

We took the analysis a stage further to see whether the proportion of mothers who
thought children found nothing unpleasant in going to the dentist varied according
to the mother's dental attendance pattern, social class and the region in which
she lived. As can be seen in Table 10.14 there were no large systematic
variations with any of these characteristics. In fact about three-quarters of
all mothers think children do find it unpleasant. Thus the mothers who attach a
certain amount of importance to dental health have not necessarily convinced
themselves that children will find a trip to the dentist pleasant, any more than
have those mothers whose experience is mostly based on visits stimulated by
dental trouble.

Comparing the variations in Table 10.14 with those in Table 10.13 shows that the
mothers own feelings about going to the dentist have a closer relationship with
her attitude to how children feel than do her own dental attendance pattern or
other background characteristics.

Table 10.14

Proportion of mothers who think children find nothing unpleasant about going to the dentist by characteristics of mother

Characteristics of mother		Proportion of mothers who think children find nothing unpleasant about going to the dentist, for children aged							
		5+		8+		12+		14+	
Dental attendance pattern	Regular	24%	407	24%	230	12%	165	15%	288
	Occasional	13%	101	36%	58	12%	52	16%	86
	Irregular	22%	309	24%	140	21%	127	21%	252
	Edentulous	15%	93	26%	98	16%	96	16%	241
Social class	I, II & III non-manual	21%	283	25%	177	14%	165	16%	284
	III manual	20%	441	28%	227	16%	174	16%	396
	IV and V	25%	158	24%	108	21%	92	23%	176
Region	The North	19%	312	25%	173	13%	140	18%	294
	Midlands and East Anglia	14%	195	23%	109	16%	88	20%	197
	Wales and the South West	27%	151	25%	80	16%	77	20%	143
	London and the South East	26%	264	29%	170	19%	146	14%	252

We asked the mothers to elaborate on what it was they thought children found unpleasant about going to the dentist. The most frequently mentioned source of unpleasantness was the process of having fillings, especially the dentist's drill; having injections was the next most often stated cause of unpleasantness. Beyond that more general problems were mentioned, such as 'the thought of going', 'the instruments' and 'the general discomfort'. Gas and extractions were mentioned as causing unpleasantness much less frequently than were fillings. Specific causes of unpleasantness such as 'the sight of blood', 'the dentists' (or nurses') white coat', 'the stories that pass between children at school', 'the other patients', were not very frequently given by mothers although they were graphically described by those who did. Mothers of children of different ages gave very similar answers on the whole, although among the mothers of fourteen year olds there was an increase in the proportion who said that it was the waiting that was unpleasant. Table 10.15 gives the detailed results as to what was responsible for the unpleasantness.

Table 10.15

What mothers think children find most unpleasant about going to the dentist

Things mentioned as being unpleasant for children	Children aged			
	5+	8+	12+	14+
Nothing	21%	26%	16%	18%
Fillings (the drill)	23%	26%	28%	24%
Injections	13%	14%	16%	15%
Gas	6%	7%	5%	5%
Extractions	3%	4%	4%	3%
Waiting	6%	6%	9%	13%
The dental chair	5%	4%	7%	5%
General discomfort	10%	9%	8%	8%
The thought of going	12%	10%	11%	11%
The instruments	13%	9%	12%	10%
The stories	2%	2%	1%	1%
Blood	3%	2%	2%	2%
Manner of dentist	4%	3%	2%	3%
White coats	2%	2%	1%	2%
Other patients	1%	1%	2%	1%
Base	922	532	451	886

We also asked the mothers what it was that they themselves found unpleasant. Earlier we showed that the mother's own general feelings about visits to the dentist were related to how she thought children felt and in Table 10.16 we look in more detail to see if a similar relationship exists for the actual causes of unpleasantness. In this table we show, for those mothers who themselves found a particular aspect unpleasant compared with those that did not, the proportion who thought children found that aspect unpleasant. Since there was little variation between mothers of children of different ages we have presented this more detailed analysis for the five and fourteen year olds only.

Table 10.16

Proportion of mothers who think children find certain aspects of going to the dentist unpleasant, by mother's own feelings

Mother's views on various aspects of her own dental visits	Children aged	
	5+	14+
	Proportion of mothers who think children find nothing unpleasant about going to the dentist	
Nothing unpleasant	34% 143	30% 184
Something unpleasant	18% 774	14% 697
	Proportion of mothers who think children find fillings (the drill) unpleasant	
Fillings unpleasant	40% 248	51% 164
Fillings not unpleasant	15% 669	18% 717
	Proportion of mothers who think children find injections unpleasant	
Injections unpleasant	27% 206	31% 162
Injections not unpleasant	9% 712	11% 719
	Proportion of mothers who think children find waiting at the dentist unpleasant	
Waiting unpleasant	22% 105	42% 127
Waiting not unpleasant	4% 812	8% 754

Mothers who found particular aspects of a visit to the dentist unpleasant themselves were much more likely to say that those things caused unpleasantness for children than were mothers who did not mention them as a source of unpleasantness for themselves. For instance only 18% of the mothers of fourteen year olds who did not themselves think fillings were unpleasant said that fillings made a visit to the dentist unpleasant for a child, whereas among the mothers who mentioned fillings as making their own dental visits unpleasant 51% said that fillings made dental visits unpleasant for children. This is only one illustration but for all the major aspects which were suggested the mother was much more likely to mention them as unpleasant for children if she herself found them unpleasant.

11 Mother's views on the dental care of her child

In Chapter 10 we discussed mothers' general attitudes towards dentistry and their knowledge about various aspects of decay and dental development. In the interview these issues were discussed as they affected children in general, not in terms of the mother's own child. In this chapter we investigate some particular issues such as preferences for various forms of treatment, and estimated treatment need, which are related to the mother's own child.

11.1 Mother's preference for fillings or extractions

We asked each mother whether, if her child had a bad baby back tooth, she would prefer such a tooth to be filled or extracted. We also asked her what her preference would be if the bad tooth was a back permanent tooth.* There were marked differences in preference according to whether the tooth concerned was a deciduous tooth or a permanent tooth. About half the mothers said that they would prefer a bad back baby tooth extracted whereas only one in ten said they would prefer a bad back permanent tooth extracted (see Table 11.1). It is particularly unfortunate in view of these varying attitudes towards the treatment of teeth in the two dentitions that many mothers are not apparently aware that back permanent teeth usually erupt around the age of six (see Section 10.2).

Table 11.1

Mother's preference for filling or extraction for her child, for deciduous and permanent back teeth

Mother's preference for treatment		Children aged			
		5+	8+	12+	14+
		%	%	%	%
Back baby tooth	Filled	42	38	36	37
	Extracted	49	52	55	55
	Other	9	10	9	8
		100	100	100	100
		%	%	%	%
Back permanent tooth	Filled	88	88	87	85
	Extracted	9	9	9	11
	Other	3	3	4	4
		100	100	100	100
	Base	922	532	451	886

* In the interview we also asked about a bad front permanent tooth but since the answers were very similar to those for a bad back permanent tooth we have confined the presentation to the comparison of back teeth, from the two different dentitions.

It is likely that the mother's treatment preference for her child is related to her own attitudes, in particular her own dental attendance pattern. Table 11.2 shows the proportion of mothers who preferred restoration and extraction for back deciduous teeth and for back permanent teeth. The preferences of the mothers did not vary very much according to the age of the child, but varied considerably with attendance pattern. Taking mothers of five year olds as an illustration the results show that among mothers who were regular dental attenders 58% would prefer a bad deciduous back tooth to be filled, compared with only 28% of mothers who only go to the dentist when they have some kind of trouble. Conversely among mothers (of five year olds) who were irregular attenders, as many as 66% said they would prefer a bad back deciduous tooth extracted compared with 29% of regular attenders who preferred extraction for a deciduous back tooth. It is of interest that even among regular dental attenders over a quarter of mothers preferred extraction for the bad back deciduous tooth.

Table 11.2

Preference for treatment for bad back teeth by mother's dental attendance pattern

Mother's dental attendance pattern	Children aged							
	5+		8+		12+		14+	
	Proportion of mothers preferring bad back baby tooth filled rather than extracted							
Regular	58%	407	50%	230	56%	165	56%	288
Occasional	34%	101	47%	58	38%	52	42%	86
Irregular	28%	309	23%	140	20%	127	28%	252
Edentulous	26%	93	25%	98	25%	96	23%	241
	Proportion of mothers preferring bad back baby tooth extracted rather than filled							
Regular	29%	407	37%	230	31%	165	32%	288
Occasional	56%	101	43%	58	49%	52	49%	86
Irregular	66%	309	69%	140	77%	127	66%	252
Edentulous	65%	93	69%	98	67%	96	71%	241
	Proportion of mothers preferring bad back permanent tooth filled rather than extracted							
Regular	94%	407	92%	230	94%	165	95%	288
Occasional	91%	101	97%	58	90%	52	93%	86
Irregular	80%	309	86%	140	80%	127	79%	252
Edentulous	83%	93	75%	98	81%	96	77%	241
	Proportion of mothers preferring bad back permanent tooth extracted rather than filled							
Regular	2%	407	4%	230	1%	165	1%	288
Occasional	5%	101	-	58	8%	52	2%	86
Irregular	18%	309	13%	140	16%	127	17%	252
Edentulous	12%	93	21%	98	13%	96	18%	241

In terms of the permanent dentition more than nine out of ten mothers who were regular attenders preferred restoration for permanent back teeth. Even among mothers who were themselves less dentally conscious about their own teeth, or had already lost them, over three-quarters said that they would prefer restorative treatment for bad back permanent teeth. When viewed from the other standpoint, that is those who positively stated a preference for extraction, the difference in attitudes of mothers with different dental attendance patterns is fairly marked, for only one or two per cent of regular attenders said they preferred extraction for the child's bad back permanent teeth, whereas among irregular attenders 18% of mothers of five year olds preferred extraction. Although the irregular dental attenders who preferred extraction for permanent teeth were in a minority they nevertheless form a sizeable sub-group (6% of all mothers of five year olds), whose children will, in all probability receive little parental guidance in matters concerning oral hygiene and dental health.

We pursued the issue of mother's preferences for treatment a stage further to see whether or not the dental treatment received by the child, as shown by the dental examination, was associated at all with the mother's expressed preferences. This analysis can only be carried out in terms of fillings received, for the proportion of deciduous teeth extracted rather than exfoliated is not known, and the proportion of permanent teeth extracted is not indicative of the number of permanent teeth being left, unrestored, until extraction is needed. For this comparison we take the condition of the lower left second deciduous molar ('e') among five year olds and eight year olds as an indicator of the treatment of back deciduous teeth, and we take the lower left first permanent molar ('six') in twelve year olds and fourteen year olds as an indicator of the treatment of back permanent teeth.

Table 11.3

Proportion of particular teeth filled or filled and decayed, by mother's attendance pattern and treatment preference

Mother's attendance pattern and treatment preference		Proportion of lower left 'e's filled† in children aged				Proportion of lower left '6's filled† in children aged			
Regular attender preferring:		5+		8+		12+		14+	
Child's bad back baby tooth:	filled	26%	235	41%	116	–		–	
	extracted	15%	119	22%	84	–		–	
Child's bad back permanent tooth:	filled	–		–		63%	155	72%	273
	extracted	–		–		*	1	*	3
Irregular attender preferring:									
Child's bad back baby tooth:	filled	15%	87	18%	32	–		–	
	extracted	8%	205	16%	96	–		–	
Child's bad back permanent tooth:	filled	–		–		48%	101	52%	200
	extracted	–		–		28%	20	42%	41

† *filled or filled and decayed*

Among the five year olds there is a threefold difference between the proportion of children with a filled lower left 'e' according to whether their mothers were regular attenders and expressed a preference for filling such a tooth or whether their mothers were irregular attenders who expressed a preference for extraction (26% filled compared with 8% filled). Among mothers of five year olds who were regular attenders and preferred a bad back baby tooth extracted 15% had the lower left 'e' filled, which was the same proportion as among irregular mothers who would prefer the tooth filled. Thus among the five year olds, mother's attendance pattern and preferences were associated with the treatment received for the lower left 'e'.

Among the eight year olds the picture was somewhat different in so far as the group which was outstandingly different in terms of treatment received were those eight year olds whose mothers were regular dental attenders and preferred deciduous back teeth to be filled. Among this group 41% of lower left 'e's were filled. This was nearly twice as many children with that tooth filled as among those whose mother, although a regular attender, preferred deciduous teeth extracted (22% filled) and more than twice for the children whose mothers were irregular attenders, whatever their preferences (18% and 16% filled).

In terms of the permanent teeth we can only compare three groups, since very few mothers who were regular attenders preferred extraction for permanent teeth. Among twelve year olds whose mothers were regular attenders and who preferred fillings for permanent back teeth 63% had their lower left six filled while among twelve year olds whose mothers were irregular attenders but who preferred filling for their child's back permanent teeth 48% had their lower left six filled. For those whose mothers were irregular attenders and preferred extraction of bad back permanent teeth 28% had their lower left six filled. Among the fourteen year olds the rank order was the same (72%, 52%, 42%) although the magnitude of the difference between children whose mothers were irregular attenders but whose preferences were different had been reduced.

Survey data cannot tell us whether mothers get the treatment for their child which they prefer, or prefer the treatment which their child receives. The results certainly indicate that the children of the more dentally aware mothers have a considerable advantage for a long term dentate future, if it is assumed that restorative dentistry in childhood is a good investment. At the other extreme the evidence is not completely discouraging in so far as a proportion of children are receiving restorative treatment despite having no particular encouragement from home.

Since we find that the attitude of the mother to extractions and fillings is associated to some extent with the treatment which the child receives it is of interest to look in detail at the reasons that the mothers gave as to why they preferred a particular type of treatment. (Some mothers gave more than one reason). The reasons given were different for the two dentitions and are shown in Table 11.4.

The two main reasons given for preferring baby back teeth to be filled rather than extracted were firstly that it was better for the development of the permanent teeth (57%, 56%, 61%, 62% respectively for the four groups of mothers) and secondly that it was best to keep the baby teeth as long as possible (without mentioning the effect on the development of the permanent dentition), which was the reason given by about a third of mothers who preferred fillings. Another reason given for preferring fillings was the specific problem of the child not being able to chew if the teeth were extracted. Relatively few mothers who preferred deciduous teeth to be filled gave the negative reason that extractions are frightening.

Table 11.4

Mother's reasons for preferring particular treatment

Mother's main reasons for preferring baby back teeth to be filled rather than extracted	Children aged			
	5+	8+	12+	14+
Better for development of teeth	57%	56%	61%	62%
Better kept as long as possible	34%	35%	31%	30%
Keeping baby teeth helps chewing	16%	8%	14%	17%
Extractions are frightening	6%	8%	7%	3%
Base	384	200	162	325
Mother's main reasons for preferring baby back teeth to be extracted rather than filled				
Pointless to fill since teeth fall out	57%	58%	60%	51%
Get rid of pain with least trouble	40%	35%	31%	35%
Children don't like having fillings	17%	14%	13%	12%
Better for development of teeth	13%	13%	15%	21%
Do not believe in fillings	9%	12%	5%	7%
Base	447	279	246	484
Mother's main reasons for preferring permanent back teeth to be filled rather than extracted				
Helps preserve teeth	91%	94%	91%	92%
Extraction affects eating	19%	19%	24%	27%
Extraction affects appearance	11%	11%	10%	11%
False teeth unsatisfactory	5%	5%	6%	7%
Extraction affects development	3%	5%	10%	7%
Extractions are unpleasant	2%	1%	1%	1%
Base	807	465	389	750
Mother's main reasons for preferring permanent back teeth to be extracted rather than filled				
Fillings don't last, cause trouble	59%	51%	57%	60%
Don't like (believe in) fillings	35%	33%	28%	21%
Extractions stop pain	25%	15%	15%	21%
Bad teeth lead to bad breath	5%	4%	13%	9%
Base	78	50	38	94

Among the mothers who preferred extraction for deciduous teeth over half (57%, 58%, 60%, 51%) said they felt it was pointless to fill teeth which were going to fall out anyway. Over a third said they preferred it because extraction gets rid of pain with the least trouble. A number of mothers who preferred extraction said this was because children do not like having fillings (17%, 14%, 13%, 12%). Some mothers thought that the extraction of bad deciduous teeth helped the development of the permanent teeth, often in so far as the disease would not then be transmitted.

When giving the reasons for preferring permanent teeth to be filled the vast majority of mothers who held this view said this was to preserve the teeth since, unlike the deciduous dentition, they were not going to be replaced. Nine out of ten mothers preferring filling for permanent teeth gave this reason for their preference, the other reasons taking a very secondary place. There was among these secondary reasons considerable emphasis put on the effect of extraction on appearance and function.

Among the mothers who said they would prefer extractions for permanent teeth there was a strong anti-filling attitude. Over half (59%, 51%, 57%, 60%) said that fillings did not last and caused a lot of trouble. Quite a number (35%, 33%, 28%, 21%) said they did not like or believe in having fillings. Accompanying this antipathy towards restorative treatment was the reason for preferring extraction that extractions stop pain and prevent future pain. The strength of feeling expressed against fillings and the obviously high association of dentistry and pain emphasizes once again the differences in dental attitudes and experience that different groups in the community have.

11.2 Mother's preference for anaesthetics

We asked the mothers whether, if their child had to have a tooth extracted, they would prefer this to be done with gas or with an injection. In the following analyses, the term injection refers to a local anaesthetic in the mouth, unless otherwise stated. On the question of anaesthetics for extractions the mother's views differed according to the age of the child (see Table 11.5). Among mothers of five year olds 51% said they would prefer gas, this proportion declined to 29% of mothers of fourteen year olds. The decline in preference for gas was accompanied by an increase in the preference for injection (in the gum) from 36% of the mothers of five year olds to 53% of mothers of fourteen year olds preferring that method. Some mothers said that they preferred an intravenous injection, and some said they had no opinion and would either leave it to the dentist or, especially among mothers of fourteen year olds, would leave any preference for anaesthetic to be expressed by the child.

Table 11.5

Mother's preference for anaesthetic if child had to have an extraction

Type of anaesthetic preferred by mother	Children aged			
	5+	8+	12+	14+
	%	%	%	%
Gas	51	47	34	29
Injection	36	41	48	53
Intravenous injection	6	5	7	7
Leave it to the dentist	4	3	3	2
Leave it to the child	-	1	4	7
Others	3	3	4	2
	100	100	100	100
Base	922	532	451	886

We examined whether the preference for different forms of anaesthetic varied according to the mother's characteristics, and found that the variation that occurred for mothers of children of different ages persisted but that in addition the proportion of mothers who preferred extraction by gas was lowest among the mothers who were regular dental attenders, those in the top social class group, and those who lived in London and the South East, although regional differences were not apparent among the mothers of fourteen year olds. The proportion preferring gas was highest among mothers who were irregular attenders or had already lost all their natural teeth, those in the lowest social class group and those who lived in the North or the Midlands and East Anglia (see Table 11.6).

Table 11.6

Proportion of mothers preferring gas for extraction by characteristics of mother

Characteristics of mother		Proportion of mothers preferring gas for extraction for children aged							
		5+		8+		12+		14+	
Dental attendance pattern	Regular	45%	407	47%	230	27%	165	19%	288
	Occasional	47%	101	40%	58	31%	52	29%	86
	Irregular	60%	309	47%	140	38%	127	32%	252
	Edentulous	57%	93	50%	98	40%	96	37%	241
Social class	I, II & III non-manual	45%	283	42%	177	29%	165	22%	284
	III manual	53%	441	47%	227	37%	174	31%	396
	IV and V	58%	158	51%	108	35%	92	33%	176
Region	The North	56%	312	54%	173	43%	140	33%	294
	Midlands and East Anglia	53%	195	50%	109	44%	88	29%	197
	Wales and the South West	53%	151	39%	80	29%	77	28%	143
	London and the South East	47%	264	43%	170	23%	146	26%	252

As with the earlier discussion on preference for dental treatment we were interested to know whether the mother's preferences for different types of anaesthetic were related at all to the anaesthetic experience that the child had previously had. Again, of course, the survey data merely indicates whether any association exists, it cannot determine whether the mother's preference precedes the treatment or vice-versa. For this analysis we compare four different groups of mothers, those who are regular dental attenders themselves and would prefer gas as anaesthetic for the child, those who are regular attenders and would prefer an injection for the child, those who are irregular attenders and would prefer gas, and those who are irregular attenders and prefer injection. In Table 11.7 we show, for each group of mothers, the proportion of children who are said to have experienced at least one extraction by gas, and the proportion who are said to have had at least one extraction by injection.

Table 11.7

Children's anaesthetic experience by mother's dental attendance pattern and anaesthetic preference

Mother's attendance pattern and anaesthetic preference	Children aged							
	5+		8+		12+		14+	
	Proportion of children who have had gas							
All mothers	19%	922	49%	532	59%	451	58%	886
Regular, prefers gas	26%	182	57%	107	65%	45	55%	54
Regular, prefers injection	9%	163	31%	98	42%	89	46%	183
Irregular, prefers gas	23%	186	61%	66	65%	49	63%	80
Irregular, prefers injection	12%	87	24%	55	41%	58	48%	124
	Proportion of children who have had an injection							
All mothers	5%	922	19%	532	37%	451	38%	886
Regular, prefers gas	2%	182	7%	107	16%	45	12%	54
Regular, prefers injection	7%	163	29%	98	49%	89	44%	183
Irregular, prefers gas	2%	186	5%	66	20%	49	17%	80
Irregular, prefers injection	2%	87	20%	55	31%	58	38%	124

Overall there was little difference between the proportion of children who had experienced the two types of anaesthetic according to their mother's dental attendance pattern, as long as the mothers had similar anaesthetic preferences; that is the mothers who were regular dental attenders appeared to have no extra advantage in relating anaesthetic preference and anaesthetic experience. This is in contrast to the results concerning preference for restoration as against extraction where attendance pattern and preference in combination were of greater impact than preference alone.

There was, however, a strong association between the mother's expressed preference for one or other form of anaesthetic and the child's anaesthetic experience. The association was more dominant among mothers who preferred extraction by gas. Among the eight year olds a half or more of the children whose mothers preferred gas had had extraction by gas, less than a tenth had had extraction by injection.

Among the children of mothers who preferred injection, a significantly higher proportion except among the five year olds had had extraction by injection and a significantly lower proportion of all ages had had extraction by gas, thus showing an association between the mother's views and the child's experience. Nevertheless among the children of mothers who said they preferred injection the proportion of children who had had extraction by injection hardly ever exceeded the proportion who had had extraction by gas.

We asked the mothers who preferred gas for extraction why this was and the major reason given was that it was better for the child to be unconscious (see Table 11.8). The explanation for this preference for unconsciousness included a widely held view that it was better for the child to have no memory of the treatment as such and that, for the younger children especially, it was better for them not to be able to get restless. The second most common reason for preference for gas was in fact, a dislike of injections, nearly a third of mothers who preferred gas said the child was (or would be) afraid of injections. A smaller proportion disliked injections on the grounds that they hurt. A number of mothers felt that there were fewer after-effects with gas than injections, and some mothers preferences were stated to be based on past experience of gas.

Table 11.8

Mother's reasons for preferring gas for extraction

Mother's main reasons for preferring gas for extractions	Children aged			
	5+	8+	12+	14+
Better to be unconscious	77%	72%	65%	66%
Afraid of injections	29%	31%	33%	29%
Gas has fewer after-effects	9%	11%	18%	18%
Child has had gas before	6%	14%	11%	20%
Easier for dentist to treat	9%	6%	5%	4%
Injections hurt	8%	5%	4%	4%
Base	472	247	153	256

Among mothers who preferred injections for extractions the most frequently mentioned reason was that gas has unpleasant after-effects which was mentioned by a half or more of mothers who preferred injection for extraction (Table 11.9). The second most frequently mentioned reason for preferring injection was the children's fear of being unconscious. In addition some mothers mentioned fear associated specifically with the mask, and the smell of gas. A little less than one in ten, on average, said that they preferred injection because they thought that gas involves some risks. A little over one in ten said they preferred injection because the child had experience of injections, while some mothers preferred injection because they felt it was quicker.

Table 11.9

Mother's reasons for preferring injection for extraction

Mother's main reasons for preferring injection for extraction	Children aged			
	5+	8+	12+	14+
Gas has unpleasant after-effects	49%	58%	59%	58%
Fear of gas (unconsciousness)	42%	32%	38%	37%
Fear of mask, smell of gas	25%	15%	13%	11%
Has always had injection	10%	11%	13%	14%
Gas has risks	7%	12%	11%	9%
Injection is quicker	8%	4%	6%	4%
Base	328	220	217	466

Most of the mothers who preferred injections gave reasons which were not in fact positive reasons for having injections but reasons why they would not like gas. Among mothers who preferred gas many gave positive reasons, one of which was the aspect which caused the other mothers to reject gas, that is the fact that the child is made unconscious. In Section 10.6 we showed what mothers thought children find most unpleasant about going to the dentist and we saw that injections came fairly high on the list, and from the lack of positive reasons given for preferring injections for extraction it is clear that mothers recognise that injections are only preferrable in the context of the alternatives available.

11.3 Mother's estimate of her child's current treatment need

We asked each mother to say whether, if her child went to the dentist the next day, she thought any dental treatment would be needed and if so whether she thought this would involve any fillings or any extractions. Table 11.10 shows that over half of the mothers said their child would need no dental treatment if he or she went to the dentist the following day (61%, 58%, 59%, 56% for the four groups of mothers).

The survey dental examination, being based on visual diagnosis gives a conservative estimate of current treatment need. Even so we have shown that for children of these ages the proportion who had no current decay at the time of the dental examination was 37%, 22%, 39% and 38% respectively. The mothers were obviously over optimistic in their dental outlook. Even though some of the mothers were optimistic other mothers were prepared to say that they thought their child would need at least one extraction if he went to the dentist tomorrow. There were 10%

of mothers of five year olds, 9% of mothers of eight year olds, 7% of mothers of twelve year olds and 6% of mothers of fourteen year olds who said they thought extractions would be necessary.

Table 11.10

Mother's estimate of treatment need if child went to dentist tomorrow

Mother's estimate of treatment need	Children aged			
	5+	8+	12+	14+
	%	%	%	%
No fillings, no extractions	61	58	59	56
Some fillings, no extractions	15	18	17	22
No fillings, some extractions	6	4	4	3
Some fillings, some extractions	4	5	3	3
Other answers and "don't know"	14	15	17	16
	100	100	100	100
Base	922	532	451	886
Proportion of children with no active decay at the examination	37%	22%	39%	38%

The problems which ensue from the mother's estimate of the child's current need are very different according to whether or not she believes a treatment need exists. First we look at the problem if she believes no treatment need exists. Table 11.11 shows what proportion of mothers of different characteristics said their child currently needed no treatment of the type required for decay. Mothers who are themselves regular dental attenders and mothers in the top social class group were more likely than other mothers to say their children currently had no need of treatment.

Table 11.11

Proportion of mothers estimating child to need no treatment by characteristics of mother

Characteristics of mother		Proportion of mothers estimating child to need no treatment for children aged							
		5+		8+		12+		14+	
Dental attendance pattern	Regular	73%	407	71%	230	71%	165	67%	288
	Occasional	57%	101	61%	58	61%	52	62%	86
	Irregular	52%	309	49%	140	54%	127	54%	252
	Edentulous	51%	93	52%	98	60%	96	54%	241
Social class	I, II & III non-manual	71%	283	69%	177	65%	165	63%	284
	III manual	59%	441	60%	227	60%	174	58%	396
	IV and V	56%	158	52%	108	61%	92	54%	176
Region	The North	62%	312	60%	173	65%	140	59%	294
	Midlands and East Anglia	58%	195	62%	109	54%	88	56%	197
	Wales and the South West	62%	151	62%	80	60%	77	62%	143
	London and the South East	64%	264	61%	170	66%	146	59%	252

To test the accuracy of the mother's estimate we compared the number of teeth with active decay (in either dentition) that were found at the survey dental examination for those children whose mothers stated that they currently needed no treatment. The results are given in Table 11.12. Except for the mothers of eight year olds about half of the mothers who were regular dental attenders and said their children needed no fillings or extractions were in agreement with the dental examination findings; mothers of eight year olds were less accurate with only a third of those said by the mother to have no treatment need having no decay recorded at the examination. Less than one in ten children of those mothers, who were regular attenders and said their child needed no treatment, were found to have five or more teeth with active decay. There was always less than 50% agreement between the mothers who were irregular or occasional dental attenders and the results of the dental examination. In fact for the eight year olds only one in four mothers who were irregular attenders and said their child needed no treatment agreed with the results of the dental examination while the children of another quarter of these mothers were actually found to have five or more teeth with active decay.

Table 11.12

The decay situation among children estimated by their mothers to need no treatment, by mother's dental attendance pattern

Mother's dental attendance pattern	Children aged							
	5+		8+		12+		14+	
	Proportion of children with no decay at the examination among those estimated (by their mothers) to need no treatment							
Regular	57%	296	35%	164	52%	118	50%	193
Occasional	49%	57	41%	35	30%	32	43%	53
Irregular	47%	163	27%	68	39%	68	47%	136
Edentulous	27%	47	21%	51	47%	58	37%	129
	Proportion of children with five or more decayed teeth at the examination among those estimated (by their mothers) to need no treatment							
Regular	9%	296	11%	164	7%	118	5%	193
Occasional	8%	57	13%	35	-	32	1%	53
Irregular	15%	163	23%	68	8%	68	12%	136
Edentulous	27%	47	20%	51	14%	58	5%	129

A mother who erroneously thinks that a child needs no treatment and therefore takes no action is one problem which faces those trying to provide an effective dental service, but a mother stating that she thinks her child needs some teeth extracted and taking no action is a rather different problem. As with the previous analysis, we tested from the dental examination data whether the mothers who said their children currently needed extractions were correct in their assessments. The examination provided two sources of comparison. We did not expect that mothers would necessarily be distinguishing between decayed teeth that could be treated and those which the examiner assessed as unrestorable. So firstly we show in Table 11.13 the number of teeth with active decay that were found among children said by their mothers to be currently in need of extraction. Among the five and eight year olds over 90% of the children had some decay, and for 64% of the five year olds and 51% of the eight year olds five or more teeth had active decay. Thus for the age group where deciduous teeth were still contributing a considerable part to the child's dental situation these mothers were nearly all right at least in as far as there was decay present. Among the older children 80% of those said to be in need of extraction had some decay, with 28% of the twelve year olds and 44% of the fourteen year olds having five or more teeth involved. Thus again the vast majority of the mothers who said their child needed extractions appeared at least to be aware of decay.

Table 11.13

Number of teeth with active decay* among children estimated by their mothers to need some extractions

Number of teeth with active decay*	Children estimated (by their mothers) to need one or more teeth extracted, aged			
	5+	8+	12+	14+
	%	%	%	%
None	4	6	17	18
1-4	32	43	55	38
Five or more	64	51	28	44
	100	100	100	100
Base	97	48	33	53

*Decayed or filled and decayed

In Table 11.14 we show what proportion of the children had at least one tooth that the dentist classified as unrestorable. This was so for 83% of the five year olds, 80% of the eight year olds, 53% of the twelve year olds and 54% of the fourteen year olds whose mothers said they needed extractions. The high figure for the five year olds and eight year olds reflects the fact that the deciduous dentition is still involved to a considerable extent, and the drop to 53% and 54% reflects the change to the permanent dentition.

Table 11.14

Number of unrestorable teeth among children estimated by their mothers to need some extractions

Number of unrestorable teeth	Children estimated (by their mothers) to need one or more teeth extracted, aged			
	5+	8+	12+	14+
	%	%	%	%
None unrestorable	17	20	47	46
Some unrestorable	83	80	53	54
	100	100	100	100
Base	97	48	33	53

The results demonstrate that the children whose mothers said they were currently in need of extraction were on the whole in need of treatment and in many cases in need of extractions. Even among the older children where the proportion who had some unrestorable teeth was lower, over 80% had some current decay.

As only half of mothers who are regular attenders, and fewer of mothers with other attendance patterns were correct when they said that their child did not currently need treatment for decay, and as most of the children whose mothers said that they needed extractions were certainly in need of treatment but not apparently getting it even though the need was known, then it is clear that for neither group is it wise to rely on the mother's estimate of treatment need to initiate the child's next dental visit.

11.4 Mother's estimate of her child's dental future

As a conclusion to the analysis of the mother's preferences and expectations for her child we wanted the mothers to make some assessment of what they thought the future held. Towards the end of the interview we asked the mother to project her thoughts forward to when the child was grown-up, and to say at what age she thought he might need to have full dentures. We asked her to make the estimate within ten year bands, that is ".. in his twenties, thirties, forties .." and so on.

Among mothers of five year olds 17% thought their children would need full dentures in their twenties or thirties. In the other age groups there were as many pessimistic mothers, the proportions being 14%, 13% and 15%. At the other end of the age scale about 30% of mothers thought their child might not need full dentures until he was in his sixties, or perhaps never at all.

Table 11.15
Mother's estimate of child's dental future

Mother's estimate of age at which child will need full dentures	Children aged			
	5+	8+	12+	14+
	%	%	%	%
20's	6 ⎫ 17	4 ⎫ 14	4 ⎫ 13	4 ⎫ 15
30's	11 ⎭	10 ⎭	9 ⎭	11 ⎭
40's	22	23	20	22
50's	20	25	24	22
60's	12	10	12	10
Never	18	14	19	19
Don't know	11	14	12	12
	100	100	100	100
Base	922	532	451	886

With a question such as this there was quite a lot of hope or fear mingled with the estimates. Many of the hopes and fears would have been influenced not only by the child's dental troubles so far but with the mother's own attitude and experience. In Tables 11.16 and 11.17 we show how the mother's estimates of the child's dental future varied with the mother's own characteristics. In the first table we show the proportion who estimated that their child would need full dentures relatively early in adult life (in his twenties or thirties) and in the second the proportion of mothers who thought such a need would not arise until the child was in his sixties, or might never arise at all.

Table 11.16

Proportion of mothers estimating their child will need full dentures in his twenties or thirties by characteristics of mother

Characteristics of mother		Proportion of mothers estimating child will need full dentures in his twenties or thirties for children aged			
		5+	8+	12+	14+
Dental attendance pattern	Regular	8% 407	5% 230	5% 165	6% 288
	Occasional	13% 101	7% 58	14% 52	11% 86
	Irregular	23% 309	23% 140	16% 127	19% 252
	Edentulous	32% 93	26% 98	20% 96	24% 241
Social class	I, II & III non-manual	6% 283	5% 177	12% 165	10% 284
	III manual	20% 441	20% 227	17% 174	17% 396
	IV and V	21% 158	14% 108	8% 92	16% 176
Region	The North	17% 312	14% 173	14% 140	16% 294
	Midlands and East Anglia	25% 195	19% 109	16% 88	18% 197
	Wales and the South West	18% 151	14% 80	17% 77	17% 143
	London and the South East	8% 264	11% 170	7% 146	11% 252

The mothers who were regular dental attenders were the least likely to estimate full denture need for their children in their twenties or thirties, but for the other attendance patterns such a low expectation was not uncommon. A fifth of mothers who were irregular attenders gave their children a dentate future no longer than that, and among mothers who had already lost all their own teeth a quarter expected their children to get no further than their twenties or thirties without a similar need. A similar kind of variation occurred with mothers from different social class groups, a smaller proportion of those in the top group feeling that a need for full dentures for their child would arise as early as in his twenties or thirties. As far as region was concerned there was generally less expectation of early total tooth loss among mothers in London and the South East than elsewhere. This variation is of considerable interest since these expectations echo the regional variation in tooth loss before thirty found in the earlier survey of adult dental health.*

Table 11.17 shows the variation in the proportion of mothers who were much more opti 'stic about their child's dental future, that is the proportion who thought the child would be in his sixties or more or would perhaps never need full dentures. This estimate may include a considerable amount of wishful thinking rather than realistic forecasting, but by looking at the variations between mothers with

---

* Adult Dental Health in England and Wales in 1968 by P G Gray, J E Todd, G L Slack, J S Bulman (HMSO).

different attitudes one can see how for some groups the thought of anyone reaching sixty without having full dentures was very much a minority view. For example among the mothers of five year olds the proportion estimating 'sixty or never' was as high as 41% among mothers who were regular dental attenders themselves, but as low as 14% among those who had already become edentulous.

Table 11.17
Proportion of mothers estimating their child will need full dentures in his sixties or never by characteristics of mother

Characteristics of mother		Proportion of mothers estimating child will need full dentures in his sixties or never for children aged							
		5+		8+		12+		14+	
Dental attendance pattern	Regular	41%	407	37%	230	43%	165	44%	288
	Occasional	30%	101	30%	58	36%	52	34%	86
	Irregular	23%	309	16%	140	21%	127	22%	252
	Edentulous	14%	93	7%	98	25%	96	17%	241
Social class	I, II & III non-manual	45%	283	37%	177	41%	165	41%	284
	III manual	23%	441	20%	227	25%	174	24%	396
	IV and V	29%	158	18%	108	24%	92	22%	176
Region	The North	26%	312	21%	173	32%	140	23%	294
	Midlands and East Anglia	27%	195	20%	109	25%	88	20%	197
	Wales and the South West	32%	151	19%	80	34%	77	38%	143
	London and the South East	39%	264	34%	170	34%	146	37%	252

As one might expect from Table 11.16, we see, in Table 11.17, that the top social class group had the greatest proportion of those with a high expectation for the dentate future of their children, and generally more mothers living in London and the South East had high expectations for their child's dentate future.

The effect of the expectations of one generation for the next being so closely associated with their own experience highlights the problems associated with bringing about a change in outlook towards dental health, especially since a considerable part of the step from natural teeth to dentures for adults appears to be influenced by factors other than the dental condition of the individual remaining teeth.*

* Adult Dental Health in Scotland 1972 by J E Todd and A Whitworth (HMSO), Chapter 10.

12 The child's dental background

12.1 Dental treatment experience

A child's accumulated dental experience cannot be ascertained from a dental examination alone, so we used part of the interview with the mother to find out from her the range of dental treatment that her child had so far experienced. The natural starting point for dental experience is to investigate what proportion of children have never, in fact, been to a dentist. The proportion is naturally related to age being 29% of five year olds, 9% of eight year olds, 3% of twelve year olds and 3% of fourteen year olds. Thus beyond the age of about five very few children manage to avoid goint to the dentist. In Table 12.1 we examine the variation in the proportion of children who have never been to the dentist according to various characteristics of the child and his background.

Table 12.1

Proportion of children who have never been to the dentist, by background characteristics

Background characteristics		Proportion who have never been to the dentist of children aged							
		5+		8+		12+		14+	
	All children	29%	922	9%	532	3%	451	3%	886
Sex	Boys	30%	468	8%	276	3%	229	5%	438
	Girls	28%	455	10%	256	3%	222	3%	448
Mother's	Regular	11%	407	3%	230	1%	165	1%	288
dental	Occasional	30%	101	9%	58	4%	52	2%	86
attendance	Irregular	50%	309	20%	140	7%	127	6%	252
pattern	Edentulous	32%	93	9%	98	4%	96	3%	241
Social	I, II & III non-manual	18%	283	3%	177	1%	165	1%	284
class	III manual	32%	441	9%	227	4%	174	2%	396
	IV and V	40%	158	20%	108	4%	92	10%	176
Region	The North	30%	312	9%	173	5%	140	4%	294
	Midlands and East Anglia	37%	195	14%	109	4%	88	3%	197
	Wales and the South West	23%	151	4%	80	3%	77	3%	143
	London and the South East	26%	264	8%	170	2%	146	4%	252

There was no difference between boys and girls in the proportion of children who had never been to the dentist. There was, as one might well expect, a considerable variation according to the mother's dental attendance pattern. Among five year olds whose mothers were themselves regular dental attenders only 11% of the children had never been to the dentist compared with 30% of those with mothers who attend for an occasional check-up, 32% of children whose mothers had already lost all their natural teeth, and 50% of children whose mothers only go to the dentist when they have trouble with their teeth. One possible explanation for the big difference between the edentulous mothers and the irregular attenders is that the former have themselves had treatment, albeit rather radical which means that they have been in contact with the dental services which may have influenced them to take their children, whereas the mothers who are irregular attenders may have had less contact themselves with the dental services, and the contact which they have had may not have led to a full course of treatment. Among the eight year olds as with the five year olds it is, again, the group of children whose mothers are irregular dental attenders who are by far the most likely to have never been to a dentist. Among the older children dental problems, if nothing else, have assured that few children, whatever their mother's dental attendance pattern, had not been to the dentist.

The variations with social class reflect the same kind of variations as with mother's attendance pattern, which is of course related to social class. The variations in the proportion of children who have never been to the dentist in the different regions is not strikingly different.

We asked the mothers of five year olds who had never been to the dentist whether there was any particular reason for this. Not surprisingly the most frequently mentioned reason was that the child had not had toothache or any other kind of trouble and so it had not, as yet, been necessary.

We examined the dental condition of the five year olds who had never yet been to the dentist and found, as indicated by the mothers, that they had less evidence of decay than average. Among the children who had been to the dentist, 24% had no known decay experience whereas among those who had not been, 38% had no known decay experience.

Some of the children who had been to the dentist had not yet needed any treatment in terms of fillings or extractions. This was the case for 26% of five year olds. Only 7% of eight year olds had been to the dentist but needed no treatment and this proportion fell to 3% among the twelve and fourteen year olds. In Table 12.2 we show how the proportion of children who saw a dentist but needed no treatment for decay varied for different background characteristics. For all backgrounds it was only among the five year olds that there was an appreciable proportion who had attended but needed no treatment. The differences between boys and girls were small, but five year olds whose mothers were regular dental attenders were much more likely to have attended but needed no treatment (37%) than were the five year olds whose mothers were irregular attenders (13%). Similarly there were considerable variations with social class. Variations between regions were small compared to those found between the social classes or dental attendance patterns. By the age of eight only a small minority of children had been seen by a dentist and not needed treatment. It is therefore of more interest for the older groups to concentrate on the kind of treatment that children have received.

Table 12.2

Proportion of children who have been to a dentist but have never had fillings or extractions, by background characteristics

Background characteristics		Proportion who have been to a dentist but never had fillings or extractions of children aged							
		5+		8+		12+		14+	
	All children	26%	922	7%	532	3%	451	3%	886
Sex	Boys	24%	468	8%	276	3%	229	3%	438
	Girls	28%	455	6%	256	2%	222	2%	448
Mother's	Regular	37%	407	10%	230	2%	165	2%	288
dental	Occasional	31%	101	9%	58	-	52	6%	86
attendance	Irregular	13%	309	4%	140	5%	127	4%	252
pattern	Edentulous	14%	93	4%	98	-	96	1%	241
Social	I, II & III non-manual	38%	283	10%	177	3%	165	3%	284
class	III manual	20%	441	7%	227	2%	174	3%	396
	IV and V	24%	158	2%	108	1%	92	2%	176
Region	The North	24%	312	5%	173	2%	140	3%	294
	Midlands and East Anglia	22%	195	5%	109	1%	88	3%	197
	Wales and the South West	25%	151	11%	80	3%	77	2%	143
	London and the South East	31%	264	9%	170	2%	146	3%	252

Table 12.3 shows the proportion of children who according to their mother, had had at least one extraction. Among five year olds about a quarter were said to have already had experience of extractions. Two-thirds of eight year olds were said to have had some teeth extracted, as were three-quarters of twelve year olds and fourteen year olds. Thus extraction of teeth is by no means a rare experience, the majority of children having had at least one extraction by the age of eight. Extractions are not confined to any particular group of children, for even those

Table 12.3

Proportion of children who have ever had any extractions by background characteristics

Background characteristics		Proportion who have ever had any extractions for children aged							
		5+		8+		12+		14+	
	All children	24%	922	64%	532	78%	451	77%	886
Sex	Boys	27%	468	64%	276	79%	229	75%	438
	Girls	20%	455	64%	256	78%	222	79%	448
Mother's	Regular	22%	407	62%	230	75%	165	75%	288
dental	Occasional	26%	101	57%	58	86%	52	71%	86
attendance	Irregular	23%	309	60%	140	73%	127	75%	252
pattern	Edentulous	36%	93	73%	98	87%	96	86%	241
Social	I, II & III non-manual	17%	283	62%	177	76%	165	74%	284
class	III manual	28%	441	66%	227	82%	174	80%	396
	IV and V	23%	158	59%	108	79%	92	77%	176
Region	The North	28%	312	73%	173	81%	140	81%	294
	Midlands and East Anglia	24%	195	64%	109	87%	88	79%	197
	Wales and the South West	21%	151	60%	80	71%	77	78%	143
	London and the South East	19%	264	56%	170	76%	146	70%	252

whose mothers are regular dental attenders, or who are in the top social class
group, do not escape the experience of extraction. Nevertheless the children most
at risk for extraction experience are those whose mothers have themselves experienced full clearance, a result suggesting a certain acceptability of extraction among
this group.

Surprisingly there is a more systematic variation in extraction experience when all
factors are ignored except region. For all age groups except the twelve year olds
there is a significant difference between the proportion of children who had had
at least one extraction in the North as compared with London and the South East.

Table 12.4

Proportion of children who have ever had any fillings by background characteristics

Background characteristics		Proportion who have ever had any fillings for children aged							
		5+		8+		12+		14+	
	All children	34%	922	65%	532	84%	451	83%	886
Sex	Boys	33%	468	63%	276	82%	229	78%	438
	Girls	36%	455	67%	256	86%	222	86%	448
Mother's	Regular	46%	407	77%	230	94%	165	91%	288
dental	Occasional	28%	101	68%	58	88%	52	82%	86
attendance	Irregular	23%	309	56%	140	75%	127	78%	252
pattern	Edentulous	31%	93	51%	98	75%	96	78%	241
Social	I, II & III non-manual	38%	283	74%	177	89%	165	93%	284
class	III manual	35%	441	64%	227	82%	174	80%	396
	IV and V	22%	158	56%	108	82%	92	71%	176
Region	The North	31%	312	60%	173	79%	140	78%	294
	Midlands and East Anglia	29%	195	54%	109	81%	88	79%	197
	Wales and the South West	39%	151	71%	80	85%	77	85%	143
	London and the South East	40%	264	74%	170	90%	146	88%	252

Having discussed the variation in extraction experience we next turn to the level
of restorative experience, that is the proportion of children said by the mother
to have had at least one filling. It is perhaps some encouragement to find that a
greater proportion of children, at each age, had filling experience than had
extraction experience. A third of five year olds were said to have had a filling,
as were two-thirds of eight year olds and over four-fifths of twelve and fourteen
year olds. Table 12.4 shows how experience of restorative dentistry varied between
children with different backgrounds. Unlike the position with respect to
extractions the children of mothers who were regular dental attenders had always
experienced more restorative dentistry, whichever age group one looks at. Among
five year olds 46% of those whose mothers were regular attenders were said to
have had some restorative experience compared with only 23% of those whose
mothers were irregular attenders. The comparable figures among the twelve year
olds were 94% and 75% having had restorative experience. There were similar
variations between the experience of children of different social class groups.
There was also a difference in restorative experience of the child according to
the region in which he or she lived. Wales and the South West, and London and
the South East were the two regions which generally had the highest proportion
of children with experience of restorative dentistry.

12.2 Mother's choice of dental service

A child can obtain dental treatment from several different sources, and can choose and change between the services provided. The two main services available are the General Dental Service of the National Health Service and the School Dental Service. The choice between services is, of course, influenced by their relative resources and availability. As well as providing treatment, the School Dental Service is responsible for school inspections, and in fact has far fewer treatment outlets than are available through the General Dental Service. We asked mothers which of the services had been used by the child, why that service had been chosen and whether any changes between services had taken place. In those cases where the child had not yet been to the dentist we asked the mother which was the service she would be most likely to take the child to when she had to make the choice.

Table 12.5
Dental services chosen for child

Dental services chosen for child	Children aged			
	5+	8+	12+	14+
General Dental Service	72%	74%	77%	77%
Private treatment	1%	3%	3%	2%
School Dental Service	29%	39%	44%	48%
Under five clinic*	2%	3%	4%	2%
Dental hospital	2%	6%	9%	10%
Forces	-	-	1%	-
Base	922	532	451	886

Local authority clinic.

Initially, we look in Table 12.5, at what proportion of children of each group had been or would be taken to each of the kinds of service available. Nearly three-quarters of mothers had chosen the General Dental Service for the child. Very few children indeed had ever had private treatment. The proportion who had ever chosen to use the School Dental Service increased from 29% among five year olds to 48% among fourteen year olds. A few children had been taken to Local Authority Dental Clinics for the under fives. The proportion of children who had ever been to a Dental Hospital for treatment increased from 2% of the five year olds to 10% of the fourteen year olds. In this table the percentages exceed one hundred when added since some children had attended more than one type of service.

The General Dental Service and the School Dental Service, between them accounted for the vast majority of the dental attention received by children and we continue the analysis of the type of service used confining ourselves to these two. Some children had been treated within both services and in Table 12.6 we show the proportion who had solely used one or other of the main services and those who had tried both.

Among the five year olds we have already seen that a fairly high proportion have not yet been to the dentist (see Table 12.1). For these children the mother stated which service she was most likely to use. In these cases, by definition, the mother would only have mentioned one service. Obviously as the child grows older then the chances of changing the type of dentist he goes to increase, and we see that the proportion of children who have experienced both the General Dental Service and the School Dental Service rises to a quarter of the fourteen year olds. The table also shows that a half or more of the children of each age group had been

to the General Dental Service only, whereas a fifth of children had been to the
School Dental Service only. Thus the major load of children's dental treatment
is being borne by the General Dental Service.

Table 12.6

Choice from main dental services

Choice from main dental services	Children aged			
	5+	8+	12+	14+
	%	%	%	%
General Dental Service only	67	59	55	51
School Dental Service only	24	25	21	22
Both	5	14	22	26
Neither	4	2	2	1
	100	100	100	100
Base	922	532	451	886

In the first instance the choice of the dental service that the child uses must be
made by the mother and so we investigate whether mothers with different
characteristics were more or less likely to choose different dental services. The
analysis is simplified if we confine it to those children who have selected and
stayed with one of the major dental services. Table 12.7 shows the proportion of
children for whom the mother has chosen, and not changed from, the General Dental
Service whereas Table 12.8 shows the proportion who have chosen, and not changed
from, the School Dental Service.

Table 12.7

Proportion of children for whom mother has chosen, and not changed from, the General
Dental Service, by mother's characteristics

Characteristics of mother		Proportion for whom mother has chosen, and not changed from, the G.D.S. for children aged							
		5+		8+		12+		14+	
Dental attendance pattern	Regular	82%	407	71%	230	72%	165	70%	288
	Occasional	68%	101	62%	58	53%	52	45%	86
	Irregular	49%	309	42%	140	40%	127	42%	252
	Edentulous	65%	93	52%	98	48%	96	41%	241
Social class	I, II & III non-manual	79%	283	69%	177	64%	165	66%	284
	III manual	64%	441	55%	227	50%	174	47%	396
	IV and V	58%	158	54%	108	48%	92	40%	176
Region	The North	71%	312	59%	173	54%	140	49%	294
	Midlands and East Anglia	59%	195	52%	109	44%	88	44%	197
	Wales and the South West	68%	151	58%	80	53%	77	48%	143
	London and the South East	69%	264	64%	170	63%	146	62%	252

The proportion of mothers who had chosen the General Dental Service for her child
and never changed from it was higher among those who were themselves regular
dental attenders than was the case for mothers with any other dental attendance

pattern. As many as seven out of ten of the children of mothers who were regular dental attenders were in this position. Fewer than half of the children whose mothers were irregular attenders had always been to the General Dental Service. A similar kind of variation occurred with social class, a higher proportion of children of the top social class group being taken to and staying with the General Dental Service. Among the children aged twelve or more a higher proportion chose and stayed with the General Dental Service among those who lived in London and the South East than elsewhere.

Table 12.8

Proportion of children for whom mother has chosen, and not changed from, the School Dental Service, by mother's characteristics

Characteristics of mother		Proportion for whom mother has chosen, and not changed from, the S.D.S. for children aged							
		5+		8+		12+		14+	
Dental attendance pattern	Regular	10%	407	10%	230	5%	165	9%	288
	Occasional	21%	101	24%	58	21%	52	20%	86
	Irregular	42%	309	45%	140	37%	127	31%	252
	Edentulous	26%	93	32%	98	28%	96	28%	241
Social class	I, II & III non-manual	13%	283	13%	177	15%	165	11%	284
	III manual	27%	441	28%	227	23%	174	25%	396
	IV and V	33%	158	30%	108	28%	92	30%	176
Region	The North	21%	312	24%	173	23%	140	24%	294
	Midlands and East Anglia	35%	195	40%	109	40%	88	28%	197
	Wales and the South West	20%	151	16%	80	18%	77	21%	143
	London and the South East	22%	264	19%	170	10%	146	16%	252

In Table 12.8 we examine the relationship between mother's dental attendance pattern and the choice of the School Dental Service for the child.

The mothers who are most likely to choose the School Dental Service for their children and remain with it are those who are themselves irregular dental attenders. For the four age groups the proportions of children who have always used the School Dental Service among those whose mothers are irregular attenders are 42%, 45%, 37% and 31% respectively, whereas among children whose mothers are regular dental attenders the comparable proportions are 10%, 10%, 5% and 9%. Similarly with social class, the children in the top social class group were the least likely to have always been to the School Dental Service. In terms of regional variation the results for the Midlands and East Anglia were of particular interest. For the five, eight and twelve year olds a significantly higher proportion of children had been to and stayed with the School Dental Service. This was not so for the fourteen year olds in that region.

In terms of mother's attendance pattern and social class it is clear that the two main dental services are meeting the demands of different parts of the community, with the School Dental Service more likely to be seeing the children from the least dentally conscious backgrounds. We asked the mothers why they chose the service they did and the reasons which they gave also underline the difference in composition of the two groups. The reasons for choosing the General Dental Service are given in Table 12.9, those for choosing the School Dental Service are given in Table 12.10.

Table 12.9

Reasons for choosing the General Dental Service

Reasons for choosing the General Dental Service	Children for whom mother has chosen, and not changed from, G.D.S., aged			
	5+	8+	12+	14+
Took child to own dentist	62%	62%	65%	60%
Started visits before school	20%	21%	22%	22%
Dislike School Dental Service	25%	29%	27%	30%
Nearer, more convenient	14%	10%	16%	13%
Did not know of School Service	9%	6%	2%	3%
Base	622	313	247	455

Among the children who have been to, and stayed with, the General Dental Service, the most frequent reason for the mother's choice was that she took the child to her own dentist. This was given as a reason by 60% of the mothers and reflects very strongly the characteristics of the mothers themselves. A fifth of the mothers said the reason for their choice was that the child started going to the dentist before school age, and about a quarter said that they preferred not to use the School Dental Service.

Table 12.10

Reasons for choosing the School Dental Service

Reasons for choosing the School Dental Service	Children for whom mother has chosen, and not changed from, the S.D.S., aged			
	5+	8+	12+	14+
Notified from school	22%	32%	47%	40%
Nearer, more convenient	26%	32%	29%	33%
S.D.S. good with children	33%	28%	14%	21%
Other siblings go there	22%	13%	9%	8%
Base	221	132	96	195

The reasons given by the mothers who chose the School Dental Service and had not changed from it were completely different. No particular reason given appeared to be dominant. A high proportion of mothers said they chose the School Dental Service because they were notified from school, 22%, 32%, 47% and 40% for the four age groups respectively. This reason reflects the mother's own dental attitudes since it implies that the child did not go to the dentist before school age and that the mother did not consider that she had any particular loyalties to any other dentist. A reason that was expressed among mothers who chose the School Dental Service, but which did not occur extensively among those who chose the General Dental Service, was that the service chosen was good with children. This again probably reflects the familiarity of the mothers with the dental services. For the mothers who chose the School Dental Service any dentist was likely to be unfamiliar, in which case to think that dentists in the school service are going to be better with children is fairly reasonable since they have chosen that field of dentistry. For those who chose the General Dental

Service the majority were continuing an existing arrangement and merely extending the family network.

We have mostly limited the detailed analysis in this section to the two groups of children for whom one or other of the main dental services had been chosen and no changes made. Among the children who had used both services the majority said they made just one change. Among the children aged five and eight most movement was occurring from the General Dental Service to the School Dental Service, whereas in the two older age groups the position was reversed so that among the fourteen year olds most of the changes were from the School Dental Service to the General Dental Service.

For the children who had been to the dentist we asked the mothers whether their child would be going back to the same dentist or practice again, and how far away he was from the child's home. About nine out of ten mothers were not anticipating that the child would change dentist (although in the event this could happen). The major reason given for a known impending change was that the family had moved since the last dental visit.

There was no variation for the different age groups in how far away the dentist was from the child's home. About 40% of mothers of five year olds said the dentist was less than a mile away, 30% said he was one or two miles away, about 15% said he was three or four miles away and just under 10% said the dentist was five miles or more from the child's home. We also asked the mothers whether anyone else in the family went to the same dentist. In terms of the attendance of the rest of the family we examined the survey results for the two groups of children who had been to only one of the main dental services, that is either the General Dental Service, or the School Dental Service, and in Table 12.11 we show to what extent the child's attendance was part of a family pattern for those whose mothers had chosen the General Dental Service and stayed with it.

Table 12.11

Who else in the family goes to the same dentist, for children who have been to and not changed from the General Dental Service?

Who else in the family goes there?	Children who have been to, and not changed from, the General Dental Service, aged			
	5+	8+	12+	14+
	%	%	%	%
No one	8	8	4	12
Other children	6	9	13	14
Mother and other children	13	17	12	11
Father and other children	1	3	3	2
Parents and other children	57	53	63	55
Mother	9	7	4	4
Father	2	1	1	1
Parents	4	2	–	1
	100	100	100	100
Base	479	291	240	441

For nine out of ten of the children who have always been to the General Dental Service other members of their family go to the same dentist or practice, for over half of these children this meant both father and mother and other children. Such family involvement provides a good basis for making dental health a matter of concern and interest for the whole family, providing motivation and continuous contact.

In Table 12.12 we show what proportion of the children who have always been to the School Dental Service have other members of the family who go to the same dentist (or clinic). By definition there is not, of course, the same opportunity for parental involvement that exists within the General Dental Service and so for a third of these children it was found that no one else in the family went to the same dentist.

Table 12.12
Who else in the family goes to the same dentist for children who have been to and not changed from the School Dental Service?

Who else in the family goes there?	Children who have been to, and not changed from, the School Dental Service, aged			
	5+	8+	12+	14+
	%	%	%	%
No one	39	36	35	41
Other children	61	64	65	59
	100	100	100	100
Base	110	108	88	179

The family involvement that exists for the children using different services even though the variation is inevitable, highlights again the difference in the composition of the two groups and the environments within which the children's dental attitudes are formed.

12.3 School dental inspections
Part of the function of the School Dental Service is to carry out dental inspections in schools in order to monitor the state of dental health among children. As a result of such an inspection a note may be sent home with the child if the dentist has found any indication of decay. The note advises the mother to seek dental attention for the child. She is entirely free, of course, to choose which dental service the child will go to and in fact whether treatment will be sought or not. The dental examination for this survey was itself carried out in schools with the cooperation of the School Dental Service but with a rather more detailed examination than is practical in the normal situation of school inspections. We asked the mothers whether, excluding the special inspection done for the survey, the children had previously been dentally examined in school. The mother's answers are shown in Table 12.13 and as one might expect, the five year olds, in their first year at school, are least likely to have so far had a school inspection. Even among this youngest age group 39% had in fact been examined. Among the eight year olds three-quarters were said to have been inspected at least once, which was the case for 88% of the twelve year olds and 87% of the fourteen year olds.

Table 12.13

Has child ever had a school dental inspection?

Whether child has ever had a school dental inspection	Children aged			
	5+	8+	12+	14+
	%	%	%	%
Yes	39	77	88	87
No	54	16	9	8
Don't know	7	7	3	5
	100	100	100	100
Base	922	532	451	886

The proportion of mothers who said the child had never been dentally inspected at school ranged from 54% of the five year olds to 16% of the eight year olds to 9% of the twelve year olds and 8% of the fourteen year olds. Thus some children escaped the inspection procedure completely or alternatively the inspection procedure escaped the notice of some mothers completely. A relatively small proportion of mothers said they did not know whether the child had had a school dental inspection or not.

In Table 12.14 we examine whether or not there was any regional variation in the proportion of children who had ever been examined at school. The first part of the table shows the proportion who, the mother said, had been seen; the second part shows the proportion who, the mother said, had never been seen. Among the five year olds the proportion of children who had been inspected was high in Wales and the South West, compared to the other regions. Among the five, eight and twelve year olds the proportion who had never been seen in school was high in the Midlands and East Anglia compared with other regions, being significantly higher than each of the other regions among the twelve year olds.

Table 12.14

Has child ever had a school dental inspection, by region

Region	Children aged							
	5+		8+		12+		14+	
	Proportion who had had at least one school dental inspection, of children aged							
The North	36%	312	78%	173	86%	140	89%	294
Midlands and East Anglia	35%	195	68%	109	76%	88	87%	197
Wales and the South West	52%	151	88%	80	93%	77	89%	143
London and the South East	37%	264	76%	170	94%	146	84%	252
	Proportion who, mother says, had never had a school dental inspection							
The North	55%	312	13%	173	8%	140	9%	294
Midlands and East Anglia	61%	195	26%	109	20%	88	8%	197
Wales and the South West	43%	151	10%	80	5%	77	8%	143
London and the South East	53%	264	17%	170	4%	146	10%	252

In the School Dental Service it has always been a difficult compromise to balance
limited resources between inspection and treatment. The regional variations in
inspection, especially the proportion of children said never to have been inspected,
are therefore of particular interest when compared with the regional variation in
the proportion of children who have been to and stayed with the School Dental Service
for their treatment (see Table 12.8). However it must be remembered that the regions
include many local authorities each of which is responsible for organising its own
School Dental Service; any regional variations which exist show the resultant effect
of all the services in that region which may well not be homogeneous in their
policies.

We have so far discussed whether the mother thinks the child has ever had a school
dental inspection but of course for the older children this covers a fairly long
period of time. We therefore, in addition, asked the mother to say how long ago the
child's last school dental examination had been. The results are given in Table
12.15.

Table 12.15
How long ago was child's last dental inspection?

How long ago was last inspection?	Children aged			
	5+	8+	12+	14+
	%	%	%	%
Never	54	16	9	8
Don't know	11	21	16	25
Three years or more	-	4	12	16
Two years, less than three	-	7	11	8
A year, less than two	3	15	17	14
Under a year ago	32	37	35	29
	100	100	100	100
Base	922	532	451	886

About a third of mothers estimated that the last dental inspection their child had
was under a year ago, and among the children aged eight and twelve about a half of
mothers said the last inspection had been less than two years ago. Nearly a quarter
of the mothers of twelve and fourteen year olds said their last school dental
inspection had been more than two years ago.

The most important consequence of a school dental inspection is, of course, that
the dentist sends a note home to the mother if he considers that the child needs
dental attention. We asked all the mothers whether or not the child had ever
brought such a note home. Among five year olds, many of whom had not yet had a
school dental inspection, 13% of mothers said they had received a note, among eight
year olds 34% of mothers had received a note, among twelve year olds the proportion
was 42% and for fourteen year olds the proportion was 37%. Thus although the
proportion of mothers who said their child had been examined at school was 39%, 77%,
88% and 87% a very much lower proportion said that they had ever received a note
advising them to seek treatment. The reasons for this disparity could be that the
child had no treatment need when inspected, the note system was not operated, the
child was not an efficient postman, or that the mother did not remember receiving

the note. The survey results have shown the unlikelihood of a high proportion of
the children being found to be dentally fit in which case it might seem prudent
to investigate alternative follow-up procedures.

Table 12.16

Has child ever brought a note home from school, by background characteristics

Background characteristics		Proportion who have ever brought a note home from school, of children aged							
		5+		8+		12+		14+	
Mother's dental attendance pattern	Regular	11%	407	31%	230	33%	165	30%	288
	Occasional	18%	101	29%	58	50%	52	46%	86
	Irregular	14%	309	38%	140	51%	127	40%	252
	Edentulous	14%	93	42%	98	39%	96	41%	241
Social class	I, II & III non-manual	10%	283	33%	177	40%	165	28%	284
	III manual	13%	441	36%	227	48%	174	41%	396
	IV and V	16%	158	32%	108	40%	92	41%	176
Region	The North	14%	312	37%	173	40%	140	42%	294
	Midlands and East Anglia	14%	195	31%	109	54%	88	43%	197
	Wales and the South West	12%	151	34%	80	36%	77	33%	143
	London and the South East	12%	264	34%	170	40%	146	29%	252
Type of dentist	Always G.D.S.*	10%	479	28%	291	32%	240	28%	441
	Always S.D.S.*	20%	110	42%	108	52%	88	48%	179

* G.D.S.—General Dental Service; S.D.S.—School Dental Service

We also examined (see Table 12.16) whether the proportion of mothers who said that
they had received a note from school varied with factors such as the mother's
attendance pattern, social class, region and the type of dental service used by
the child. The mothers who were themselves regular dental attenders were less
likely to have received a note from school than were the other mothers, but of
course this is the group in which one is likely to find better dental care among
the children, and evidence that dental attention is being sought. The same kind
of variation occurred with social class, this again being a reflection of the
higher concentration in the top social class group of mothers who are regular
dental attenders themselves. Among the five and eight year olds there was no
regional variation in the proportion of mothers who had received a note from school
but among the older children more of the mothers in the North and the Midlands and
East Anglia said they had received notes from school.

One factor which was systematically associated with the proportion of mothers who
had ever received a note was the dental service which the child used. We have
already seen that the choice of the School Dental Service was more likely for the
less dentally aware mothers whose choice of dentist was in some cases prompted by
a note from school. It is more likely for this group to be relying on and needing
the notification which the school inspection system provides.

Among the mothers who said they had received a note from school about their child's
need for dental attention, eight out of ten said that the child saw a dentist
within a month. Of those whose children did not see a dentist within a month of
the note there were three main reasons given by the mothers for leaving it for the
time being: that they did not think it was necessary as there appeared to be no
sign of any trouble; that the child was too frightened to go, or that they left it
to the next regular check-up time.

13 Visiting the dentist

The circumstances of the child's visits to the dentist and the child's attitude
to the occasion must be of fundamental importance in determining the treatment
which he receives and his dental outlook for the future. In this chapter we
concentrate on three areas of interest, the child's first dental visit or course
of visits, the child's most recent dental visit or course of visits, and the
mother's description of how she thinks the child feels about various aspects of
visiting the dentist. By definition therefore, the information in this chapter
is about children who have been to the dentist.

13.1 The child's first dental visit

We asked the mothers some fairly detailed questions about the very first dental
visit that their child had made. Answering such questions may have been rather
difficult for the mothers of the older children for whom the first visit may have
taken place many years earlier, but there is little indication from the results
that the mothers could not recall the event.

The mothers were asked why the child had been taken to the dentist the very first
time. The most frequent reason given was to get the child accustomed to going to
the dentist (34%, 32%, 26%, and 21% for the four age groups respectively). Other
major reasons were that the child went for a check-up (26%, 22%, 19%, 17%), or the
child had toothache (16%, 19%, 20%, 22%), or because the mother was anxious about
something and wanted to ask advice (12%, 16%, 16%, 16%). Among five year olds who
had been to the dentist, the proportion of first visits that had been prompted by
a note from school was understandably lower than for the other age groups (6%,
12%, 15%, 17%), this was mainly due to the fact that many of the five year olds
had not yet had a school inspection and secondly that the note as a stimulus for
the first visit was more likely to be the case among children whose first dental
visit was to occur after the age of five. It is obvious from the older groups
that the note from school plays an important part among those whose first dental
visit had not occurred before school age. The details of the reasons given for
the child's first dental visit are given in Table 13.1.

In Chapter 10 we reported the general views of mothers as to when first to take
children to the dentist. In 16% of cases (see Table 10.10) mothers thought that
the first time the child had toothache was soon enough. We find from Table 13.1
that the proportion of children whose first visit was in fact stimulated by toothache was very close to the level that might have been predicted from the attitudes
of the mothers.

Table 13.1

Reasons for the child's first dental visit

Reasons for first dental visit	Children who have been to the dentist, aged			
	5+	8+	12+	14+
Get child used to dentist	34%	32%	26%	21%
Check-up	26%	22%	19%	17%
Toothache	16%	19%	20%	22%
Mother wanted advice	12%	16%	16%	16%
Note from school	6%	12%	15%	17%
Someone else going	6%	4%	4%	6%
Base	*656*	*484*	*435*	*855*

Perhaps the two extremes of reasons given for the first dental visit are 'to get the child used to going to the dentist,' and 'the child had toothache.' The former implies no expectation of imminent treatment need whilst the latter is prompted by an urgent treatment need. In Table 13.2 we show for mothers of different dental attendance patterns what proportion of the children's first visits were aimed at familiarising the child with the dental process in the least painful way. About half of mothers of children aged five, eight and twelve who were themselves regular attenders said they first took their child to the dentist to get him or her used to going. Among the fourteen year olds this proportion was lower (38%). It is not possible to tell whether this difference indicates that over time there has been a change in attitudes among mothers who are regular attenders, or whether over time the mother's memory of the first visit has become blurred. No other attendance pattern group included such a high proportion who took their children for that reason. In fact among mothers who were themselves irregular attenders, hardly more than 10% said that on the first occasion they took their child to familiarise him with going to the dentist. Mothers who occasionally go for a check-up, and those who had already lost all their teeth included a higher proportion (than did the irregulars) of mothers who first took their child to get him used to it; however these proportions were not nearly as high as among the mothers who were regular attenders.

Table 13.2

Proportion of children whose first visit was to get them used to going to the dentist, by mother's dental attendance pattern

Mother's dental attendance pattern	Proportion whose first visit was to get them used to the dentist, of children who had been to the dentist, aged							
	5+		8+		12+		14+	
Regular	49%	*362*	51%	*224*	51%	*164*	38%	*286*
Occasional	21%	*71*	26%	*53*	12%	*50*	23%	*84*
Irregular	12%	*155*	11%	*113*	9%	*118*	11%	*237*
Edentulous	20%	*64*	19%	*89*	12%	*92*	10%	*233*

In Table 13.3 we examine how the proportion of children whose first dental visit was prompted by toothache varied according to the mother's dental attendance

pattern. Only about 10% of mothers who were regular attenders said that their
child's first dental visit had been because of toothache. Among mothers who were
irregular attenders or had already lost all their teeth between a quarter and a
third said that for their child, toothache had been the reason for the first visit.

Table 13.3

Proportion of children whose first visit was because of toothache,
by mother's dental attendance pattern

Mother's dental attendance pattern	Proportion whose first dental visit was because of toothache of children who had been to the dentist, aged							
	5+		8+		12+		14+	
Regular	7%	362	9%	224	9%	164	12%	286
Occasional	18%	71	14%	53	9%	50	16%	84
Irregular	33%	155	32%	113	26%	118	27%	237
Edentulous	36%	64	32%	89	36%	92	30%	233

We also asked how old the child had been when he or she first went to the dentist.
The results are shown in Table 13.4. At the bottom of the table we show the
proportion of children, at each age, who were said never to have been to the
dentist. Among the children who have already had the experience of going to the
dentist, there is a higher proportion among the five year olds who went at the age
of three or less. However the children aged five who have not yet been to the
dentist will be making their first visit at the age of five or more. If one allows
for the eventual introduction to dentistry of all those who have not yet been, then
the difference between the age groups is much reduced. Even so, there appears to
be a higher proportion of the five year olds whose first dental visit took place at
the age of three or less compared to the fourteen year olds. It is difficult to say
whether this is due to a change in dental attitudes or the effect of asking the
mothers of the older children to remember the first dental visit over a longer
period of time.

Table 13.4

Age at which child first went to the dentist

Age at first visit	Children who have been to the dentist, aged			
	5+	8+	12+	14+
	%	%	%	%
Three or under	57	43	36	31
Four	27	20	17	18
Five or more	16	37	47	51
	100	100	100	100
Base	656	484	435	855
Proportion of children who have never been to the dentist (Table 12.1)	29% 922	9% 532	3% 451	3% 886

One illustration of the kind of introduction that a child has had to dentistry is the type of treatment he received on his first dental visit. In Table 13.5 we show for all children who had been to the dentist what proportion had needed no fillings or extractions, the proportion who had had some extractions and the proportion who had had some fillings on that first occasion. Two-thirds of five year olds and about a half of eight, twelve and fourteen year olds had had neither fillings nor extractions as a result of their first dental visit. Among the twelve and fourteen year olds a third had had some extractions as a result of their first visit. This was so for only 26% of the eight year olds and 17% of the five year olds who had been to the dentist, but of course those whose first dental visit had not yet taken place might eventually succeed in making the figures comparable. The proportion of children whose first dental visit had resulted in their having some fillings was about 15% for all age groups.

Table 13.5

Dental treatment received as result of first visit

Treatment received at first visit	Children who have been to the dentist, aged			
	5+	8+	12+	14+
No fillings no extractions	65%	56%	52%	47%
Some extractions	17%	26%	32%	36%
Some fillings	15%	16%	16%	15%
Base	*656*	*484*	*435*	*855*

It is thus probable that for about a third of children their first dental experience is one of extraction. Such an experience is, of course, most likely to occur amongst those whose dental attitudes do not allow for any anticipation of dental trouble. In order to examine the effect on the kind of treatment that the child first experiences, we show in Table 13.6 what treatment the child received as the result of his first dental visit, for those children whose introduction to dentistry was stimulated by toothache. For over three-quarters of the children whose first dental visit was prompted by toothache their first experience of dentistry was extraction. Although about one-fifth of the five and eight year olds (fewer of the older age groups) had some fillings, many of these children experienced extraction and no restorative treatment.

Table 13.6

Dental treatment received when first dental visit was because of toothache

Treatment received at first visit	Children whose first visit was because of toothache, aged			
	5+	8+	12+	14+
No fillings no extractions	2%	3%	4%	4%
Some extractions	75%	78%	84%	86%
Some fillings	21%	23%	15%	10%
Base	*115*	*93*	*84*	*183*

13.2 The child's most recent dental visit

Although the circumstances of the first dental visit provide a useful insight into the kind of introduction that children have to dentistry it is perhaps even more illuminating to examine the details of the child's most recent dental visit. As with the analysis about the first occasion we start by examining what the reason was for the most recent visit. Three main reasons were given, that the child went for a check-up, that the child had toothache or some kind of trouble, or that the mother had received a note from school. The detailed results are given in Table 13.7.

Table 13.7

Reason for most recent dental visit

Reason for most recent dental visit	Children who have been to the dentist, aged			
	5+	8+	12+	14+
	%	%	%	%
Check-up	61	63	63	65
Trouble	27	22	20	22
Note from school	7	12	11	9
Other reasons	5	3	6	4
	100	100	100	100
Base	*656*	*484*	*435*	*855*

Nearly two-thirds of the mothers said that the child's most recent visit had been for a check-up, between a fifth and a quarter said the visit had resulted from some kind of dental trouble and in about one in ten cases the mother said the visit had been prompted by a note from school. There was little variation between the reasons given for children of different ages. The reason given for the child's most recent visit provides the best single estimate of how the child's dental attendance pattern is developing. It is therefore of considerable interest to examine the extent to which the child's behaviour reflects that of his or her mother. In Table 13.8 we show the proportion of children whose most recent dental visit was for a check-up according to the dental attendance pattern of the mother.

Table 13.8

Proportion of children whose most recent visit was for a check-up by mother's dental attendance pattern

Mother's dental attendance pattern	Proportion whose most recent visit was for a check-up among children who have been to the dentist, aged							
	5+		8+		12+		14+	
Regular	76%	*362*	76%	*224*	75%	*164*	80%	*286*
Occasional	52%	*71*	58%	*53*	73%	*50*	73%	*84*
Irregular	42%	*155*	46%	*113*	46%	*118*	52%	*237*
Edentulous	39%	*64*	56%	*89*	60%	*92*	55%	*233*

Among mothers who were themselves regular dental attenders, three-quarters said that the child's most recent dental visit had been for a check-up. Among the mothers who occasionally go to the dentist for a check-up, three-quarters of those of children aged twelve and fourteen said the child last went for a check-up, but the proportion was just over a half for the five and eight year olds. This may be the result of greater priority being given to permanent teeth. The proportion of mothers who are irregular attenders themselves who said the child's most recent dental visit was for a check-up ranged from 42% to 52% and the mothers who were edentulous were fairly similar, ranging from 39% to 60%. Although it was encouraging to see that about a half or more of children whose mothers were not regular attenders were said to have been for a check-up last time, the children of regular attenders were considerably more likely to have attended last time for a check-up.

In Table 13.9 we examine the other extreme in attendance pattern terms, that is the proportion of children whose last visit was prompted by dental trouble, again showing the variations according to the mother's attendance pattern. Among five year olds who had been to the dentist the proportion whose last visit had been stimulated by dental trouble ranged from 16% to 36% to 42% and 45% according to whether the mother was a regular attender, an occasional attender, only visited the dentist when having trouble, or had already become edentulous. There was thus nearly a threefold difference in the proportion of children who last went with trouble according to the dental attendance pattern of the mother. Although among the other age groups the variation was not as great, it still ranged from a little over 10% among children whose mothers are regular attenders to a third of children whose mothers visit when they have trouble or are already edentulous.

Table 13.9

Proportion of children whose most recent visit was because of trouble by mother's dental attendance pattern

Mother's dental attendance pattern	Proportion whose most recent visit was because of trouble among children who have been to the dentist, aged							
	5+		8+		12+		14+	
Regular	16%	362	13%	224	11%	164	11%	286
Occasional	36%	71	23%	53	10%	50	15%	84
Irregular	42%	155	33%	113	31%	118	28%	237
Edentulous	45%	64	28%	89	25%	92	31%	233

The previous two tables have shown that there is a significant tendency for the children of mothers who are regular attenders to show signs of becoming regular attenders themselves and for the children of mothers who are not regular attenders, especially of those who are edentulous or who only go to the dentist when they have trouble,to exhibit no signs of acquiring a good dental attendance pattern for them- selves. Another aspect from which one can examine the developing attendance pattern of the child is to relate the reason for the child's last visit to the reason for the first visit. In Table 13.10 we show the proportion of children whose last visit was for a check-up according to whether their first visit was to get accustomed to going to the dentist, for a check-up or because of toothache or a note from school.

Among children whose first visit to the dentist was in advance of dental need, three-quarters or more gave a check-up as the reason for the most recent visit, on the other hand, among children whose first visit was stimulated by expressed need (either toothache or a note), the proportion whose most recent visit was for a check-up ranged from 24% to 51%; the situation was better for the older children than the younger ones, and although the level of change from lack of anticipation to anticipation is perhaps encouraging, there nevertheless remains a considerable disparity between the children whose dental experience began with dental care in mind and those whose experience began with dental trouble.

Table 13.10

Proportion of children whose most recent dental visit was for a check-up, according to the reason for their first dental visit

Reason for child's first dental visit	Proportion whose most recent visit was for a check-up among children who have been to the dentist, aged							
	5+		8+		12+		14+	
Get child used to dentist	78%	225	81%	156	76%	114	86%	178
Check-up	80%	173	72%	105	77%	82	77%	146
Toothache	30%	115	35%	93	46%	86	49%	184
Note from school	24%	42	39%	56	44%	64	51%	147

In Table 13.11 we show the situation in reverse, that is the proportion of children whose most recent dental visit was stimulated by dental trouble, according to the reason for their first dental visit. Among the five and eight year olds whose first visit was because of toothache, 62% and 52% respectively visited the dentist last time because of trouble. These figures are particularly high because some of the five and eight year olds whose dental habits leave something to be desired may only have been to the dentist once, thus providing perfect correlation between the reasons for their first and last visits. This problem should not influence the twelve and fourteen year old groups and for these ages there is a significant tendency for the children whose first visit was because of toothache to have most recently been because of trouble, 33% for twelve year olds and 38% for fourteen year olds compared to 8% and 7% of children whose first visit was to get used to going to the dentist.

Table 13.11

Proportion of children whose most recent dental visit was because of trouble according to the reason for their first dental visit

Reason for child's first dental visit	Proportion whose most recent visit was because of trouble among children who have been to the dentist, aged							
	5+		8+		12+		14+	
Get child used to dentist	13%	225	11%	156	8%	114	7%	178
Check-up	14%	173	19%	105	16%	82	13%	146
Toothache	62%	115	52%	93	33%	86	38%	184
Note from school	26%	42	7%	56	22%	64	22%	147

It is clear that some of the variations in dental attitudes and dental patterns of behaviour are established very early in life and that although there is some suggestion that a certain amount of 'conversion' takes place, the group of children who are introduced in early life, to a system of regular dental care remain largely steadfast, at least according to their mothers.

In Chapter 12 we showed the range of dental services selected for the child, and described the variations in the choices according to the mother's characteristics. We now examine the reason for the child's most recent dental visit in relation to the dental service which is used. As in the earlier analysis we confine the presentation to the two groups of children who have been to and not changed from each of the two main services. Table 13.12 shows the reason for the last visit for children who have always been to the General Dental Service.

Table 13.12

Reason for most recent dental visit for children who have been to and not changed from the General Dental Service

Reason for most recent dental visit	Children who have been to and not changed from the G.D.S., aged			
	5+	8+	12+	14+
	%	%	%	%
Check-up	69	72	74	78
Trouble	24	21	15	17
Note from school	2	4	4	1
Other	5	3	7	4
	100	100	100	100
Base	479	291	240	441

About three-quarters of those who had always been to the General Dental Service were said to have been for a check-up last time. For the five year olds and eight year olds a quarter and a fifth respectively were said to have gone because of dental trouble. Among the older age groups only 15% and 17% of children were said to have gone last time because of trouble. Fewer than five percent of those who have always been to the General Dental Service were prompted to go last time because of a note from school.

Table 13.13 shows the reasons for the most recent dental visit for children who have always been to the School Dental Service. Among the five year olds the predominant reason for attendance was dental trouble (40%), a third of the five year olds were said to have gone for a check-up and a fifth went because of receiving a note from school. The reasons for the last visit of the five year olds who have always been to the School Dental Service are probably rather atypical of the reasons for the most recent visits of the older children, since for the five year olds who use the School Dental Service, the most recent visit is likely to have also been the first. Among the older children a smaller proportion of most recent visits were stimulated by dental trouble and a higher proportion were for a check-up. The proportion of children going for check-ups for their last visit to the school dentist never reaches the level exhibited among children who have always been to the General Dental Service (see Table 13.12). The older age groups suggest that the note from school plays a large part in stimulating dental attendance among those who are accustomed to using the School Dental Service.

Table 13.13

Reason for most recent dental visit for children who have been to and not changed from the School Dental Service

Reason for most recent dental visit	Children who have been to and not changed from the S.D.S., aged			
	5+	8+	12+	14+
	%	%	%	%
Check-up	35	43	42	40
Trouble	40	21	27	27
Note from school	21	29	26	29
Other	4	7	5	4
	100	100	100	100
Base	*110*	*108*	*88*	*179*

Since different people have different interpretations of what constitutes regular attendance and children have a variable timespan in terms of when they have dental trouble we next look at the question of how long ago the most recent visit to the dentist took place (see Table 13.14). We examine this in terms of the proportion of children who had not been to the dentist at all in the last six months, in the last year, and in the last two years.

Table 13.14

Proportion of children who had not been to the dentist recently, among those who have been to the dentist

Child had not been to the dentist in the last	Among children who have been to the dentist, the proportion who have not been recently, aged			
	5+	8+	12+	14+
Six months	25%	30%	34%	40%
One year	6%	9%	17%	21%
Two years	1%	2%	6%	12%
Base	*656*	*484*	*435*	*855*

Among five year olds who had at some time been to the dentist, a quarter of them had not been in the last six months, 6% had not been in the last year and only 1% had not been in the last two years. Among the eight year olds with experience of going to the dentist, 30% were said not to have been in the past six months, 9% were said not to have been in the last year and 2% were said not to have been in the last two years. (In these two age groups there were quite a number of children who had not been to the dentist at all - see Chapter 12.) Among twelve year olds who had been to the dentist at least once, a third had not been in the last six months, 17% had not been in the last year and 6% had not been in the last two years. It was among the fourteen year olds that we found the highest proportion of children who, although they had been to the dentist at some time, had not been recently; 40% were said not to have been in the last six months, 21% had not been in the last year, and 12% had not been within the last two years.

The length of time between dental visits is highly likely to vary according to the reason for the child's dental attendance, and so in Table 13.15 we show the proportion of children whose most recent visit had not been within the last six months, year or two years according to the reason for the last visit. The table has three sections each showing the results for one time period.

Table 13.15

Proportion of children who have not been to the dentist recently, according to the reason for their most recent visit

Reason for child's last dental visit	Children who have been to the dentist, aged							
	5+		8+		12+		14+	
	Proportion who have not been to the dentist in the last six months							
Check-up	19%	401	18%	304	24%	272	31%	554
Trouble	34%	177	51%	104	52%	85	53%	185
Note from school	15%	44	58%	56	78%	48	74%	78
	Proportion who have not been to the dentist in the last year							
Check-up	3%	401	4%	304	8%	272	12%	554
Trouble	8%	177	22%	104	32%	85	37%	185
Note from school	4%	44	18%	56	45%	48	54%	78
	Proportion who have not been to the dentist in the last two years							
Check-up	-	401	1%	304	3%	272	6%	554
Trouble	1%	177	6%	104	14%	85	26%	185
Note from school	-	44	2%	56	17%	48	33%	78

It is difficult to interpret the results for the five year olds since many of them have had their first dental visit within the time period we are discussing and have therefore not yet established a pattern of dental behaviour. Among the older children there were large differences in the proportion who had not been to the dentist within the last six months. Of the children whose last visits were for a check-up, one in five eight year olds, one in four twelve year olds and one in three fourteen year olds had not been in the last six months, compared with a half of those whose last visit was because of trouble and three-quarters of the twelve and fourteen year olds whose last visit had been prompted by a note from school.

In the second section of the table we show the proportion of children who had not been to the dentist in the last year. Again the results for the five year olds are affected by their brief experience, but there are marked variations with the reason for the last dental visit among the other age groups; among the fourteen year olds the proportions were 12% for those whose last visit was for a check-up, 37% for those whose last visit was because of dental trouble and 54% for those whose last visit resulted from a note from school. The third section of the table shows the proportion of children who had not been to the dentist within the last two years. In the dental life of the child, two years is a long period and this is reflected in the survey results as the proportions both for the five and eight year olds were small. Among the twelve and fourteen year olds there were again large variations according to dental attitude and behaviour. Among the fourteen year olds 6% of those whose last visit was for a check-up, 26% of those whose last visit had been because of dental trouble and 33% of those whose last visit had been because of a note from school, had not been to the dentist in the last two years. The two last mentioned groups are relatively small in numbers but nevertheless they reflect a very different dental way of life from that of the children who go for dental check-ups.

Table 13.16
Proportion of children who had not been to the dentist recently, according to the dental service they use

Child has been to and never changed from the	Children who have been to the dentist, aged							
	5+		8+		12+		14+	
	Proportion who have not been to the dentist in the last six months							
General Dental Service	23%	479	21%	291	23%	240	32%	441
School Dental Service	32%	110	53%	108	64%	88	56%	179
	Proportion who have not been to the dentist in the last year							
General Dental Service	6%	479	8%	291	9%	240	14%	441
School Dental Service	5%	110	16%	108	37%	88	38%	179
	Proportion who have not been to the dentist in the last two years							
General Dental Service	1%	479	3%	291	4%	240	9%	441
School Dental Service	-	110	2%	108	18%	88	24%	179

In addition we looked at the question of how long ago the last visit had been made in relation to the type of dental service used (see Table 13.16). As with earlier analyses using this information, we have confined ourselves to the two groups of children who have tried one or other of the main services and remained with it. For the children using the General Dental Service, less than a quarter of those aged five, eight and twelve had not been to the dentist within the past six months, for the fourteen year olds the proportion was a third. For the children who attended the School Dental Service, the proportion who had not been in the past six months was over a half for all except the five year olds for whom it was a third. Thus the combined effects of the majority of irregular attenders using the School Dental Service and the children who are regular attenders going less frequently than regular attenders who use the General Dental Service lead to a slower cycle of treatment within the School Dental Service. In order to examine more closely the interaction of the types of patient and types of service we have pursued this particular issue further. Confining ourselves to the fourteen year olds we show in Table 13.17 what proportion of children had not been to the dentist for varying periods according to both the dental service used and the two main reasons for the most recent dental visit.

Table 13.17

Proportion of fourteen year olds who had not been to the dentist recently, according to the reason for their last visit and dental service they used

Child had not been to the dentist in the last	Fourteen year olds who have been to the dentist whose most recent dental visit was			
	For check-up		Because of trouble	
	Only been to G.D.S.*	Only been to S.D.S.*	Only been to G.D.S.*	Only been to S.D.S.*
Six months	28%	40%	54%	57%
One year	9%	23%	41%	40%
Two years	5%	12%	30%	29%
Base	344	71	75	48

* G.D.S. - General Dental Service; S.D.S. - School Dental Service.

For fourteen year olds whose mothers said they had been last time for a check-up the proportion who had not been at all in the last six months was 28% for those who had only ever been to the General Dental Service, but 40% for those who had only ever been to the School Dental Service. The proportion of children who had not been for over a year was 9% for those who had always been to the General Dental Service, but 23% for those who had always been to the School Dental Service. Thus there was a frequency difference in visits for check-ups between the two services. There was, on the other hand, no difference in the proportion of children who had not been to the dentist within the last six months, one year and two years between the services among children whose last visit was because they had some dental trouble.

Throughout this section the survey results have shown that the reason for the child's most recent dental visit provides a considerable insight to the child's dental way of life. In Table 13.18 we show the type of treatment that was received as a result of the last dental visit and then in Table 13.19 we show the extent to which the type of treatment varied with the reason for attendance.

Table 13.18

Treatment received at the most recent dental visit

Treatment received at most recent dental visit	Children who have been to the dentist, aged			
	5+	8+	12+	14+
No fillings no extractions	45%	33%	31%	34%
Some extractions	19%	25%	20%	16%
Some fillings	32%	42%	43%	43%
Base	651	482	429	849

Among five year olds who had been to the dentist 45% had neither fillings nor extractions as a result of their last visit. Among the older children, a third had neither fillings nor extractions last time. As a result of their last visit 19% of five year olds, 25% of eight year olds, 20% of twelve year olds and 16% of fourteen year olds who had been to the dentist had some extractions. Among the five year olds with some experience of going to the dentist a third had some fillings last time they went; among the older children 40% had some fillings as a result of their most recent visit to the dentist.

When one looks at the type of treatment that the mother says the child had last time he or she went to the dentist according to the reason for going, one finds there are some very large variations indeed. The first section of Table 13.19 shows the proportion of children who had neither fillings nor extractions. It was only among the children who went for a check-up last time that this proportion was of an appreciable size. About two-thirds of five year olds who went for a check-up had neither fillings nor extractions, and nearly a half of the older children who went for a check-up had neither fillings nor extractions last time.

Table 13.19
Treatment received at most recent dental visit, according to reason for last visit

Reason for last dental visit	Children who have been to the dentist, aged							
	5+		8+		12+		14+	
	Proportion who received no fillings and no extractions on last dental visit							
Check-up	64%	401	48%	304	46%	272	48%	554
Trouble	6%	177	2%	104	1%	85	2%	185
Note from school	19%	44	15%	56	10%	48	7%	78
	Proportion who received some extractions on last dental visit							
Check-up	3%	401	8%	304	9%	272	4%	554
Trouble	57%	177	65%	104	61%	85	50%	185
Note from school	24%	44	44%	56	20%	48	21%	78
	Proportion who received some fillings on last dental visit							
Check-up	29%	401	44%	304	42%	272	42%	554
Trouble	34%	177	36%	104	34%	85	44%	185
Note from school	54%	44	46%	56	74%	48	64%	78

As one might expect, hardly any of the children whose last visit was prompted by dental trouble had neither fillings nor extractions. Among the children whose last visit was stimulated by a note from school, 19% of five year olds, 15% of eight year olds, 10% of twelve year olds and 7% of fourteen year olds had neither fillings nor extractions when they went to the dentist. This result suggests that among the younger children, either school inspections are referring those with problems other than decay, or the mother was not aware of the treatment carried out, or there was a professional difference of opinion as to the treatment need of the child.

The second section of the table shows the proportion of children who had some extractions last time and as one might expect, the children whose visits were prompted by dental trouble were the most likely to have had extractions. This was so for 57%, 65%, 61% and 50% of the age groups respectively. Among the children whose last visit was for a check-up, only 3%, 8%, 9% and 4% respectively had

extractions. The children who went to the dentist because of a note from school
were in an intermediate position in terms of having extractions, 24%, 44%, 20% and
21%, having had some teeth out last time.

The final section of the table shows the proportion of children who had some
fillings last time they went to the dentist. These results need to be interpreted
bearing in mind the earlier sections of the table. Remembering that two-thirds of
the five year olds and a half of the other age groups whose last visit was for a
check-up had had neither fillings nor extractions, then the addition of the
proportion who had some fillings (29%, 44%, 42%, 42%) largely accounts for the
whole group. Among the children who last went to the dentist with some kind of
trouble, a fairly similar proportion had some fillings (34%, 36%, 34% and 44%), but
in this case virtually none of the children had no treatment for decay, the majority
having extractions only. In terms of fillings it is particularly interesting to
look at the children whose most recent dental visit was because of a note from
school. By definition these children were considered to be in some dental need,
and also by definition they were not prompted into attendance by pain and discomfort. It was in this group that, overall, the highest proportion of children had
some fillings, a proportion that was, except for the eight year olds, significantly
higher than that for children who had gone to the dentist because of toothache or
trouble. The results thus show that among children for whom action is taken before
the advent of pain, the position with respect to restorative dentistry appeared
to be much more encouraging.

It is clear that variations in dental attitudes play a fundamental part in
determining the dental future that children have. The effects of such variations
are visible even among the youngest children and remain so through the age groups,
thus forming the basis of later variation among adults.

13.3 The child's attitude to dental visits

We asked the mother about various aspects of visiting the dentist and what her
child's attitudes were to these things. Although an interview with the mother
restricts us to what she believes the child to feel, and this may not in all cases
be a true reflection of how the child actually feels, nevertheless we felt that
the questions would throw some light on what sort of occasion the mother anticipates
when a dental visit for her child is imminent. As with the two preceding sections,
the analysis is confined to children who have been to the dentist.

We asked the mothers whether they thought the child minded going to the dentist
on the very first occasion, and whether or not the child minds going now. More
than eight out of ten children were said not to have minded going the first time.
Among the children aged eight, twelve and fourteen a slightly higher proportion
were said to mind going now than had minded going the first time (see Table 13.20).

Table 13.20

Proportion of children who mind going to the dentist

		Children who have been to the dentist, aged			
		5+	8+	12+	14+
First visit		%	%	%	%
	Minded	12	14	14	17
	Did not	88	86	86	83
		100	100	100	100
Nowadays		%	%	%	%
	Minds	14	22	23	25
	Does not	86	78	77	75
		100	100	100	100
	Base	656	484	435	855

In Table 13.21 we examined whether the child's aversion to the dentist was related to various background characteristics. In addition to the background characteristics generally used in the analysis, we look at whether the mother said she herself minds going to the dentist. There was little systematic variation with the mother's own attitude, the reason for the child's most recent dental visit or the type of dental service used although there were some isolated cases of significant differences.

Table 13.21

Proportion of children who mind going to the dentist nowadays, by background characteristics

Background characteristics		Proportion who mind going to the dentist, of children who have been to the dentist, aged							
		5+		8+		12+		14+	
Mother's	Minds	18%	444	22%	240	30%	206	28%	390
attitude	Does not	12%	477	22%	291	18%	242	23%	492
Reason for	Check-up	9%	401	23%	304	22%	272	21%	554
child's	Trouble	26%	177	21%	104	28%	85	33%	185
last visit	Note from school	19%	44	16%	56	33%	48	37%	78
Type of dentist	Always G.D.S*	12%	479	24%	291	21%	240	25%	441
been to	Always S.D.S*	21%	110	20%	108	25%	88	26%	179

* G.D.S. - General Dental Service; S.D.S. - School Dental Service.

We asked the mother whether she, herself, generally goes to the dentist with the child or not. For the five and eight year olds 92% of mothers said they usually go, with 91% and 88% saying that they went last time. Among the older children a lower proportion said they usually went with the child. For twelve year olds 78% said they usually go and 67% said they went last time, and for the fourteen year olds 58% said they usually go and 50% said they went last time. Thus even amongst the oldest children a half of the mothers say they accompany the child to the dentist (see Table 13.22).

Table 13.22

Whether mother usually goes to the dentist with the child

Whether mother goes with child	Children who have been to the dentist, aged			
	5+	8+	12+	14+
	%	%	%	%
Mother usually goes	92	92	78	58
Does not	8	8	22	42
	100	100	100	100
	%	%	%	%
Mother went last time	91	88	67	50
Did not	9	12	33	50
	100	100	100	100
Base	656	484	435	855

We asked all the mothers how they thought the child felt in the waiting room and it appeared that the older children were more nervous than the younger ones. For the five year olds three-quarters of the mothers said the child did not worry in the waiting room, but for the fourteen year olds only a half of the mothers thought the child did not worry. Nearly 10% of the twelve and fourteen year olds were said to be very nervous in the waiting room (see Table 13.23).

Table 13.23

How the mother thinks child feels in the waiting room

How mother thinks child feels in the waiting room	Children who have been to the dentist, aged			
	5+	8+	12+	14+
	%	%	%	%
Does not worry	75	61	46	50
Nervous	18	30	42	37
Very nervous	3	6	9	9
Don't know	4	3	3	4
	100	100	100	100
Base	656	484	435	855

We examined how the children felt in the waiting room by the reason for the child's last visit and the type of dentist the child was accustomed to. Among the five year olds and fourteen year olds, the highest proportion of children who were thought not to worry in the waiting room were those whose last visit was for a check-up. For the twelve year olds there was no appreciable difference with the reason for the most recent dental visit. Except for the five year olds, among whom more had no treatment need, there was no difference between children accustomed to using the two main services in how they felt in the waiting room.

Table 13.24

Proportion of children who are thought not to worry in the waiting room by background characteristics

Background characteristics		Proportion of children who are thought not to worry in the waiting room, aged							
		5+		8+		12+		14+	
Reason for	Check-up	82%	401	62%	304	47%	272	54%	554
child's last	Trouble	65%	177	50%	104	43%	85	38%	185
dental visit	Note from school	59%	44	74%	56	35%	48	39%	78
Type of dentist	Always G.D.S.*	79%	479	60%	291	48%	240	52%	441
been to	Always S.D.S.*	67%	110	63%	108	51%	88	50%	179

* G.D.S. - General Dental Service; S.D.S. - School Dental Service.

We asked the mother how she thought the child behaved in the dental chair and three-quarters thought the child was well behaved (see Table 13.25). About one in ten thought the child was nervous but co-operative. The proportion of children thought, by the mother, to be unco-operative in the chair decreased with age, being 8%, 7%, 4% and 3% for the four groups respectively. The proportion of mothers who said they did not know how the child behaved in the dental chair was highest for the oldest children. There were no variations in how the mother thought the child behaved according to the reason for the visit or the type of service used.

Table 13.25

How the mother thinks the child behaves in the dental chair

How the mother thinks the child behaves in the dental chair	Children who have been to the dentist, aged			
	5+	8+	12+	14+
	%	%	%	%
Well behaved	78	76	81	79
Nervous, no trouble	8	10	9	7
Unco-operative	8	7	4	3
Don't know	6	7	6	11
	100	100	100	100
Base	656	484	435	855

We have seen earlier (Chapter 10) that most mothers do not find a visit to the dentist pleasant, nor do they think that children find it pleasant, but on the other hand not many mothers say that their child has had a particularly unpleasant experience at the dental surgery. We asked the mothers whether their child had ever had an unpleasant experience and the reply was in the affirmative for 9% of five year olds, 16% of eight year olds, 19% of twelve year olds and 21% of fourteen year olds. The results are shown in Table 13.26. There is obviously more opportunity for an unpleasant experience to occur as exposure increases and it is therefore not surprising that the proportion of children that have been to the dentist who have had an unpleasant experience increases through the age groups. There was no variation in the proportion who have had an unpleasant experience according to the reasons for their most recent visit or the type of service they use.

Table 13.26

Has the child ever had any unpleasant experience at the dentist's surgery

Any unpleasant experiences		Children who have been to the dentist, aged			
		5+	8+	12+	14+
		%	%	%	%
	Yes	9	16	19	21
	No	91	84	81	79
		100	100	100	100
	Base	*656*	*484*	*435*	*855*

We asked the mothers concerned what it was that caused the unpleasant experience and there were four main reasons given: the drill, the injection, having gas, and the manner of the dentist. Thus for those children where a particularly unpleasant experience had occurred the causes of the problem were, in most cases, the same kind of things as were said by mothers to cause unpleasantness in general for them and for children (see Section 10.6).

We asked the mothers whether they felt their child would need encouragement to go to the dentist next time and for the most part they did not think so. The proportion who thought they would was 14% of five year olds, 13% of eight year olds, 10% of twelve year olds and 12% of fourteen year olds. The encouragement the mothers would give would be to say that it was for the child's own good and that everyone had to go, or they would just take him, and with the younger children a certain amount of bribery and coercion was suggested.

Having asked the mother several questions on how she thought the child felt about going to the dentist and whether there were likely to be any problems about going next time, we asked her how, in fact, she would decide when it was time for the child to go to the dentist again. Table 13.27 shows the answers the mothers gave and demonstrates an apparently high level of organisation on the part of the mothers and the dentists. In 12% - 16% of cases the dentist was said to send a reminder, in 7% - 10% of cases the dentist was said to send an actual appointment, in a quarter of cases an appointment was fixed at the end of the last treatment. For about a quarter of the five year olds and less than a fifth of the eight, twelve and fourteen year olds the mother said that the child went at a regular interval and so she knew when the next time would be, (although the interval varied from four months to a year). For just over 10% of the children who had been to the dentist at least once, the mother said that the next dental visit would be the next time the child had toothache, and for 11% - 18% the mother said the child would go again next time she received a note from school.

Table 13.27

How will you decide when it is time for child to go again?

How mother decides it is time for child's next dental visit	Children who have been to the dentist, aged			
	5+	8+	12+	14+
Child goes regularly	24%	19%	17%	19%
Dentist sends reminder	16%	15%	16%	12%
Dentist sends appointment	10%	8%	9%	7%
Appointment made last time	23%	24%	24%	24%
When has toothache	10%	12%	11%	12%
When gets note from school	11%	18%	17%	18%
Base	656	484	435	855

Among the indicators for the timing of the next dental visit the most detrimental from the point of view of the child's dental health must be 'the next time he or she has toothache' and 'waiting for the next note from school.' We have already seen the likely treatment outcome that will result from avoiding any dental attendance until prompted by toothache, and we have also seen the length of time that has passed for many children since the last known school inspection. In Table 13.28 we show the proportion of mothers stating that they will use one of these two indicators as a method of deciding when the child will next go to the dentist according to the reason the child last went to the dentist.

Table 13.28

Proportion of mothers taking toothache and note from school as indications of need for treatment, by reason for child's most recent dental visit

Reason for child's most recent dental visit	Children who have been to the dentist, aged							
	5+		8+		12+		14+	
	Proportion of mothers who say next dental visit will be next time child has toothache							
Check-up	3%	401	5%	304	5%	272	6%	554
Trouble	24%	177	36%	104	28%	85	31%	185
Note from school	2%	44	10%	56	14%	48	14%	78
	Proportion of mothers who say next dental visit will be next time receive note from school							
Check-up	5%	401	10%	304	10%	272	11%	554
Trouble	16%	177	18%	104	25%	85	18%	185
Note from school	33%	44	56%	56	56%	48	65%	78

The first section of the table shows the proportion of mothers saying that the child will next go to the dentist the next time he has toothache. For the children whose last visit was for a check-up the proportion is 6% or less. For the children whose last visit was prompted by a note from school the proportion who said they would wait until the child had trouble was 14% or less; but for the children whose last attendance had been prompted by trouble the proportion was 24% among the five year olds, 36% among the eight year olds, 28% among the twelve year olds and 31% among the fourteen year olds. There was thus a high proportion of mothers of children whose last visit had been the result of dental trouble whose stated intention was to repeat the same pattern in the future.

The second section of the table shows the proportion of mothers who said that the child's next attendance would be when the mother next got a note from school. Among children whose last visit was for a check-up not more than 11% of mothers said this. Among children whose last visit was because of trouble 25% or less said that the child would next go to the dentist as a result of a note from school. Among those whose last visit had been prompted by such a note from school the position was entirely different. In this case the proportion of mothers who said that they were relying on a note from school to show that it was time to go to the dentist again was 33% for the five year olds, 56% for the eight year olds, 56% for the twelve year olds and 65% for the fourteen year olds.

There are thus some groups of children whose dental behaviour is closely associated with parental attitudes that do little to promote the dental well being of the child. Anyone aiming to provide adequate services for these children faces a formidable task in trying to counter such dental deprivation.

14 Toothbrushing

The topic of toothbrushing is always one of interest in dental surveys and, unfortunately, it is also one of the most difficult on which to get accurate and detailed information. An obvious factor, when one is asking questions about toothbrushing, is the frequency with which it is done, and it would then seem comparatively easy to relate this to the child's dental health and dental background. However, frequency of toothbrushing is a fairly blunt tool for analysis since the range is small and most children came within the 'twice-a-day' category. There is also the problem of reliability of the response since, on this topic, the dentally acceptable replies are well known by most people. We therefore asked a wide range of questions about various aspects of toothbrushing, which included frequency, in order to try to overcome these problems. We begin by discussing some of the wider issues of the mother's attitudes towards the subject.

14.1 Attitudes towards toothbrushing

The mothers were asked whether they thought children should be encouraged to brush their teeth and it was no surprise to find that 99% of them said that they should. We asked them why they held this view and the vast majority said it was important because it helped to preserve the teeth from disease. Other reasons are shown in Table 14.1 but, as it can be seen, none attained the importance of the role of toothbrushing in preserving the teeth.

Table 14.1

Reasons why a mother should encourage a child to brush his teeth

Mother's reason why children should be encouraged to brush their teeth	Children aged			
	5+	8+	12+	14+
Preserves teeth	87%	88%	88%	86%
Sweetens breath	10%	10%	12%	14%
For appearance's sake	12%	12%	15%	12%
Good for the gums	6%	7%	7%	5%
Good habit, teaches care	10%	8%	6%	7%
Base	922	532	451	886

With toothbrushing having such a high estimated value among mothers we were interested to know at what age they thought children should first be encouraged to brush their teeth. About three-quarters of the mothers thought that it should be before the age of three, the opinions of these mothers being equally divided between 'at the age of two' and 'before the age of two'. The results are given in Table 14.2 and show that the mothers' attitudes varied a little for the different age groups with slightly fewer mothers of fourteen year olds saying that children ought to be encouraged to start brushing their teeth before the age of three.

Table 14.2

At what age should children first be encouraged to brush their teeth?

Mother's estimates of age at which a child should start to brush his teeth	Children aged			
	5+	8+	12+	14+
	%	%	%	%
Under two	40	35	39	32
Two	38	40	35	38
Three	15	15	16	19
Four	4	6	6	7
Five or more	3	4	4	4
	100	100	100	100
Base	922	532	451	886

It is thus apparent that most mothers think children should acquire the habit of toothbrushing at a very early age, in fact at an age at which the child would not have developed sufficient physical co-ordination to be able to perform the task competently by himself. We therefore asked the mothers at what age they thought children would be able to brush their teeth properly by themselves (see Table 14.3). The mothers made some allowance for the very young children but even so three-quarters of them estimated that by the age of six a child would be able to brush his own teeth competently. This is a rather unfortunate over-estimation by the mothers as most dentists believe that even many adults find difficulty in cleaning their teeth efficiently.

Table 14.3

At what age should children be able to brush their teeth properly by themselves?

Mother's estimate of age at which a child can brush his teeth properly	Children aged			
	5+	8+	12+	14+
	%	%	%	%
Under three	7	9	11	10
Three	19	15	16	15
Four	22	22	22	22
Five	26	27	27	30
Six	13	13	11	12
Seven	6	5	8	5
Eight or more	7	9	5	6
	100	100	100	100
Base	922	532	451	886

Against this background of the general attitudes of mothers towards toothbrushing we investigated the pattern of behaviour of the child whom we selected in the sample. Firstly, of course, we asked whether or not the child ever brushed his teeth and found that in 98% of cases he did. We then asked how often he did it and the results are given in Table 14.4 The distribution of frequencies was very similar for all age groups although slightly more fourteen year olds were said to brush their teeth more than twice a day than children in the other age groups. The most common frequency was twice a day with over half of the children coming in this category. About a third of the children were said to brush their teeth once a day so overall, nine out of ten children were said to brush their teeth at least once a day.

Table 14.4

How often are the teeth brushed?

Frequency of toothbrushing	Children aged			
	5+	8+	12+	14+
	%	%	%	%
Three or more times a day	5	5	6	8
Twice a day	51	52	55	60
Once a day	33	33	31	24
Less than once a day	11	10	8	8
	100	100	100	100
Base	922	532	451	886

The mothers were asked what time of day the children brushed their teeth and, as one might anticipate, the two most favoured times were in the morning and last thing at night. The most frequent time given was last thing at night because the times in the morning were subdivided into before and after breakfast. Three-quarters of the children were said to clean their teeth last thing at night and over half were said to clean them after breakfast (see Table 14.5).

Table 14.5

At what time of day are the teeth brushed?

Time of day for toothbrushing	Children aged			
	5+	8+	12+	14+
Before breakfast	10%	10%	15%	23%
After breakfast	50%	49%	52%	44%
In the morning	12%	17%	17%	19%
After meals	7%	6%	6%	9%
Before bed, at night	75%	76%	73%	76%
When he feels like it	2%	1%	2%	1%
Variable times	7%	6%	6%	7%
Base	922	532	451	886

We asked the mothers whether they checked that the child had brushed his teeth and, if so, how often they did this. The proportion of mothers who checked at all varied considerably with age, ranging from 81% of the mothers of five year olds to 34% of the mothers of fourteen year olds. In Table 14.6 we show how frequently those mothers, who said they checked at all, did so. For mothers of children in the two younger age groups, who said that they checked, over two-thirds said that they did so at least once a day. This high frequency of checking was not maintained by the mothers of the older children fewer than half saying they checked that often.

Table 14.6

Frequency with which mothers who check toothbrushing do so

How often mothers check toothbrushing	Children whose mothers check toothbrushing, aged			
	5+	8+	12+	14+
	%	%	%	%
At least twice a day	24	14	8	6
Once a day	52	51	39	40
Once a week	22	31	41	41
Now and again	2	4	12	13
	100	100	100	100
Base	748	395	243	304
Proportion of mothers who check toothbrushing	81% 922	73% 532	54% 451	34% 886

However, it is likely that the effectiveness of any checking is determined not by the frequency with which it is done but rather by the methods used, so we asked those mothers who said that they checked on toothbrushing how they did it. The methods used varied considerably according to the age of the child. The most direct method of checking mentioned was for the mother to clean the child's teeth herself, and this was mentioned by 11% of the mothers who said they checked their five year olds' teeth and 2% of those who said they checked their eight year olds' teeth. The most common method of checking among the mothers of five year olds was to be present while the child cleaned his teeth. This method declined in popularity over the four age groups (38%, 24%, 15% and 14% respectively). For the five, eight and twelve year olds a third of the mothers who said that they checked on toothbrushing said they did so by looking at the teeth to see if they were clean, but this method was only mentioned by 19% of the mothers of fourteen year olds. As the child becomes older the mother who checks does so more often by asking the child; only 14% of the mothers who checked their five year olds did so by asking, whereas among the fourteen year olds 47% of the mothers checked this way. Among the oldest children this was by far the most common form of checking. It is doubtful whether asking about an action is as effective a check as looking at the result but there was obviously a decline in the more direct methods of checking with age. Similarly the remaining methods, that is checking the toothbrush, smelling toothpaste on the child's breath, hearing the toothbrushing and getting the toothbrush down for the child, although perhaps more discrete are not likely to show whether the teeth were properly cleaned. The detailed results for methods of checking toothbrushing are given in Table 14.7

Table 14.7

Methods used by mothers to check toothbrushing

How does mother check toothbrushing?	Children whose mothers check toothbrushing, aged			
	5+	8+	12+	14+
Cleans child's teeth	11%	2%	-	-
Is present, watches	38%	24%	15%	14%
Looks at teeth	33%	38%	34%	19%
Asks	14%	28%	40%	47%
Checks toothbrush has been used	7%	11%	13%	26%
Smells toothpaste on breath	11%	14%	9%	4%
Hears toothbrushing	1%	2%	3%	4%
Gets brush down	6%	6%	4%	1%
Base	748	395	243	304
Proportion of mothers who check toothbrushing	81% 922	73% 532	54% 451	34% 886

Having looked at the mother's attitudes to toothbrushing in general we now turn to the relationship between toothbrushing and the child's dental background. For this analysis we use the frequency of toothbrushing as an indicator of the mother's attitudes and the child's habits as regards toothbrushing.

14.2 Toothbrushing and dental background

Table 14.8 shows the relationship between the child's frequency of toothbrushing and the mother's dental attendance pattern. Among the five and eight year olds, the proportion of children said to brush their teeth at least twice a day was highest, as one would expect, among the children whose mothers were regular attenders. However, among the twelve and fourteen year olds, although the proportion for the regular attenders was still higher than that for the irregular attenders, it was not significantly different from the proportion for children of edentulous mothers. This apparent anomaly could be due to the fact that whereas it is unlikely for a mother of a five or eight year old to have already lost all

Table 14.8

Frequency of toothbrushing according to mother's dental attendance pattern

Mother's dental attendance pattern	Children aged			
	5+	8+	12+	14+
	Proportion who brush their teeth twice a day or more			
Regular	67% 407	70% 230	70% 165	75% 288
Occasional	54% 101	57% 58	53% 52	66% 86
Irregular	46% 309	42% 140	54% 127	58% 252
Edentulous	30% 93	47% 98	63% 96	71% 241
	Proportion who brush their teeth less than once a day			
Regular	4% 407	5% 230	2% 165	3% 288
Occasional	10% 101	3% 58	8% 52	11% 86
Irreulgar	19% 309	16% 140	17% 127	15% 252
Edentulous	9% 93	17% 98	7% 96	7% 241

her teeth and yet have previously cared for them, a mother of a twelve or fourteen year old, especially where that child is the youngest of several, could reasonably be at an age where edentulousness does not necessarily imply lack of care. In the second part of Table 14.8 we show the other extreme with respect to toothbrushing, the proportion of children who were said to brush their teeth less than once a day. This proportion was relatively small except among those children whose mothers were irregular dental attenders and the younger children of edentulous mothers.

In Table 14.9 we examine whether the dental behaviour of the child, as indicated by the reason for his most recent dental attendance, shows any relationship with toothbrushing. As with the previous table we find that the highest proportion of children said to brush their teeth twice a day or more is among those whose dental behaviour reflects the greatest interest in dental care. Whatever the age of the child, those whose most recent dental visit had been for a check-up were the most likely to brush their teeth twice or more per day. Those whose most recent visit had been prompted by trouble or by a note from school were more likely to brush their teeth less than once a day than the other children (see Table 14.9).

Table 14.9

Frequency of toothbrushing by reason for child's most recent dental visit

Reasons for child's most recent dental visit	Children aged							
	5+		8+		12+		14+	
	Proportion who brush their teeth twice a day or more							
Check-up	68%	401	64%	304	65%	272	73%	554
Trouble	56%	177	45%	104	50%	85	56%	185
Note from school	57%	44	51%	56	56%	48	56%	78
	Proportion who brush their teeth less than once a day							
Check-up	4%	401	6%	304	6%	272	6%	554
Trouble	15%	177	23%	104	19%	85	13%	185
Note from school	10%	44	11%	56	8%	48	14%	78

The relationship shown between the dental attendance patterns of both the mother and the child, and the child's toothbrushing habits demonstrates that those who carry out one main aspect of dental care, that is regular dental check-ups, are more likely also to practise another, that is frequent toothbrushing, than are those that do not.

14.3 Toothbrushing and dental health

At the beginning of the chapter on toothbrushing we showed how nearly all mothers considered toothbrushing to be important, saying that it preserved the teeth and prevented disease. Since this view was so widely held it is of interest to see what kind of relationship we find in the survey data between toothbrushing frequency and dental health. In Table 14.10 we show four different indicators of current dental health, the proportion of children with some current decay, the proportion with some gum inflammation, the proportion with some debris and the proportion with some calculus.

Table 14.10
Toothbrushing and dental health

Frequency of toothbrushing	Children aged							
	5+		8+		12+		14+	
	Proportion with some current dental decay							
Three times a day or more	61%	44	75%	24	65%	25	56%	72
Twice a day	61%	469	74%	276	57%	241	59%	508
Once a day	66%	297	79%	172	66%	133	65%	202
Less than once a day	67%	98	87%	52	72%	36	67%	72
	Proportion with some gum inflammation							
Three times a day or more	20%	44	55%	24	55%	25	46%	72
Twice a day	24%	469	53%	276	47%	241	50%	508
Once a day	24%	297	63%	172	60%	133	58%	202
Less than once a day	42%	98	64%	52	66%	36	75%	72
	Proportion with some debris							
Three times a day or more	39%	44	59%	24	59%	25	43%	72
Twice a day	37%	469	64%	276	60%	241	53%	508
Once a day	36%	297	75%	172	68%	133	57%	202
Less than once a day	50%	98	73%	52	78%	36	80%	72
	Proportion with some calculus							
Three times a day or more	1%	44	-	24	28%	25	24%	72
Twice a day	6%	469	12%	276	26%	241	33%	508
Once a day	3%	297	17%	172	27%	133	33%	202
Less than once a day	3%	98	17%	52	36%	36	41%	72

There appeared to be a weak relationship between the frequency of toothbrushing and the presence of current decay but, as we shall see, this relationship was probably due to the fact that those children who brush their teeth fairly frequently are also the children who go to the dentist regularly.

In contrast there was a marked difference between the proportion of children with gum inflammation according to how often they brushed their teeth and this was so for each age-group. It was the group of children who were said to brush their teeth less than daily who usually made the biggest contribution to the variation, and who were in the worst position dentally. A similar result was found for debris. There was a significant difference in the proportion of children with debris according to their reported toothbrushing frequency, with those brushing less than once a day being in the worst situation.

Very few of the five year olds were found to have calculus but among the eight and twelve year olds where it was more prevalent, there is some suggestion of a relationship with toothbrushing. This becomes more evident for the fourteen year olds among whom the differences were found to be significant.

We have seen in Section 14.2 that toothbrushing and dental attendance are themselves related, and it is therefore possible that the relationship between toothbrushing and dental health is reflecting dental attendance pattern variations. In order to see whether the variations of dental health with toothbrushing are independant of dental attendance we examined the information for the fourteen year olds in more detail. We separated the children whose last dental visit was for a check-up from those whose last visit was because of dental trouble or a note from school and re-tested the variations between dental health and toothbrushing. The results are shown in Table 14.11.

Table 14.11

Toothbrushing, dental health and the reason for the most recent dental visit among fourteen year olds

Frequency of toothbrushing	Children aged fourteen			
	Most recent dental visit			
	Check-up		Trouble or note from school	
	Proportion with some current decay			
Three times a day or more	43%	41	74%	23
Twice a day	56%	358	73%	115
Once a day	59%	115	79%	75
Less than once a day	56%	30	79%	33
	Proportion with some gum inflammation			
Three times a day or more	37%	41	59%	23
Twice a day	49%	358	54%	115
Once a day	55%	115	59%	75
Less than once a day	70%	30	76%	33
	Proportion with some debris			
Three times a day or more	40%	41	50%	23
Twice a day	51%	358	56%	115
Once a day	51%	115	65%	75
Less than once a day	67%	30	88%	33
	Proportion with some calculus			
Three times a day or more	28%	41	18%	23
Twice a day	32%	358	37%	115
Once a day	33%	115	32%	75
Less than once a day	36%	30	44%	33

It can be seen from Table 14.11 that any relationship that appeared to exist between current decay and frequency of toothbrushing is completely overshadowed by that existing between the proportion of children with current decay and attendance pattern. There was, on the other hand, a significant difference in the proportion of children with gum inflammation and the proportion with debris according to how often they brushed their teeth, both for those who last attended for a check-up and those who did not. As far as the presence of calculus was concerned there was a trend with toothbrushing for the children who had last been for a check-up but this trend was not big enough, given the sample sizes, to show a significant difference. Among those whose last visit to the dentist had been prompted by dental trouble or a note from school the differences in the proportion of children with calculus, according to toothbrushing frequency were significant. Thus in general the association between the frequency of toothbrushing and the gum conditions exists independently of the attendance pattern of the child.

The fact that no marked difference was established between frequency of toothbrushing and current decay cannot be interpreted to mean that there is no association between toothbrushing and decay, but only that the indicators used (current decay and reported frequency of toothbrushing) showed no association. It may be that these indicators were not sufficiently sensitive, since associations have been found between toothbrushing and debris, and between debris and decay.

15 Toothache

We have seen in earlier chapters that for some mothers and some children the advent of toothache is the first indication of any need to go to the dentist. The pain and discomfort of toothache may well highlight such visits and give them more emphasis within the framework of all dental visits than is their due in terms of frequency. We therefore spent some time in the interview talking to the mothers about toothache and the circumstances surrounding any occasions on which the child had had toothache.

15.1 The event of toothache

Among the children in the three oldest age groups about a half were said to have suffered from toothache once or more. For the five year olds, who had not yet had as much time to have toothache, two-thirds had never experienced it and a third had already had toothache at least once. It is of interest to look at the proportion of children who were said to have had toothache twice or more, in so far as this suggests that the first occasion did not result in a long term effort to stop the same situation happening again. Among five year olds 12% of children were said to have had toothache twice or more. The comparable figure for eight year olds was 19%, for twelve year olds 24% and fourteen year olds 22%. Thus for quite a high proportion of children, especially among the older ones, having toothache did not prove to be a successful deterrent for the future. The detailed results for the number of times the children had toothache are given in Table 15.1.

Table 15.1

Number of times child has had toothache

Number of times had toothache	Children aged			
	5+	8+	12+	14+
	%	%	%	%
Never	67	52	49	51
Once	21	29	27	27
Twice	7	11	15	13
Three times	3	6	5	6
Four or more times	2	2	4	3
	100	100	100	100
Base	922	532	451	886

We asked the mothers how long the toothache lasted the first time. In about a fifth of cases, although slightly more for the five year olds, it lasted less than half a day, but in more than 10% of cases it lasted a week or more. Very few mothers were unable to give an estimate of the amount of time that had been involved. We examined the data on how long the toothache had lasted on the second occasion for those children who had had toothache more than once, and the variations in length of time were similar to the first attack. Since there was no evidence that subsequent occasions were different, we present the length of time the child had toothache on the first occasion only in Table 15.2.

Table 15.2
How long did the toothache last, the first time?

How long did the toothache last the first time?	Children who have had toothache, aged			
	5+	8+	12+	14+
	%	%	%	%
Less than half a day	28	20	24	20
Half a day, less than two days	30	36	35	36
Two days, less than a week	26	31	29	30
A week or more	15	11	9	12
Don't know	1	2	3	2
	100	100	100	100
Base	303	256	231	431

A bout of toothache does not necessarily result in a visit to the dentist, so we asked the mothers whether or not they had taken their child after the first or second attack of toothache. In the vast majority of cases toothache did result in a visit to the dentist. Nearly nine out of ten children were taken with their first bout and among the eight, twelve and fourteen year olds just over 80% of the second attacks also resulted in dental visits, although this proportion was slightly lower (70%) for the five year olds who had experienced a second attack of toothache.

Table 15.3
Proportion of children for whom toothache resulted in a dental visit

	Proportion who went to the dentist to see about the toothache, of children aged							
	5+		8+		12+		14+	
The first occasion	86%	303	86%	256	88%	231	87%	431
The second occasion	69%	100	81%	89	83%	103	84%	181

On the first occasion of toothache the aching tooth was, in the majority of cases, extracted. This was so for a half of the children aged five who had had toothache, and for two-thirds of the older children who had had toothache. The aching tooth was filled in about a fifth of cases for all age groups. For about a quarter of five year olds the aching tooth was neither filled nor extracted. In some cases this was because the child did not see a dentist and in others the visit to the dentist did not result in such treatment. For the older children only about one in ten aching teeth were neither extracted nor filled.

We examined the outcome for the aching tooth among those children who had had a second attack of toothache, and found the results to be very similar except among the five year olds. As we have already shown those five year olds who had suffered twice or more were less likely to be taken to the dentist on the second occasion and thus the mothers were more likely to say that the child needed no treatment. Since the first two occasions appeared, on the whole, similar in terms of what happened to the tooth we confine the presentation to the figures for the first occasion only (see Table 15.4).

Table 15.4

What happened to the aching tooth on the first occasion?

What happened to the aching tooth?	Children who had toothache, aged			
	5+	8+	12+	14+
Nothing	25%	11%	11%	13%
Tooth extracted	50%	70%	67%	64%
Tooth filled	20%	17%	18%	23%
Base	303	256	231	431

We asked the mothers who took their children to the dentist as a result of the first attack of toothache whether or not they had had any difficulty in getting the toothache treated. Nine out of ten mothers said they did not have any difficulty while one in ten said that they did. The two main problems for those who had difficulty were either that they had to try several dentists before they were successful, or that they had to wait for an appointment, which sometimes meant waiting till the next session in which the dentist was going to carry out extractions with gas. The question about difficulties in getting treatment was only asked of those mothers who were successful in taking their child to the dentist and so we do not know whether any of the mothers who did not take their child to the dentist were influenced by actual or anticipated difficulties in doing so. We examined the comparable information for the second occasion of toothache and the position was similar, so, as with the other topics, we present in Table 15.5 the data for the first occasion of toothache only.

Table 15.5

Was there any difficulty in getting the toothache treated on the first occasion?

Was there any difficulty in getting the toothache treated?	Children who went to the dentist to see about the first attack of toothache, aged			
	5+	8+	12+	14+
	%	%	%	%
No	89	88	91	86
Had to try several dentists	4	4	4	6
Had to wait for appointment	4	4	3	5
Other answers	3	4	2	3
	100	100	100	100
Base	226	214	201	374

15.2 Toothache and the child's dental background

In Table 15.6 we show the proportion of children who were said to have never had toothache according to the child's background characteristics. Proportionately more five, eight and twelve year olds were found never to have had toothache if their mothers were regular dental attenders. In the fourteen year olds there was less variation according to the mother's attendance pattern but the children of edentulous mothers were less likely (as in all age groups) to have never had toothache.

Table 15.6
Proportion of children who never had toothache, by background characteristics

Background characteristics		Proportion who never had toothache of children aged							
		5+		8+		12+		14+	
Mother's	Regular	76%	407	57%	230	58%	165	57%	288
dental	Occasional	66%	101	58%	58	38%	52	62%	86
attendance	Irregular	62%	309	43%	140	46%	127	49%	252
pattern	Edentulous	46%	93	48%	98	42%	96	41%	241
Social	I, II & III non-manual	77%	283	59%	177	56%	165	61%	284
class	III manual	64%	441	48%	227	43%	174	48%	396
	IV and V	60%	158	50%	108	46%	92	45%	176
Region	The North	66%	312	49%	173	48%	140	49%	294
	Midlands and East Anglia	63%	195	53%	109	43%	88	40%	197
	Wales and the South West	65%	151	52%	80	53%	77	49%	143
	London and the South East	73%	264	55%	170	51%	146	64%	252
Reason for child's	Check-up	74%	401	60%	304	52%	272	58%	554
most recent dental	Trouble	23%	177	13%	104	24%	85	24%	185
visit	Note	66%	44	54%	56	57%	48	47%	78

As one would expect from the association with the mother's dental attendance pattern, children in the top social class group, whatever their age, were consistently more likely to have never had toothache. There was little regional variation although a generally higher proportion of children from London and the South East than elsewhere had never experienced toothache, a difference which was significant among the fourteen year olds. As regards the reason for the child's most recent dental visit it was no surprise to find that children whose last dental visit was prompted by trouble were the least likely to be free from toothache experience.

Table 15.7 shows the other end of the spectrum, that is the proportion of children who were said to have had toothache twice or more according to their background characteristics. Children whose mothers were edentulous were more often found to have had toothache twice or more as were the eight, twelve, and fourteen year olds of mothers with an irregular dental attendance pattern. No variation was found according to social class except among the twelve year olds where children in the top social class group were least likely to have had toothache twice or more. Regional variation was again slight. Among eight year olds, children from the North were more often found to have had recurrent toothache than children in the Midlands and East Anglia, while among the fourteen year olds, children in London and the South East were the least likely to have had several bouts. As one would

expect from Table 15.6 it was the children whose last dental visit was precipitated
by trouble that were found to be most frequently beset by recurrent toothache.

Table 15.7

Proportion of children who had had toothache twice or more by background
characteristics

Background characteristics		Proportion who had had toothache twice or more, of children aged							
		5+		8+		12+		14+	
Mother's	Regular	8%	407	15%	230	19%	165	17%	288
dental	Occasional	12%	101	13%	58	24%	52	16%	86
attendance	Irregular	13%	309	25%	140	24%	127	25%	252
pattern	Edentulous	24%	93	23%	98	35%	96	26%	241
Social	I, II & III non-manual	10%	283	15%	177	18%	165	18%	284
class	III manual	12%	441	22%	227	28%	174	23%	396
	IV and V	12%	158	18%	108	27%	92	23%	176
Region	The North	12%	312	24%	173	24%	140	24%	294
	Midlands and East Anglia	10%	195	14%	109	28%	88	25%	197
	Wales and the South West	12%	151	18%	80	22%	77	24%	143
	London and the South East	11%	264	18%	170	24%	146	15%	252
Reason for child's	Check-up	9%	401	14%	304	20%	272	17%	554
most recent dental	Trouble	29%	177	40%	104	46%	85	40%	185
visit	Note	14%	44	20%	56	21%	48	23%	78

Although the children in the most dentally aware groups were less likely to have
had toothache, they were by no means free from it. For example, among fourteen
year olds 17% of those whose last visit to the dentist had been for a check-up
had had toothache twice or more, and 42% had had toothache at least once.

16 Mother's awareness of accidental damage

We asked all the mothers whether their child had ever had a fall or some other accident that damaged the teeth. We asked these questions in terms of the child's total experience so far, and included accidents to any teeth in either dentition. Firstly we describe the details that the mother gave about such accidents and how they happened, and in the second section we examine whether the children classified by the dentist as having traumatised incisors at the time of the examination were said by the mother to have had some kind of accident or not.

16.1 Accidents involving the teeth

Compared with toothache, accidents involving the teeth were relatively infrequent, and, for the vast majority of children who had experienced them, such accidents had only happened once. The proportion said to have had an accident was 15% among five year olds, 13% among eight year olds, 18% among twelve year olds and 17% among fourteen year olds (see Table 16.1).

Table 16.1

Number of times child has had an accident and damaged his teeth

Number of times child has had an accident and damaged his teeth	Children aged			
	5+	8+	12+	14+
	%	%	%	%
Never	85	87	82	83
Once	14	12	17	16
Twice or more	1	1	1	1
	100	100	100	100
Base	922	532	451	886

We asked the mothers how the accident had happened and in Table 16.2 it can be seen that most accidents were due to the child falling over or running into a stationary object. A particularly high proportion of mothers of five year olds gave this as the cause of their child's accident but at this age other kinds of accidents such as falling off moving objects, playing, or fighting were not so frequently mentioned as they were for the older children. It is interesting to note that playing or fighting was more frequently mentioned by mothers of fourteen year olds than for any other age groups. Fewer than one in ten of the accidents occurred when the child was playing an organised sport.

Table 16.2

How did the accident happen?

How did the accident happen?	Children who have damaged their teeth, aged			
	5+	8+	12+	14+
	%	%	%	%
Fell over* stationary object	78	58	60	58
Fell off* moving object	11	26	19	12
Playing, fighting	4	11	9	19
Playing a team sport	–	4	7	6
Eating something	6	1	5	4
Other	1	–	–	1
	100	100	100	100
Base	138	70	83	152

Including 'ran into'.

The most frequent kind of damage that resulted from the accidents was that some of the teeth were chipped, this was so for half the accidental damage reported among the fourteen year olds. Discolouration of the tooth was particularly frequent among the five year olds, reflecting that any damage to the teeth for this age group would have involved the deciduous teeth.

Table 16.3

What was the damage to the teeth?

What was the damage to the teeth?	Children who have damaged their teeth, aged			
	5+	8+	12+	14+
Tooth chipped	34%	44%	45%	50%
Tooth broken off	10%	10%	23%	21%
Tooth loosened	15%	14%	7%	6%
Tooth discoloured	22%	13%	8%	2%
Tooth knocked out of position	8%	8%	5%	8%
Tooth knocked out	8%	6%	6%	4%
Tooth knocked into gum	6%	6%	6%	5%
Bruised/cut gum	7%	6%	–	4%
Tooth fractured/cracked	4%	–	4%	8%
Other	4%	4%	5%	4%
Base	138	70	83	152

We asked the mothers which dentition had been involved, and among the younger children, as one would expect, a high proportion of the accidents had involved deciduous teeth (see Table 16.4). Among the twelve and fourteen year olds a third of the accidents we were told about had involved deciduous teeth and two-thirds had involved permanent teeth. Approximately two-thirds of accidents resulted in a visit to the dentist for children of all age groups.

Table 16.4

Which dentition was involved in the accident, and did the child see a dentist?

Which dentition was involved in the accident?		Children who have damaged their teeth, aged			
		5+	8+	12+	14+
		%	%	%	%
	Deciduous	100	70	37	30
	Permanent	-	30	63	69
	Both	-	-	-	1
		100	100	100	100
Did the child see a dentist?		%	%	%	%
	Yes	58	72	69	64
	No	42	28	31	36
		100	100	100	100
	Base	138	70	83	152

As with the questions about toothache, we asked the mothers whether, when they took the child to the dentist because of the accident, they had any difficulty in getting treatment. Again the question was only asked in those cases where the child had been to the dentist. The results were very similar to those for toothache (see Chapter 15). Overall fewer than one in ten mothers who went to the dentist found any difficulty in getting treatment and the difficulties found were again divided between having to try several dentists or having to wait for an appointment (see Table 16.5).

Table 16.5

Was there any difficulty getting treatment?

Was there any difficulty getting treatment?	Children who have damaged their teeth and seen a dentist about it, aged			
	5+	8+	12+	14+
	%	%	%	%
No	94	90	87	93
Had to try several dentists	3	5	7	4
Had to wait for appointment	3	5	4	2
Other answers	-	-	2	1
	100	100	100	100
Base	65	47	57	96

Of the accidents reported among five year olds three-quarters did not result in any dental treatment being carried out (Table 16.6). For the other age groups just over a half of the accidents resulted in dental treatment. The range described indicates how widely treatment for accidental damage varies, needing to be specific to the damage caused.

Table 16.6

What treatment was needed?

What treatment was needed?	Children who have damaged their teeth, aged			
	5+	8+	12+	14+
None	74%	48%	39%	46%
Left for later treatment	2%	9%	14%	16%
Tooth filed	1%	2%	7%	5%
Tooth extracted	13%	24%	16%	9%
Tooth filled	-	-	2%	3%
Tooth crowned/capped	-	2%	8%	10%
Nerve taken out	-	-	2%	1%
Tooth came out on its own	7%	7%	6%	5%
Xray	2%	8%	6%	3%
Brace	1%	-	2%	2%
Denture	-	2%	-	2%
Other	2%	3%	6%	4%
Base	138	70	83	152

16.2 Mother's awareness of accidental damage compared with the survey findings

The questions in the interview included any accidental damage that had occurred to either dentition during the child's lifetime. The dental examination, however, only included information about those incisors present at the time of the survey. Thus the data from the interview and the examination are comparable only in so far as the trauma found by the examiner might be expected to be included within the accidental damage reported by the mother. In Table 16.7 we show for the children who had traumatised incisors according to the dental examination what proportion of mothers said her child had had an accident which damaged his teeth. For all age groups there was approximately only 50% agreement between what the mother had said and the dental examination findings.

Table 16.7

Proportion of mothers who said child had damaged his teeth, among children whom the dentist had classified as having traumatised incisors

Whether mother said child had damaged his teeth	Children classified as having traumatised incisors, aged			
	5+	8+	12+	14+
	%	%	%	%
Some damage	48	43	55	52
No damage	52	57	45	48
	100	100	100	100
Base	75	39	81	143

It is hard to believe that any major event concerning the teeth, especially the incisors, was not known to the mothers and so we re-examined the range of trauma that the dentists recorded for the dental examination. In Chapter 5 we showed that fractures of the enamel, the least severe level of damage included in the survey, accounted for the majority of teeth classified as traumatised. For the children where the dentist and mother were in disagreement we examined what kind of trauma had been recorded. Among the five year olds 70% were classified as having discolouration or fractured enamel only, among the eight year olds 87% had fractured enamel only, among the twelve year olds 66% had fractured enamel only and a further 24% had fractured enamel and dentine. Among the fourteen year olds 77% had fractured enamel only. Thus the discrepancies over accidental damage to front teeth between the dentists and the mothers arose for the most part over the mothers not recognising the least severe of the categories included in the dental examination.

17 Mother's views on orthodontics

In Chapter 8 we gave the orthodontic findings from the dental examination. During the interview we asked mothers some fairly general background questions on how they felt about orthodontics and we also asked them specifically whether their child had ever had any orthodontic irregularity and whether anything had been done about it. Initially we discuss the general outlook of mothers towards the question of orthodontics and later we relate what the mother said about her child's condition to what the dentist recorded at the survey examination.

17.1 Attitudes towards orthodontics

Having introduced the problem that some children have crooked or protruding teeth we asked the mothers how important they felt the correction of such anomalies to be. Table 17.1 gives the results in detail and shows that three-quarters of mothers said that it was very important to straighten teeth; a further 20% said that straightening teeth was fairly important. Thus in the context of a general question, orthodontic treatment was very acceptable.

It has been suggested that mothers might feel differently about orthodontic treatment according to whether it was a boy or a girl who needed it. Although we did not ask the question directly, we recorded any spontaneous answers expressing this view and in fact about 10% of mothers said that they considered it of more importance if a girl had an orthodontic problem.

Table 17.1

Mother's views on importance of orthodontic treatment

How important is it to straighten crooked or protruding teeth in children?	Children aged			
	5+	8+	12+	14+
	%	%	%	%
Very important	73	73	73	75
Fairly important	21	20	21	18
Not very important	4	4	3	3
Depends (on how bad it is)	2	3	3	4
	100	100	100	100
Base	*922*	*532*	*451*	*886*

We investigated whether the proportion of mothers who thought that it was very important to straighten teeth varied according to the mother's characteristics such as dental attendance pattern, social class and region, but there was no systematic variation with any of these factors.

Considering the low proportion of children who had received orthodontic treatment compared to the orthodontic need found by the survey dental examiners (see Chapter 8), a very high proportion of mothers said they thought it was very important to carry out orthodontic treatment where it was necessary. In order to ascertain whether there was any misunderstanding about orthodontic treatment which might explain this big disparity we asked the mothers whether they thought that orthodontic treatment for children would be free or not. The vast majority of mothers thought that any such treatment would be free, so it was not any thought of financial involvement which affected the level of unmet treatment (see Table 17.2).

Table 17.2
Whether mother thought orthodontic treatment would be free for children or not

Mother thinks orthodontic treatment would be	Children aged			
	5+	8+	12+	14+
	%	%	%	%
Free for children	86	89	92	92
Not free	8	6	4	3
Don't know	6	5	4	5
	100	100	100	100
Base	922	532	451	886

We were also interested to find out whether mothers had any idea of how long a child might need to wear a brace as a result of orthodontic treatment. Although this time varies between children and for different orthodontic needs, we wanted to see how many mothers thought it would take less than six months. We felt that if a large proportion of mothers grossly underestimated the length of time that appliance therapy takes then this would indicate that their feelings about orthodontic treatment had a fairly unrealistic and uninformed basis. In fact the proportion of mothers who thought a brace would need to be worn for less than six months was not very high (13%, 12%, 14%, and 13%). Understandably on a question which impinged on rather detailed dental knowledge, a quarter of the mothers said they did not know how long a brace would need to be worn. We would conclude that although some mothers could not give an estimate of how long a brace would be worn, only one in eight gave a time so short as to suggest that they perhaps had the wrong impression of how much time orthodontic appliance therapy involved.

Table 17.3

Mother's estimate of how long a child would need to wear a brace

How long mother thinks a brace would be needed to straighten a child's teeth	Children aged			
	5+ %	8+ %	12+ %	14+ %
Less than six months	13	12	14	13
Six months, less than a year	25	24	26	25
A year, less than two years	23	23	19	22
Two years or more	14	13	13	13
Don't know	25	28	28	27
	100	100	100	100
Base	922	532	451	886

17.2 Mother's assessment of child's orthodontic condition

After discussing some of the orthodontic issues in general we asked the mother whether her child had ever had any problem with teeth that were crossed over, crowded together, sticking out or any other similar problem. This question was related to the child's lifetime experience and so would include not only any problem which was present now, but also those that had been rectified by treatment before the dental examination. We have confined the analysis of the mother's description of the child's orthodontic position to the children aged twelve and fourteen since any anomaly should by that age have become apparent.

Table 17.4 shows that, according to their mothers, 44% of the twelve year olds and 43% of the fourteen year olds had at some stage in their lives had some dental condition such as teeth that were crossed over, crowded together or sticking out. The biggest single factor mentioned was crowding; just over a quarter of mothers said their children had crowded teeth. Mothers were obviously not making the same level of distinction for crowding as the dental examiners, for in Chapter 8, we showed that the dentists recorded 55% of twelve year olds and 50% of fourteen year olds as having some current or potential crowding and this excludes any correction of crowding by successful treatment.

Table 17.4

Whether mother thought child had an orthodontic condition

Mother's orthodontic assessment of child	Children aged	
	12+ %	14+ %
No condition	56	57
Some condition	44	43
	100	100
Crossed over	10%	10%
Crowded together	26%	28%
Sticking out	17%	15%
Base	451	886

In fact we show in Table 17.5 the result of information obtained in the dental examination showing the proportion of children aged twelve and fourteen who had received no orthodontic treatment and according to the dental examiner needed none; those who needed treatment and had not previously had any; those who had received some orthodontic treatment but needed other or more treatment, and those who had received orthodontic treatment and currently were not in need of further treatment. The dentists estimated that 49% of twelve year olds and 51% of fourteen year olds had no orthodontic experience and no treatment need. This overall estimate of the proportion of children who never have orthodontic problems is not unlike the one made by the mother (see Table 17.4) which was 56% for twelve year olds and 57% for fourteen year olds, but later in Table 17.6 we investigate the extent to which the estimates agree for the same child. Before we leave Table 17.5 however, it is worth commenting on the proportion of children who have had some orthodontic treatment and the proportion in need of some treatment. Among the twelve year olds, 20% had had some treatment, either extractions or appliance or both; for the fourteen year olds the comparable proportion was 25%. The proportion of children who were said to need orthodontic attention was 36% among the twelve year olds and 29% among the fourteen year olds. There were some children (5% of each age group) who had previously had treatment but were said to need further treatment. Thus among the twelve year olds, the need for orthodontic treatment for children with no orthodontic treatment experience was greater than the amount of treatment already provided. Among the fourteen year olds the proportion of children in need of orthodontic treatment with no prior experience was as great as the proportion of children who had experienced orthodontic treatment.

Table 17.5

Whether child had received, or currently needed, orthodontic treatment (dental examination)

Whether child had received or currently needed orthodontic treatment	Children aged	
	12+	14+
	%	%
No previous treatment / No current need	49	51
No previous treatment / Some current need	31	24
Some previous treatment / Some current need	5	5
Some previous treatment / No current need	15	20
	100	100
Base	451	886

Although the overall estimate of children free from orthodontic problems was of the same order of magnitude whether it was the mothers or the dentists who made it, there was not always agreement between the two as to which children were involved. The first column of Table 17.6 shows the position for those children whom the dentist classified as having no orthodontic treatment need, and no previous orthodontic treatment experience. One in five mothers said these children had some orthodontic irregularities. On investigation, many of these irregularities were said by the mother to be not severe enough to warrant treatment.

Table 17.6

Whether mother and dentist agreed about orthodontic assessment

Mother's orthodontic assessment	Proportion of children who according to the dental examination had			
	No previous treatment/no current need	No previous treatment/some current need	Some previous treatment/some current need	Some previous treatment/no current need
	Children aged 12+			
	%	%	%	%
No condition	79	53	11	7
Some condition	21	47	89	93
	100	100	100	100
Base	219	139	24	69
	Children aged 14+			
	%	%	%	%
No condition	78	58	7	18
Some condition	22	42	93	82
	100	100	100	100
Base	451	206	47	177

The second column of the table shows those children whom the dentist said had no prior experience of orthodontic treatment but needed some treatment. Among this group 53% of the twelve year olds and 58% of the fourteen year olds were said by their mothers to have no orthodontic irregularities. Among the children who had previous orthodontic treatment experience, the vast majority of mothers had reported that the child had had orthodontic problems. The large difference of opinion between the dentists and the mothers about those children whom the dentists say would benefit from treatment but who have so far had none, highlights the situation in which the orthodontists find themselves. The survey results suggest that mothers simply do not recognise conditions which the dentists consider to be worthy of treatment. We illustrate this lack of recognition on the part of the mother by examining whether or not she said her child had an orthodontic problem when the dentist said the child's teeth were crowded.

On the assumption that the mother would know about any crowding among teeth she could see or any extensive crowding we selected three groups of children with such conditions and examined what proportion of the mothers said that the child had some orthodontic irregularity. Table 17.7 shows the results for the twelve year olds and fourteen year olds. Among children with crowding in the region upper 3-3, 47% of the mothers of twelve year olds and 42% of the mothers of fourteen year olds said the child had no orthodontic irregularity. The position was similar with respect to those children with crowding in the region lower 3-3, 50% of the mothers of twelve year olds and 46% of the mothers of fourteen year olds said there was no orthodontic irregularity. For the children with three or more of the six segments of the mouth crowded, the mothers' estimates were similar; half of the children were said to have no orthodontic problem. The results of Table 17.6 and

17.7 thus show that among the mothers of children who currently have orthodontic problems, many do not recognise, or admit to, the condition which the dentist has recorded.

Table 17.7

Whether mother and dentist agreed about crowding

Mother's orthodontic assessment	Proportion of children who according to the dental examination had crowding in		
	The upper middle segment (3-3)	The lower middle segment (3-3)	Three or more segments
	Children aged 12+		
	%	%	%
No condition	47	50	48
Some condition	53	50	52
	100	100	100
Base	*151*	*131*	*49*
	Children aged 14+		
	%	%	%
No condition	42	46	50
Some condition	58	54	50
	100	100	100
Base	*241*	*270*	*71*

If the initiative for treatment has to come from the mother, and mothers do not recognise, or admit to, the orthodontic conditions that the dentist would wish to treat then under present circumstances there will continue to be a considerable amount of unmet need for orthodontic treatment. We cannot tell from the survey data whether, if the mother was made aware of the dentist's estimate of treatment need, she would attach the same priority to obtaining that treatment as she implied when asked how important she felt orthodontic treatment to be, or whether on the other hand she would dispute the need for treatment.

17.3 Variations in orthodontic treatment need according to background

On the basis of the examination information we can use data about past treatment experience and current treatment need to examine whether the overall need for orthodontic treatment varies with background characteristics. Table 17.8 shows the proportion of children who have had or currently need treatment according to the mother's dental attendace pattern, social class, region and the reason for the child's most recent dental visit. There were no systematic variations in need for orthodontic treatment between children with different backgrounds.

Table 17.8

Proportion of children with evidence of some orthodontic need (past or present) by background characteristics

Background characteristics		Proportion of children with evidence of some orthodontic need (past or present), aged			
		12+		14+	
Mother's dental attendance pattern	Regular	55%	165	53%	288
	Occasional	59%	52	47%	86
	Irregular	53%	127	48%	252
	Edentulous	43%	96	46%	241
Social class	I, II, III non-manual	50%	165	48%	284
	III manual	53%	174	49%	396
	IV and V	49%	92	52%	176
Region	The North	56%	140	54%	294
	Midlands and East Anglia	55%	88	42%	197
	Wales and the South West	47%	77	51%	143
	London and the South East	48%	146	47%	252
Reason for most recent dental visit	Check-up	51%	272	50%	554
	Trouble	50%	85	44%	185
	Note from school	44%	48	42%	78

In Table 17.9 we show the variation in the proportion of children who have received some orthodontic treatment according to the child's background. In terms of receiving orthodontic treatment, the children from the most dentally aware backgrounds and those whose own dental behaviour showed an interest in dental care, were the children most likely to have had orthodontic treatment. In the four regions, the fourteen year olds in the Midlands and East Anglia were less likely to have had orthodontic treatment than were children of the same age in other regions.

Table 17.9

Proportion of children who have had orthodontic treatment by background characteristics

Background characteristics		Proportion of children who have had orthodontic treatment, aged			
		12+		14+	
Mother's dental attendance pattern	Regular	28%	165	32%	288
	Occasional	30%	52	27%	86
	Irregular	13%	127	19%	252
	Edentulous	14%	96	24%	241
Social class	I, II, III non-manual	24%	165	29%	284
	III manual	18%	174	24%	396
	IV and V	18%	92	24%	176
Region	The North	24%	140	28%	294
	Midlands and East Anglia	16%	88	19%	197
	Wales and the South West	15%	77	29%	143
	London and the South East	23%	146	26%	252
Reason for most recent dental visit	Check-up	22%	272	29%	554
	Trouble	10%	85	12%	185
	Note from school	6%	48	15%	78

Although there was some association between dental behaviour and orthodontic treatment received, by no means had all the orthodontic need amongst the most dentally aware groups been met, nor was the need of the less dentally conscious groups totally unprovided for.

17.4   Thumbsucking

Finally in this chapter on orthodontics in the context of the home background we examine whether the child who sucks his thumb is at a disadvantage in terms of orthodontic assessment and treatment need. In the first section of Table 17.10, we show the overjet of children who, the mother said, had sucked their thumbs, compared with those who had not. For all the age groups, a significantly higher proportion of thumb suckers had an overjet of five millimetres or more compared with the non-thumb suckers.

Table 17.10

Thumb sucking and overjet, need for orthodontic treatment, and previous appliance therapy

Overjet	Children aged							
	5+		8+		12+		14+	
	Sucked thumb	Did not	Sucked thumb	Did not	Sucked thumb	Did not	Sucked thumb	Did not
	%	%	%	%	%	%	%	%
Negative	I	I	4	2	I	I	-	I
Zero	3	9	I	4	-	I	I	3
1-2 mm	48	65	31	43	37	46	43	48
3-4 mm	26	20	35	34	35	40	33	33
5 mm or more	22	5	29	17	27	12	23	15
	100	100	100	100	100	100	100	100
Need for orthodontic treatment	%	%	%	%	%	%	%	%
No treatment need	80	85	37	41	45	58	69	67
Under treatment now	-	-	I	-	13	7	6	3
Current treatment need	20	15	62	59	42	35	25	30
	100	100	100	100	100	100	100	100
Previous appliance therapy					%	%	%	%
None	-	-	-	-	93	92	81	89
Some	-	-	-	-	7	8	19	11
					100	100	100	100
Base	*232*	*688*	*132*	*399*	*90*	*359*	*160*	*721*

The second section of the table shows whether the dentist considered that there was a need for orthodontic treatment. Among the five and eight year olds there was no significant difference between the treatment need of children who had sucked their thumbs and those who had not. Among the twelve year olds significantly more thumb suckers needed or were having treatment, among the fourteen year olds there was no significant difference between thumb suckers and non-thumb suckers in current treatment need but more of the former had had appliance therapy in the past.

Part III

The interaction

18   Dental background and dental health

In Chapters 10 to 17 we have used the interview information to describe the
variations of dental attitudes, behaviour and previous experience that have
contributed towards the child's dental upbringing. We have used the examination
information where this has clarified a particular issue but, until this chapter, we
have not attempted to draw together the overall picture of the child's background
and his dental condition. In order to accomplish this in a readily digestible form
we have created a composite description of the child's background based on those
aspects which the earlier chapters have suggested had the greatest impact. We have
tried to confine the classification to information that could possibly be obtained
from the child, thereby making it feasible to attempt a similar classification where
there is no opportunity to interview the mother.

The main divisions were determined by the reason for the child's most recent dental
visit and the length of time that had elapsed since that visit. Children whose
last visit was for a check-up were also subdivided according to which of the dental
services they used. From the fairly large group of children who only ever used the
General Dental Service and whose most recent visit had been within the last six
months for a check-up we selected those who also met two other criteria, that their
mothers were regular dental attenders and that their own first dental visit had
been for a check-up or to get used to going to the dentist. We labelled this group
'AI' as having met all the main requirements we had used earlier in the analysis to
indicate a good dental background. At the other extreme of the classification are
those children who, according to the mother, had never been to the dentist. For
some of these children the more appropriate description would have been that they
had seldom been to the dentist, since the survey examination revealed that a few
of them had experienced dental treatment. There were insufficient numbers to
classify the children both by the time that had elapsed since the last dental visit
and separately by whether the last visit was because of trouble or a note from
school. Consequently these two reasons for dental attendance were grouped together.
The classification thus provides a detailed estimate of the child's dental
attendance pattern and Table 18.1 shows the proportion of children who were in
each of the categories.

In addition to the detailed categories already described Table 18.1 shows three
sub-groups which give a broad indication of the child's likely future dental
attendance pattern; we refer to the first group as regular attenders, the second
group as occasional attenders and the third group as those who only go to the
dentist when they are having trouble. These are the groups that we have used
extensively in surveys of adult dental health and so, in this way, we are predict-
ing which type of attendance pattern the child is likely to develop. Among the
five year olds a fairly large proportion have not yet been to the dentist which

Table 18.1
The child's dental attendance pattern

Child's dental attendance pattern	Children aged			
	5+	8+	12+	14+
	%	%	%	%
Check-up; in last six months; G.D.S. only; A1*	17	18	15	11
Check-up; in last six months; G.D.S. only	13	17	18	17
Check-up; in last six months; mixed	3	7	10	11
Check-up; in last six months; S.D.S. only	3	5	4	5
Other††	3	4	6	4
Regular check-up	39	51	53	48
Check-up; not in last six months; G.D.S. only	7	4	7	11
Check-up; not in last six months; mixed	–	2	4	5
Check-up; not in last six months; S.D.S. only	1	4	4	3
Occasional check-up	8	10	15	19
Trouble or note; in last six months	17	14	11	12
Trouble or note; within last two years	7	15	14	9
Trouble or note; not within last two years	–	1	4	8
Never (seldom) been	29	9	3	4
Only when has trouble	53	39	32	33
	100	100	100	100
Base	922	532	451	886

† A1   *First visit was a check-up or to get used to dentist, and mother is a regular attender.*

†† *The reason for some children's last visit was specialist advice or treatment which constituted a refinement of visiting for a check-up.*

means that over half of this age group is classified as attending only when they have trouble. Among the eight, twelve and fourteen year olds about a half of children appear to have the basis of a pattern of regular dental attendance, whereas a third are only attending when they have some kind of dental trouble. The group of children defined as having the best dental background, that is the very first category in the table, was larger than might have been expected from all the restrictions imposed by the classification; it accounted for 17% of five year olds, 18% of eight year olds, 15% of twelve year olds and 11% of fourteen year olds.

In later tables when the dental condition of children in the different categories is portrayed, the proportion of children affected can be seen from Table 18.1 which then puts into perspective the relative importance of the results in terms of how they affect children as a whole.

18.1 Dental attendance pattern and overall dental need

In Chapter 9 we drew together the main dental conditions covered by the dental examination and estimated what proportion of children would benefit from the attention of a dentist or hygienist. There were three conditions involved, any of which rendered a child in need of attention, that is any decay, any gum trouble or any orthodontic treatment need. The result of this analysis was extremely depressing since, apart from the five and six year olds, over 90% of children needed attention for some reason. Among the age groups for whom we have interview data the proportions who were in need of some attention were 79% for the five year olds, 97% for the eight year olds, 94% for the twelve year olds

Table 18.2

Proportion of children with some overall dental need by child's attendance pattern

Child's dental attendance pattern	Proportion of children with some overall dental need, aged							
	5+		8+		12+		14+	
Check-up; in last six months; G.D.S. only; A1†	64%	157	97%	97	93%	68	84%	94
Check-up; in last six months; G.D.S. only	80%	114	98%	88	92%	79	85%	152
Check-up; in last six months; mixed	90%	27	100%	38	91%	43	87%	95
Check-up; in last six months; S.D.S. only	88%	27	100%	26	*	17	98%	43
Other (see Table 18.1)	71%	32	*	19	96%	27	89%	37
Regular check-up	73%	357	98%	268	93%	234	87%	421
Check-up; not in last six months; G.D.S. only	63%	62	96%	23	87%	30	91%	97
Check-up; not in last six months; mixed	*	3	*	11	*	16	98%	44
Check-up; not in last six months; S.D.S. only	*	11	95%	20	*	18	93%	28
Occasional check-up	69%	76	96%	54	91%	64	93%	169
Trouble or note; in last six months	90%	154	94%	75	97%	52	93%	107
Trouble or note; within last two years	87%	63	98%	78	95%	61	96%	82
Trouble or note; not within last two years	*	2	*	7	100%	20	93%	73
Never (seldom) been	80%	266	98%	48	*	15	100%	31
Only when has trouble	84%	485	97%	208	97%	148	95%	293
All children	79%	922	97%	532	94%	451	91%	886

† A1= First visit was a check-up or to get used
to dentist, and mother is a regular attender.

Table 18.3

Proportion of children with some gum trouble by child's attendance pattern

Child's dental attendance pattern	Proportion of children with some gum trouble, aged							
	5+		8+		12+		14+	
Check-up; in last six months; G.D.S. only; A1†	39%	157	74%	97	75%	68	68%	94
Check-up; in last six months; G.D.S. only	39%	114	80%	88	74%	79	69%	152
Check-up; in last six months; mixed	52%	27	84%	38	68%	43	69%	95
Check-up; in last six months; S.D.S. only	46%	27	91%	26	*	17	88%	43
Other (see Table 18.1)	42%	32	*	19	82%	27	80%	37
Regular check-up	41%	357	78%	268	76%	234	72%	421
Check-up; not in last six months; G.D.S. only	38%	62	81%	23	72%	30	72%	97
Check-up; not in last six months; mixed	*	3	*	11	*	16	74%	44
Check-up; not in last six months; S.D.S. only	*	11	85%	20	*	18	73%	28
Occasional check-up	39%	76	82%	54	78%	64	73%	169
Trouble or note; in last six months	52%	154	70%	75	76%	52	79%	107
Trouble or note; within last two years	44%	63	81%	78	82%	61	78%	82
Trouble or note; not within last two years	*	2	*	7	100%	20	79%	73
Never (seldom) been	52%	266	85%	48	*	15	97%	31
Only when has trouble	51%	485	78%	208	83%	148	81%	293
All children	46%	922	79%	532	79%	451	75%	886

† A1 = First visit was a check-up or to get used
to dentist, and mother is a regular attender.

and 91% for the fourteen year olds. In this section we examine whether this
need for attention varied at all according to the child's dental attendance
pattern.

Table 18.2 shows that the variation in overall dental need between children with
different dental attendance patterns is fairly small. Even among the children with
the best record of attendance and background the proportion who, according to the
survey, would benefit from dental attention was high (64%, 97%, 93%, and 84% for
the four age groups respectively). If we look at the whole group of potential
regular dental attenders the proportions in need of some attention are 73%, 98%, 93%
and 87% respectively. Among children who attend only when they have dental trouble
or a note from school the comparable proportions were 84%, 97%, 97% and 95%. The
results thus indicate that in the terms of the survey dental examination definition
of need, the children with the best dental attendance patterns and the best dental
backgrounds did not have an overwhelming advantage. This leads us immediately
to scrutinise the various aspects of dental health which contributed to overall
dental need.

In Table 18.3 we show, for children of different attendance patterns, the
proportion who had some gum trouble, that is any gum inflammation, debris or
calculus. The proportion of children with some gum trouble was 46%, 79%, 79%, and
75% for the four age groups. For the children who were most likely to become
regular dental attenders the proportions were 41%, 78%, 76% and 72%, as compared
with 51%, 78%, 83% and 81% among the children most likely to become irregular
attenders. The children anticipated to have the greatest advantage according to
their dental attendance pattern and background were by no means free of gum trouble
although a significantly lower proportion had some gum trouble as compared with the
others. It would therefore appear that dental attendance under the present system
of dental service is not a good indicator of the likelihood of gum trouble as we
measured it.

The second aspect of the overall dental need was the need for orthodontic treatment.
We have already seen in Chapter 17 that the recognition by the mothers of current
orthodontic need is not particularly high. Of course, the need for orthodontic
treatment may reveal itself some considerable while before such treatment is
carried out, nevertheless most orthodontic treatment would be started by the time
the child was fourteen, so among that age group, at least, the results show the
level of unmet treatment need. As one can see from Table 18.4 among the eight year
olds 60% were estimated as being in need of orthodontic treatment whereas among
fourteen year olds 29% needed treatment. For the fourteen year olds orthodontic
need was found among a third of the least dentally aware group and among a quarter
of the potential regular attenders. Although the latter proportion is significantly lower it is higher than many might have expected for the group of children
with ostensibly the greatest opportunity to receive orthodontic advice and
treatment.

It is possible that in the survey dental examination the definitions laid down for
gum conditions and orthodontic need were more stringent than could be generally
applied but this was not the case for the third component of overall dental need,
active decay. We would not expect to be recording decay in the survey examination
that would be undetected in a clinical situation since the survey criteria laid
down a visual diagnosis for decay, with the use of a blunt probe for confirmation

Table 18.4

Proportion of children with some orthodontic treatment need by child's attendance pattern

Child's dental attendance pattern	Proportion of children needing some orthodontic treatment, aged							
	5+		8+		12+		14+	
Check-up; in last six months: G.D.S. only; A1†	16%	157	59%	97	29%	68	20%	94
Check-up; in last six months; G.D.S. only	15%	114	72%	88	40%	79	30%	152
Check-up; in last six months; mixed	26%	27	64%	38	35%	43	23%	95
Check-up; in last six months; S.D.S. only	12%	27	57%	26	*	17	26%	43
Other (see Table 18.1)	19%	32	*	19	29%	27	24%	37
Regular check-up	16%	357	64%	268	34%	234	25%	421
Check-up; not in last six months; G.D.S. only	18%	62	53%	23	33%	30	24%	97
Check-up; not in last six months; mixed	*	3	*	11	*	16	44%	44
Check-up; not in last six months; S.D.S. only	*	11	48%	20	*	18	28%	28
Occasional check-up	18%	76	48%	54	35%	64	30%	169
Trouble or note; in last six months	18%	154	58%	75	39%	52	27%	107
Trouble or note; within last two years	25%	63	52%	78	39%	61	39%	82
Trouble or note; not within last two years	*	2	*	7	55%	20	36%	73
Never (seldom) been	12%	266	61%	48	*	15	30%	31
Only when has trouble	16%	485	57%	208	40%	148	33%	293
All children	16%	922	60%	532	36%	451	29%	886

† _A1 = First visit was a check-up or to get used to dentist, and mother is a regular attender._

Table 18.5

Proportion of children with some active decay by child's attendance pattern

Child's dental attendance pattern	Proportion of children with some active decay, aged							
	5+		8+		12+		14+	
Check-up; in last six months; G.D.S. only; A1†	47%	157	64%	97	52%	68	46%	94
Check-up; in last six months; G.D.S. only	64%	114	76%	88	42%	79	51%	152
Check-up; in last six months; mixed	68%	27	76%	38	60%	43	52%	95
Check-up; in last six months; S.D.S. only	79%	27	75%	26	*	17	76%	43
Other (see Table 18.1)	60%	32	*	19	56%	27	50%	37
Regular check-up	58%	357	71%	268	53%	234	53%	421
Check-up; not in last six months; G.D.S. only	48%	62	73%	23	56%	30	59%	97
Check-up; not in last six months; mixed	*	3	*	11	*	16	69%	44
Check-up; not in last six months; S.D.S. only	*	11	85%	20	*	18	62%	28
Occasional check-up	52%	76	80%	54	64%	64	62%	169
Trouble or note; in last six months	80%	154	77%	75	76%	52	68%	107
Trouble or note; within last two years	82%	63	88%	78	90%	61	79%	82
Trouble or note; not within last two years	*	2	*	7	90%	20	84%	73
Never (seldom) been	71%	266	80%	48	*	15	67%	31
Only when has trouble	70%	485	82%	208	75%	148	75%	293
All children	64%	922	76%	532	62%	451	62%	886

† _A1 = First visit was a check-up or to get used to dentist, and mother is a regular attender._

purposes only. In addition, since decay is the most common dental problem and relates fairly directly to dental attendance pattern and dental background one might expect a good relationship between the child's dental attendance pattern and whether or not he had any active decay. Table 18.5 shows the proportion of children with some active decay when we examined them.

Among the five year olds 58% of those whose check-up had been recent, 52% of those whose check-up had not been recent and 70% of those who were not in the habit of going for a check-up had some active decay. Among children of this age those who had been for a recent check-up through the General Dental Service and had other additional background advantages had the lowest proportion with some active decay (47%). Although this compares favourably with the five year olds who had never been to the dentist (71% with some active decay) and with those five year olds who had been to the dentist in the last six months because of trouble or a note from school (80% with some active decay) it is still a high proportion among what should ostensibly be the most well cared for group.

Among the eight year olds one finds the highest proportion, overall, of children with active decay; 76% of eight year olds had some active decay. The proportion was as high as 71% even among children who were said to have been to the dentist for a check-up in the six months prior to the survey. Even among the group with the best dental background and habits 64% of eight year olds had some active decay. Again this was an improvement over those whose dental visits were not for check-ups among whom 82% of eight year olds had some active decay. For the five and eight year olds the deciduous dentition is, of course, making a significant contribution to the decay situation. One might anticipate that among the older children there might be a drop in the proportion found to have some active decay. The proportion of those who had been for a check-up within the last six months who had some active decay was 53% among the twelve year olds and 53% among the fourteen year olds. Among children whose check-up had taken place longer ago than six months 64% of twelve year olds and 62% of fourteen year olds had some active decay. Among those not in the habit of going for a check-up 75% of both twelve and fourteen year olds had some active decay. Thus the different dental attendance patterns showed a variation over the three main classes of a half to two-thirds to three-quarters of children with current decay.

We have looked in turn at the three component parts that contributed to the survey estimate of overall dental need, and found that for the dental need arising from decay alone there is not as much association with dental attendance as one would have liked to see. Since considerable resources are vested in the provision of dental services for children, most of which are aimed at combating decay we look in much greater detail in Section 18.2 at the variations in treatment for decay according to the child's dental attendance pattern.

18.2 Dental attendance pattern and decay

We examine generally the aspects of decay and its treatment in two ways. Firstly we look at the proportion of children with a certain level of involvement and secondly we show the average number of teeth involved with each aspect of decay and its treatment.

Table 18.6

Known decay experience and the child's attendance pattern

Child's dental attendance pattern	Proportion having ten or more teeth with known decay experience (DMF+df), of children aged							
	5+		8+		12+		14+	
Check-up; in last six months; G.D.S. only; A1†	5%	157	13%	97	7%	68	25%	94
Check-up; in last six months; G.D.S. only	10%	114	17%	88	11%	79	35%	152
Check-up; in last six months; mixed	11%	27	16%	38	7%	43	39%	95
Check-up; in last six months; S.D.S. only	–	27	17%	26	*	17	22%	43
Other (see Table 18.1)	14%	32	*	19	5%	27	32%	37
Regular check-up	8%	357	15%	268	9%	234	32%	421
Check-up; not in last six months; G.D.S. only	4%	62	4%	23	3%	30	23%	97
Check-up; not in last six months; mixed	*	3	*	11	*	16	21%	44
Check-up; not in last six months; S.D.S. only	*	11	–	20	*	18	16%	28
Occasional check-up	4%	76	2%	54	2%	64	22%	169
Trouble or note; in last six months	6%	154	6%	75	17%	52	38%	107
Trouble or note; within last two years	11%	63	7%	78	7%	61	24%	82
Trouble or note; not within last two years	*	2	*	7	5%	20	12%	73
Never (seldom) been	5%	266	3%	48	*%	15	10%	31
Only when has trouble	6%	485	5%	208	10%	148	25%	293
All children	6%	922	10%	532	8%	451	28%	886

† *A1 = First visit was a check-up or to get used to dentist, and mother is a regular attender.*

Table 18.7

Average number of teeth with known decay experience by child's attendance pattern

Child's dental attendance pattern	Average number of teeth with known decay experience (DMF+df) among children aged							
	5+		8+		12+		14+	
Check-up; in last six months; G.D.S. only; A1†	2.5	157	5.1	97	5.6	68	7.8	94
Check-up; in last six months; G.D.S. only	4.1	114	5.5	88	5.5	79	8.0	152
Check-up; in last six months; mixed	3.8	27	5.9	38	5.9	43	9.0	95
Check-up; in last six months; S.D.S. only	4.2	27	6.2	26	*	17	7.0	43
Other (see Table 18.1)	3.7	32	*	19	5.0	27	7.5	37
Regular check-up	3.3	357	5.4	268	5.6	234	8.0	421
Check-up; not in last six months; G.D.S. only	2.0	62	4.3	23	4.8	30	6.9	97
Check-up; not in last six months; mixed	*	3	*	11	*	16	7.4	44
Check-up; not in last six months; S.D.S. only	*	11	5.5	20	*	18	5.4	28
Occasional check-up	2.1	76	4.6	54	4.6	64	6.8	169
Trouble or note; in last six months	4.8	154	5.2	75	6.1	52	9.0	107
Trouble or note; within last two years	5.2	63	4.8	78	5.4	61	7.0	82
Trouble or note; not within last two years	*	2	*	7	4.9	20	5.3	73
Never (seldom) been	2.6	266	3.6	48	*	15	3.6	31
Only when has trouble	3.6	485	4.6	208	5.2	148	6.9	293
All children	3.4	922	5.0	532	5.3	451	7.4	886

† *A1 = First visit was a check-up or to get used to dentist, and mother is a regular attender.*

We begin by examining the level of known decay experience that the children have had. Table 18.6 shows the proportion of children with ten or more teeth with known decay experience and Table 18.7 shows the average number of teeth with known decay experience. The variation in total known decay experience (based on the addition of currently decayed teeth, filled teeth and extracted permanent teeth) and dental attendance pattern has two aspects of particular interest. First, children who have the fewest problems are probably likely to go to the dentist less frequently whatever their attitude to dental visits; this is borne out by the results which show that the children whose visits for check-ups are less frequent and the children who less frequently have dental trouble have a lower proportion with ten or more teeth involved with decay. Secondly, the assumption that is being made by adding together teeth that are currently decayed and those that have previously been filled is that the latter were filled at a state of decay similar to that recorded in the survey dental examination. If any of these teeth were filled at an earlier stage of decay then those children with most treatment will appear to have most disease since the equivalent tooth untreated would pass as sound on a visual diagnosis such as that used in the survey. The combined effects of disease and treatment thus result in the most dentally well cared for group of children containing the highest proportion of children with ten or more teeth involved with decay. This is particularly noticeable among the fourteen year olds where the proportion of children with ten or more teeth with known decay experience is 32% among those who have been to the dentist for a check-up within the past six months, 22% for those whose check-up was not within the last six months and 25% for those who were not in the habit of going for a check-up. Within this last group the proportion was about 10% for children who seldom go to the dentist or had not had any trouble in the last two years.

The average number of teeth involved with known decay experience illustrates the same points (see Table 18.7) and shows that by the age of fourteen the most dentally conscious children have on average about one more tooth that has been involved with decay than the less dentally conscious children.

It is therefore imperative to examine more closely the component parts of disease experience and treatment experience since together their relationship with dental care is confounded. With this in mind we turn first to examine again the situation with respect to active decay. One might well expect to find that the presence of active decay was much more closely connected with dental care and attention. In Table 18.8 we repeat for convenience the results as shown in Table 18.5, that is the proportion of children with some active decay. We commented earlier that although there is significant variation with the child's attendance pattern the proportion of children with the best attendance pattern and background who had some active decay at the time of the examination was considerably higher than one would have liked. This fact suggests that perhaps it is too high an aim to expect a substantial proportion of children having regular care at this period of their lives to be continuously free from decay. Maybe 'decay-free' is too stringent a definition and that among those children who had some active decay the numbers of teeth involved varied greatly with the child's dental attendance pattern. In Table 18.9 we show the average number of teeth that had active decay at the time of the examination. The average number of decayed teeth was 2.2 and 2.4 for five and eight year old children whose last visit had been for a check-up in the six months prior to the survey. Considering that for these five year olds 58% had some active decay and 42%

Table 18.8

Active decay and the child's attendance pattern

Child's dental attendance pattern	Proportion of children with some active decay (D+d), aged							
	5+		8+		12+		14+	
Check-up; in last six months; G.D.S. only; A1[†]	47%	157	64%	97	52%	68	46%	94
Check-up; in last six months; G.D.S. only	64%	114	76%	88	42%	79	51%	152
Check-up; in last six months; mixed	68%	27	76%	38	60%	43	52%	95
Check-up; in last six months; S.D.S. only	79%	27	75%	26	*	17	76%	43
Other (see Table 18.1)	60%	32	*	19	56%	27	50%	37
Regular check-up	58%	357	71%	268	53%	234	53%	421
Check-up; not in last six months; G.D.S. only	48%	62	73%	23	56%	30	59%	97
Check-up; not in last six months; mixed	*	3	*	11	*	16	69%	44
Check-up; not in last six months; S.D.S. only	*	11	85%	20	*	18	62%	28
Occasional check-up	52%	76	80%	54	64%	64	62%	169
Trouble or note; in last six months	80%	154	77%	75	76%	52	68%	107
Trouble or note; within last two years	82%	63	88%	78	90%	61	79%	82
Trouble or note; not within last two years	*	2	*	7	90%	20	84%	73
Never (seldom) been	71%	266	80%	48	*	15	67%	31
Only when has trouble	70%	485	82%	208	75%	148	75%	293
All children	64%	922	76%	532	62%	451	62%	886

† A1 = First visit was a check-up or to get used
  to dentist, and mother is a regular attender.

Table 18.9

Average number of decayed teeth by child's attendance pattern

Child's dental attendance pattern	Average number of decayed (D+d) teeth among children, aged							
	5+		8+		12+		14+	
Check-up; in last six months; G.D.S. only; A1[†]	1.4	157	2.1	97	1.1	68	1.2	94
Check-up; in last six months; G.D.S. only	2.9	114	2.6	88	1.0	79	1.2	152
Check-up; in last six months; mixed	2.2	27	2.4	38	1.4	43	1.5	95
Check-up; in last six months; S.D.S. only	2.8	27	3.2	26	*	17	1.9	43
Other (see Table 18.1)	3.0	32	*	19	1.8	27	1.0	37
Regular check-up	2.2	357	2.4	268	1.2	234	1.3	421
Check-up; not in last six months; G.D.S. only	1.8	62	2.7	23	1.3	30	1.9	97
Check-up; not in last six months; mixed	*	3	*	11	*	16	2.3	44
Check-up; not in last six months; S.D.S. only	*	11	3.4	20	*	18	1.7	28
Occasional check-up	1.9	76	2.9	54	1.6	64	2.0	169
Trouble or note; in last six months	3.6	154	2.5	75	2.0	52	2.1	107
Trouble or note; within last two years	4.6	63	3.6	78	2.9	61	2.7	82
Trouble or note; not within last two years	*	2	*	7	4.2	20	3.7	73
Never (seldom) been	2.5	266	3.4	48	*	15	2.4	31
Only when has trouble	3.1	485	3.2	208	2.7	148	2.7	293
All children	2.6	922	2.8	532	1.8	451	1.9	886

† A1 = First visit was a check-up or to get used
  to dentist, and mother is a regular attender.

did not, that means that among those children with decay there must have been an average of something like four teeth with active decay. Among five and eight year olds who do not go to the dentist for a check-up the average number of teeth with active decay was 3.1 and 3.2 respectively.

Among the fourteen year olds for whom only the permanent dentition was involved the average number of decayed teeth was lower. Even among this age group the average number of decayed teeth among children who had been to the dentist for a check-up within the last six months was 1.3, and again since 47% of this group had no active decay this must have been an average of two teeth per child for those who had any decay at all. Among the fourteen year olds who were not in the habit of going for dental check-ups each child had, on average, 2.7 decayed teeth. Although the least dentally aware children had more active decay than the most dentally aware the situation for the latter involved more teeth than might have been expected.

It is difficult to disentangle the relationship between attendance pattern and active decay for the children in the age groups five, eight and twelve unless deciduous and permanent teeth are examined separately. This is of particular importance if there is any likelihood that the two dentitions might receive different priority and different treatment. In Tables 18.10 to 18.13 we show separately for the two dentitions the proportion of children with some active decay and the average number of teeth involved.

Five year olds had on average 2.6 decayed deciduous teeth, the comparable figure for eight year olds was 2.0. Among the children who had been for a dental check-up within six months of the survey the average number of decayed deciduous teeth was 2.2 among five year olds and 1.8 among eight year olds; for those whose dental background did not involve dental check-ups the average number of decayed deciduous teeth was 3.1 among five year olds and 2.2 among eight year olds. Although, again, the children with the better dental habits had fewer decayed deciduous teeth many of them did not maintain a state of freedom from decay between dental visits.

As far as the permanent dentition was concerned four out of ten eight year olds, five out of ten twelve year olds and six out of ten fourteen year olds had some decayed permanent teeth at the time of the survey examination. When looked at in terms of the children with the greatest chance of being decay free through the provision of treatment we find that 34% of eight year olds, 43% of twelve year olds and 52% of fourteen year olds had some decay in permanent teeth Thus between a third and a half of children aged eight to fourteen who were said to have been for a check-up in the last six months were not free from decay in permanent teeth when we saw them. The children who do not go for dental check-ups were in a worse position with respect to decayed permanent teeth; among eight year olds 45% had some decayed permanent teeth, among twelve year olds the proportion was 66% and among fourteen year olds it was 75%. The average number of permanent teeth involved with decay is shown in Table 18.13.

The fact that a considerable proportion of the most dentally aware and well cared for children do not remain decay free between dental visits, either in terms of the deciduous or permanent dentition, raises the question of whether this is because the onset of decay is very rapid, or that being made reasonably dentally fit does

Table 18.10

Active decay in deciduous teeth and the child's attendance pattern

Child's dental attendance pattern	Proportion of children with some decayed deciduous teeth, aged							
	5+		8+		12+		14+	
Check-up; in last six months; G.D.S. only; A1†	46%	157	60%	97	18%	68	2%	94
Check-up; in last six months; G.D.S. only	64%	114	74%	88	10%	79	1%	152
Check-up; in last six months; mixed	68%	27	73%	38	22%	43	4%	95
Check-up; in last six months; S.D.S. only	79%	27	71%	26	*	17	5%	43
Other (see Table 18.1)	60%	32	*	19	20%	27	–	37
Regular check-up	57%	357	66%	268	17%	234	2%	421
Check-up; not in last six months; G.D.S. only	48%	62	69%	23	14%	30	2%	97
Check-up; not in last six months; mixed	*	3	*	11	*	16	9%	44
Check-up; not in last six months; S.D.S. only	*	11	69%	20	*	18	–	28
Occasional check-up	51%	76	70%	54	12%	64	4%	169
Trouble or note; in last six months	80%	154	69%	75	24%	52	2%	107
Trouble or note; within last two years	82%	63	82%	78	16%	61	4%	82
Trouble or note; not within last two years	*	2	*	7	37%	20	6%	73
Never (seldom) been	61%	266	76%	48	*	15	–	31
Only when has trouble	70%	485	76%	208	22%	148	3%	293
All children	63%	922	71%	532	18%	451	3%	886

† A1 = First visit was a check-up or to get used
to dentist, and mother is a regular attender.

Table 18.11

Average number of deciduous teeth with active decay by child's attendance pattern

Child's dental attendance pattern	Average number of deciduous teeth with active decay among children, aged							
	5+		8+		12+		14+	
Check-up; in last six months; G.D.S. only; A1†	1.4	157	1.6	97	0.3	68	0.1	94
Check-up; in last six months; G.D.S. only	2.8	114	2.0	88	0.2	79	–	152
Check-up; in last six months; mixed	2.2	27	1.8	38	0.3	43	0.1	95
Check-up; in last six months; S.D.S. only	2.8	27	2.5	26	*	17	0.1	43
Other (see Table 18.1)	2.9	32	*	19	0.2	27	–	37
Regular check-up	2.2	357	1.8	268	0.3	234	–	421
Check-up; not in last six months; G.D.S. only	1.8	62	2.0	23	0.1	30	–	97
Check-up; not in last six months; mixed	*	3	*	11	*	16	0.1	44
Check-up; not in last six months; S.D.S. only	*	11	2.4	20	*	18	–	28
Occasional check-up	1.9	76	2.2	54	0.2	64	–	169
Trouble or note; in last six months	3.5	154	1.9	75	0.4	52	–	107
Trouble or note; within last two years	4.6	63	2.6	78	0.2	61	0.1	82
Trouble or note; not within last two years	*	2	*	7	0.8	20	–	73
Never (seldom) been	2.5	266	2.4	48	*	15	–	31
Only when has trouble	3.1	485	2.2	208	0.4	148	–	293
All children	2.6	922	2.0	532	0.3	451	–	886

† A1 = First visit was a check-up or to get used
to dentist, and mother is a regular attender.

Table 18.12

Active decay in permanent teeth and the child's attendance pattern

Child's dental attendance pattern	Proportion of children with some actively decayed permanent teeth, aged							
	5+		8+		12+		14+	
Check-up; in last six months; G.D.S. only; A1†	1%	157	30%	97	40%	68	46%	94
Check-up; in last six months; G.D.S. only	6%	114	32%	88	38%	79	51%	152
Check-up; in last six months; mixed	-	27	31%	38	46%	43	51%	95
Check-up; in last six months; S.D.S. only	-	27	36%	26	*	17	77%	43
Other (see Table 18.1)	3%	32	*	19	41%	27	50%	37
Regular check-up	3%	357	34%	268	43%	234	52%	421
Check-up; not in last six months; G.D.S. only	2%	62	33%	23	53%	30	59%	97
Check-up; not in last six months; mixed	*	3	*	11	*	16	65%	44
Check-up; not in last six months; S.D.S. only	*	11	52%	20	*	18	62%	28
Occasional check-up	3%	76	38%	54	62%	64	61%	169
Trouble or note; in last six months	3%	154	38%	75	54%	52	68%	107
Trouble or note; within last two years	4%	63	47%	78	68%	61	78%	82
Trouble or note; not within last two years	*	2	*	7	85%	20	84%	73
Never (seldom) been	3%	266	50%	48	*	15	67%	31
Only when has trouble	3%	485	45%	208	66%	148	75%	293
All children	3%	922	39%	532	53%	451	61%	886

† A1 = First visit was a check-up or to get used to dentist, and mother is a regular attender.

Table 18.13

Average number of permanent teeth with active decay by child's attendance pattern

Child's dental attendance pattern	Average number of permanent teeth with active decay among children aged							
	5+		8+		12+		14+	
Check-up; in last six months; G.D.S. only; A1†	-	157	0.5	97	0.8	68	1.1	94
Check-up; in last six months; G.D.S. only	0.1	114	0.6	88	0.8	79	1.2	152
Check-up; in last six months; mixed	-	27	0.6	38	1.1	43	1.5	95
Check-up; in last six months; S.D.S. only	-	27	0.8	26	*	17	1.9	43
Other (see Table 18.1)	0.1	32	*	19	1.5	27	1.0	37
Regular check-up	-	357	0.6	268	1.0	234	1.3	421
Check-up; not in last six months; G.D.S. only	-	62	0.7	23	1.2	30	1.9	97
Check-up; not in last six months; mixed	*	3	*	11	*	16	2.2	44
Check-up; not in last six months; S.D.S. only	*	11	1.0	20	*	18	1.7	28
Occasional check-up	-	76	0.7	54	1.5	64	1.9	169
Trouble or note; in last six months	-	154	0.6	75	1.7	52	2.1	107
Trouble or note; within last two years	0.1	63	1.0	78	2.6	61	2.6	82
Trouble or note; not within last two years	*	2	*	7	3.4	20	3.6	73
Never (seldom) been	-	266	1.2	48	*	15	2.4	31
Only when has trouble	-	485	0.9	208	2.3	148	2.6	293
All children	0.1	922	0.7	532	1.5	451	1.9	886

† A1 = First visit was a check-up or to get used to dentist, and mother is a regular attender.

not necessarily mean being made decay free. If the latter is the case then perhaps we ought not to be surprised to find children with apparently good records of attendance with active decay.

In the examination the dentist distinguished between those decayed teeth which he considered could be restored and those that he considered to have become un-restorable. In Tables 18.14 and 18.15 we show the proportion of children with some unrestorable deciduous teeth, and some unrestorable permanent teeth.

Among five year olds 30% of children had some unrestorable deciduous teeth, among eight year olds the proportion was 38%. Among children who had been for a dental check-up in the last six months the proportion with some unrestorable deciduous teeth was 20% among five year olds and 35% among eight year olds. Among children who do not go for check-ups the comparable proportions were 38% for five year olds and 43% for eight year olds. Such a high proportion of children with unrestorable deciduous teeth must indicate that some dentists have a policy of non-intervention with the deciduous dentition except in the case of pain since even among the eight year olds who would appear to have had a long standing good dental background 28% had some unrestorable deciduous teeth.

As far as the permanent dentition was concerned the proportion of children with decayed teeth that were unrestorable was, naturally, much lower. The deciduous teeth were at the end of their life, the permanent teeth were at the beginning, therefore even though the proportions were much lower with respect to permanent teeth they were perhaps the more depressing. For children as a whole 5% of eight year olds, 12% of twelve year olds and 14% of fourteen year olds had some unrest-orable permanent teeth. Although some were found among children whose last visit had been for a check-up within six months of the survey the proportion was small (5% for twelve and fourteen year olds) compared with the children who did not go for dental check-ups. Among this latter group 21% of twelve year olds and 25% of fourteen year olds had some unrestorable permanent teeth at the time of the survey examination. Among fourteen year olds who last went to the dentist with trouble or a note from school more than two years ago as many as 36% had some unrestorable permanent teeth.

18.3 Dental attendance pattern and treatment for decay

Having investigated in some detail the distribution of current treatment need for decay we turn to examine the amount of past treatment experience among children with different attendance patterns. Initially we look at the proportion of child-ren with some filled teeth and the average number of filled teeth that they have (Tables 18.16 and 18.17).

Among the five year olds 27% had some filled teeth and this proportion varied considerably with the child's dental attendance pattern. Among children who had been to the dentist during the last six months for a check-up 43% had some filled teeth, if their check-up had been longer ago than six months 11% had some filled teeth and if they did not go to the dentist for a check-up then 19% had some filled teeth.

Table 18.14

Unrestorable deciduous teeth and the child's attendance pattern

Child's dental attendance pattern	Proportion of children with some unrestorable deciduous teeth, aged							
	5+		8+		12+		14+	
Check-up; in last six months; G.D.S. only; A1†	13%	157	28%	97	9%	68	2%	94
Check-up; in last six months; G.D.S. only	28%	114	39%	88	6%	79	1%	152
Check-up; in last six months; mixed	15%	27	42%	38	7%	43	1%	95
Check-up; in last six months; S.D.S. only	31%	27	42%	26	*	17	2%	43
Other (see Table 18.1)	26%	32	*	19	12%	27	–	37
Regular check-up	20%	357	35%	268	8%	234	1%	421
Check-up; not in last six months; G.D.S. only	23%	62	29%	23	7%	30	1%	97
Check-up; not in last six months; mixed	*	3	*	11	*	16	2%	44
Check-up; not in last six months; S.D.S. only	*	11	49%	20	*	18	–	28
Occasional check-up	21%	76	35%	54	7%	64	1%	169
Trouble or note; in last six months	49%	154	29%	75	19%	52	1%	107
Trouble or note; within last two years	47%	63	51%	78	8%	61	4%	82
Trouble or note; not within last two years	*	2	*	7	25%	20	4%	73
Never (seldom) been	28%	266	46%	48	*	15	–	31
Only when has trouble	38%	485	43%	208	15%	148	2%	293
All children	30%	922	38%	532	10%	451	2%	886

† A1 = First visit was a check-up or to get used
  to dentist, and mother is a regular attender.

Table 18.15

Unrestorable permanent teeth and the child's attendance pattern

Child's dental attendance pattern	Proportion of children with some unrestorable permanent teeth, aged							
	5+		8+		12+		14+	
Check-up; in last six months; G.D.S. only; A1†	1%	157	1%	97	2%	68	3%	94
Check-up; in last six months; G.D.S. only	1%	114	3%	88	4%	79	4%	152
Check-up; in last six months; mixed	–	27	–	38	8%	43	7%	95
Check-up; in last six months; S.D.S. only	–	27	8%	26	*	17	5%	43
Other (see Table 18.1)	–	32	*	19	12%	27	5%	37
Regular check-up	1%	357	3%	268	5%	234	5%	421
Check-up; not in last six months; G.D.S. only	–	62	6%	23	8%	30	19%	97
Check-up; not in last six months; mixed	*	3	*	11	*	16	14%	44
Check-up; not in last six months; S.D.S. only	*	11	–	20	*	18	9%	28
Occasional check-up	–	76	4%	54	15%	64	16%	169
Trouble or note; in last six months	1%	154	5%	75	16%	52	20%	107
Trouble or note; within last two years	–	63	6%	78	21%	61	26%	82
Trouble or note; not within last two years	*	2	*	7	37%	20	36%	73
Never (seldom) been	1%	266	11%	48	*	15	10%	31
Only when has trouble	1%	485	8%	208	21%	148	25%	293
All children	1%	922	5%	532	12%	451	14%	886

† A1 = First visit was a check-up or to get used
  to dentist, and mother is a regular attender.

Table 18.16

Filled teeth and the child's attendance pattern

Child's dental attendance pattern	Proportion of children with some filled (F+f) teeth, aged							
	5+		8+		12+		14+	
Check-up; in last six months; G.D.S. only; A1†	38%	157	69%	97	96%	68	95%	94
Check-up; in last six months; G.D.S. only	45%	114	73%	88	87%	79	92%	152
Check-up; in last six months; mixed	52%	27	81%	38	88%	43	96%	95
Check-up; in last six months; S.D.S. only	70%	27	87%	26	*	17	88%	43
Other (see Table 18.1)	28%	32	*	19	88%	27	88%	37
Regular check-up	43%	357	72%	268	90%	234	93%	421
Check-up; not in last six months; G.D.S. only	10%	62	49%	23	74%	30	86%	97
Check-up; not in last six months; mixed	*	3	*	11	*	16	82%	44
Check-up; not in last six months; S.D.S. only	*	11	63%	20	*	18	78%	28
Occasional check-up	11%	76	52%	54	72%	64	84%	169
Trouble or note; in last six months	45%	154	72%	75	79%	52	88%	107
Trouble or note; within last two years	25%	63	42%	78	66%	61	77%	82
Trouble or note; not within last two years	*	2	*	7	30%	20	32%	73
Never (seldom) been	2%	266	8%	48	*	15	23%	31
Only when has trouble	19%	485	43%	208	60%	148	64%	293
All children	27%	922	59%	532	77%	451	82%	886

† A1 = First visit was a check-up or to get used
   to dentist, and mother is a regular attender.

Table 18.17

Average number of filled teeth by child's attendance pattern

Child's dental attendance pattern	Average number of filled teeth (F+f) among children aged							
	5+		8+		12+		14+	
Check-up; in last six months; G.D.S. only; A1†	1.1	157	3.0	97	4.1	68	6.4	94
Check-up; in last six months; G.D.S. only	1.2	114	2.8	88	4.0	79	6.2	152
Check-up; in last six months; mixed	1.6	27	3.4	38	4.0	43	6.4	95
Check-up; in last six months; S.D.S. only	1.4	27	3.0	26	*	17	4.4	43
Other (see Table 18.1)	0.7	32	*	19	3.0	27	6.0	37
Regular check-up	1.1	357	2.9	268	3.9	234	6.1	421
Check-up; not in last six months; G.D.S. only	0.2	62	1.6	23	2.7	30	4.3	97
Check-up; not in last six months; mixed	*	3	*	11	*	16	4.3	44
Check-up; not in last six months; S.D.S. only	*	11	2.0	20	*	18	2.9	28
Occasional check-up	0.2	76	1.7	54	2.3	64	4.1	169
Trouble or note; in last six months	1.3	154	2.5	75	3.3	52	5.7	107
Trouble or note; within last two years	0.5	63	1.1	78	1.9	61	3.0	82
Trouble or note; not within last two years	*	2	*	7	0.6	20	1.0	73
Never (seldom) been	–	266	0.2	48	*	15	0.9	31
Only when has trouble	0.5	485	1.4	208	2.0	148	3.3	293
All children	0.7	922	2.2	532	3.0	451	4.8	886

† A1 = First visit was a check-up or to get used
   to dentist, and mother is a regular attender.

Table 18.18

Filled deciduous teeth and the child's attendance pattern

Child's dental attendance pattern	Proportion of children with some filled deciduous teeth, aged							
	5+		8+		12+		14+	
Check-up; in last six months; G.D.S. only; A1†	38%	157	58%	97	22%	68	3%	94
Check-up; in last six months; G.D.S. only	45%	114	54%	88	9%	79	1%	152
Check-up; in last six months; mixed	52%	27	67%	38	10%	43	3%	95
Check-up; in last six months; S.D.S. only	67%	27	58%	26	*	17	5%	43
Other (see Table)	28%	32	*	19	12%	27	1%	37
Regular check-up	43%	357	57%	268	14%	234	2%	421
Check-up; not in last six months; G.D.S. only	10%	62	36%	23	10%	30	–	97
Check-up; not in last six months; mixed	*	3	*	11	*	16	2%	44
Check-up; not in last six months; S.D.S. only	*	11	51%	20	*	18	–	28
Occasional check-up	11%	76	41%	54	9%	64	1%	169
Trouble or note; in last six months	45%	154	52%	75	14%	52	1%	107
Trouble or note; within last two years	23%	63	35%	78	5%	61	–	82
Trouble or note; not within last two years	*	2	*	7	5%	20	3%	73
Never (seldom) been	2%	266	6%	48	*	15	3%	31
Only when has trouble	18%	485	33%	208	8%	148	1%	293
All children	27%	922	46%	532	11%	451	2%	886

† A1 = First visit was a check-up or to get used
  to dentist, and mother is a regular attender.

Table 18.19

Average number of filled deciduous teeth by child's attendance pattern

Child's dental attendance pattern	Average number of filled deciduous teeth among children aged							
	5+		8+		12+		14+	
Check-up; in last six months; G.D.S. only; A1†	1.1	157	1.8	97	0.4	68	–	94
Check-up; in last six months; G.D.S. only	1.2	114	1.4	88	0.2	79	–	152
Check-up; in last six months; mixed	1.6	27	1.8	38	0.1	43	–	95
Check-up; in last six months; S.D.S. only	1.4	27	1.6	26	*	17	–	43
Other (see Table 18.1)	0.7	32	*	19	0.2	27	–	37
Regular check-up	1.1	357	1.6	268	0.2	234	–	421
Check-up; not in last six months; G.D.S. only	0.2	62	0.9	23	0.1	30	–	97
Check-up; not in last six months; mixed	*	3	*	11	*	16	–	44
Check-up; not in last six months; S.D.S. only	*	11	1.1	20	*	18	–	28
Occasional check-up	0.2	76	0.9	54	0.1	64	–	169
Trouble or note; in last six months	1.2	154	1.4	75	0.2	52	–	107
Trouble or note; within last two years	0.5	63	0.7	78	0.1	61	–	82
Trouble or note; not within last two years	*	2	*	7	–	20	–	73
Never (seldom) been	–	266	0.1	48	*	15	–	31
Only when has trouble	0.5	485	0.8	208	0.1	148	–	293
All children	0.7	922	1.2	532	0.2	451	–	886

† A1 = First visit was a check-up or to get used
  to dentist, and mother is a regular attender.

A much higher proportion of eight year olds had some filled teeth, and again the proportion varied considerably with attendance pattern, being 72% among the regular check-up children, 52% among the occasional check-up children and 43% among the irregular attenders. By the age of twelve and fourteen the vast majority of children had some filled teeth, but there was still room for considerable variation according to attendance pattern. Among fourteen year olds 93% of those who go for a regular check-up had some filled teeth, as did 84% of those who occasionally go for a check-up and 64% of those who were irregular attenders. The lower proportion for the last mentioned group was influenced by the very low filling experience among the children who seldom go to the dentist or had last had some dental trouble more than two years ago; only 23% and 32% of these children had any fillings. From Table 18.1 we can see that these two groups account for 12% of all fourteen year olds. With such little experience of restorative dentistry by the age of fourteen these children will in all probability have a very limited dental future as adults. In fact it is most likely that they will form the basis of the group who will become the young edentulous adults. The variation in restorative experience for children of different attendance patterns is made abundantly clear by the table giving the average number of filled teeth. Among the fourteen year olds the average number of filled teeth ranges from 6.4 among the children with the best dental attendance pattern and dental background to 1.0 and 0.9 among those who rarely go to the dentist.

Tables 18.18 and 18.19 show the situation with respect to filled deciduous teeth. Among children who have been to the dentist within the last six months for a check-up 43% of the five year olds and 57% of the eight year olds have some filled deciduous teeth, or conversely 57% of five year olds and 43% of eight year olds had no filled deciduous teeth. We have seen in earlier chapters that mothers do not always feel that it is worthwhile to fill deciduous teeth, and with the quite high proportion of children who have the best attendance patterns having no filled deciduous teeth it would seem that some dentists would also agree. The consequence of dentists holding this view would lead to the situation we have already seen in Table 18.14 where quite a high proportion of children, who are apparently well looked after dentally, have some unrestorable deciduous teeth. The proportion with some filled deciduous teeth is lower among the children whose dental attendance pattern is not so good but even among eight year olds who are not in the habit of going for a check-up 33% have some restorative experience with deciduous teeth.

Tables 18.20 and 18.21 show how the pattern of restorative experience for permanent teeth builds up over the years. Very few five year olds have any filled permanent teeth but 40% of eight year olds have some filled permanent teeth. For those who have recently been for a check-up the proportion is 52%, for those whose check-up was not so recent the proportion was 35% and for those who only go when they really have to 26% have some filled permanent teeth. Thus twice as many eight year olds with good dental attendance patterns have some filled teeth as is the case for eight year olds with poor attendance patterns.

By the age of twelve the proportions involved have increased considerably; 89% of the regular attenders have some filled permanent teeth, 70% of the occasional attenders and 58% of the irregular attenders have some filled permanent teeth. The children with irregular attendance patterns who have in fact been to the dentist within the previous two years are not so far behind with respect to having some

Table 18.20

Filled permanent teeth and the child's attendance pattern

Child's dental attendance pattern	Proportion of children with some filled permanent teeth, aged							
	5+		8+		12+		14+	
Check-up; in last six months; G.D.S. only; A1[†]	1%	157	44%	97	96%	68	94%	94
Check-up; in last six months; G.D.S. only	1%	114	53%	88	87%	79	92%	152
Check-up; in last six months; mixed	-	27	65%	38	85%	43	96%	95
Check-up; in last six months; S.D.S. only	4%	27	64%	26	*	17	88%	43
Other (see Table 18.1)	-	32	*	19	84%	27	88%	37
Regular check-up	1%	357	52%	268	89%	234	93%	421
Check-up; not in last six months; G.D.S. only	-	62	30%	23	74%	30	86%	97
Check-up; not in last six months; mixed	*	3	*	11	*	16	82%	44
Check-up; not in last six months; S.D.S. only	*	11	37%	20	*	18	78%	28
Occasional check-up	-	76	35%	54	70%	64	84%	169
Trouble or note; in last six months	3%	154	47%	75	77%	52	88%	107
Trouble or note; within last two years	2%	63	21%	78	66%	61	77%	82
Trouble or note; not within last two years	*	2	*	7	25%	20	32%	73
Never (seldom) been	1%	266	4%	48	*	15	23%	31
Only when has trouble	2%	485	26%	208	58%	148	64%	293
All children	1%	922	40%	532	76%	451	82%	886

† A1 = *First visit was a check-up or to get used to dentist, and mother is a regular attender.*

Table 18.21

Average number of filled permanent teeth by child's attendance pattern

Child's dental attendance pattern	Average number of filled permanent teeth among children aged							
	5+		8+		12+		14+	
Check-up; in last six months; G.D.S. only; A1[†]	-	157	1.2	97	3.8	68	6.3	94
Check-up; in last six months; G.D.S. only	-	114	1.4	88	3.8	79	6.2	152
Check-up; in last six months; mixed	-	27	1.6	38	3.9	43	6.4	95
Check-up; in last six months; S.D.S. only	-	27	1.3	26	*	17	4.3	43
Other (see Table 18.1)	-	32	*	19	2.7	27	6.0	37
Regular check-up	-	357	1.3	268	3.6	234	6.1	421
Check-up; not in last six months; G.D.S. only	-	62	0.7	23	2.6	30	4.3	97
Check-up; not in last six months; mixed	*	3	*	11	*	16	4.3	44
Check-up; not in last six months; S.D.S. only	*	11	0.9	20	*	18	2.9	28
Occasional check-up	-	76	0.8	54	2.2	64	4.1	169
Trouble or note; in last six months	-	154	1.2	75	3.1	52	5.7	107
Trouble or note; within last two years	-	63	0.4	78	1.8	61	3.0	82
Trouble or note; not within last two years	*	2	*	7	0.5	20	1.0	73
Never (seldom) been	-	266	0.1	48	*	15	0.8	31
Only when has trouble	-	485	0.6	208	1.9	148	3.3	293
All children	-	922	1.0	532	2.8	451	4.8	886

† A1 = *First visit was a check-up or to get used to dentist, and mother is a regular attender.*

Table 18.22

Missing teeth and the child's attendance pattern

Child's dental attendance pattern	Proportion of children with some permanent teeth missing due to decay, aged							
	5+		8+		12+		14+	
Check-up; in last six months; G.D.S. only; A1†	–	157	3%	97	17%	68	14%	94
Check-up; in last six months; G.D.S. only	–	114	4%	88	23%	79	23%	152
Check-up; in last six months; mixed	–	27	4%	38	19%	43	44%	95
Check-up; in last six months; S.D.S. only	–	27	5%	26	*	17	37%	43
Other (see Table 18.1)	–	32	*	19	12%	27	25%	37
Regular check-up	–	357	4%	268	21%	234	27%	421
Check-up; not in last six months; G.D.S. only	–	62	–	23	33%	30	28%	97
Check-up; not in last six months; mixed	*	3	*	11	*	16	36%	44
Check-up; not in last six months; S.D.S. only	*	11	–	20	*	18	20%	28
Occasional check-up	–	76	–	54	32%	64	29%	169
Trouble or note; in last six months	–	154	11%	75	35%	52	46%	107
Trouble or note; within last two years	–	63	6%	78	36%	61	49%	82
Trouble or note; not within last two years	*	2	*	7	12%	20	30%	73
Never (seldom) been	–	266	2%	48	*	15	14%	31
Only when has trouble	–	485	4%	208	28%	148	40%	293
All children	–	922	4%	532	25%	451	31%	886

† A1 = First visit was a check-up or to get used to dentist, and mother is a regular attender.

Table 18.23

Average number of missing teeth by child's attendance pattern

Child's dental attendance pattern	Average number of missing permanent teeth due to decay, in children aged							
	5+		8+		12+		14+	
Check-up; in last six months; G.D.S. only; A1†	–	157	–	97	0.3	68	0.4	94
Check-up; in last six months; G.D.S. only	–	114	0.1	88	0.6	79	0.6	152
Check-up; in last six months; mixed	–	27	0.1	38	0.4	43	1.1	95
Check-up; in last six months; S.D.S. only	–	27	0.1	26	*	17	0.8	43
Other (see Table 18.1)	–	32	*	19	0.3	27	0.5	37
Regular check-up	–	357	0.1	268	0.5	234	0.7	421
Check-up; not in last six months; G.D.S. only	–	62	–	23	0.8	30	0.7	97
Check-up; not in last six months; mixed	*	3	*	11	*	16	0.7	44
Check-up; not in last six months; S.D.S. only	*	11	–	20	*	18	0.7	28
Occasional check-up	–	76	–	54	0.7	64	0.7	169
Trouble or note; in last six months	–	154	0.2	75	0.8	52	1.1	107
Trouble or note; within last two years	–	63	0.1	78	0.6	61	1.3	82
Trouble or note; not within last two years	*	2	*	7	0.2	20	0.6	73
Never (seldom) been	–	266	–	48	*	15	0.3	31
Only when has trouble	–	485	0.1	208	0.6	148	1.0	293
All children	–	922	0.1	532	0.6	451	0.8	886

† A1 = First visit was a check-up or to get used to dentist, and mother is a regular attender.

restorative experience for permanent teeth. It is those children who have not been
for more than two years who would appear to be in an entirely different position.
A similar picture emerges for restorative experience for the permanent teeth of
fourteen year olds. Although the most regular attenders have the highest average
number of filled permanent teeth only those who have not been to the dentist for
very long periods have a depressingly low average. It is encouraging that the
children who have presented themselves at the dentist within the last six months
with dental trouble or because of a note from school have an average of 5.7 filled
permanent teeth compared with the average of 1.0 for those children whose last
visit, prompted by trouble or a note, was more than two years before the survey.

Since few children manage to avoid having decay then restorative or preventive
measures are the ones most likely to result in adequate reliance on natural teeth
in adult life. The alternative to restorative treatment is extraction and this is
in fact the only course of action if dental attendance is delayed until the tooth is
unrestorable. The survey dental examination did not assess whether deciduous
teeth had been extracted for decay but it did include an assessment of the
reasons why permanent teeth were missing. The examiners had four possible
categories for missing permanent teeth and they used their clinical experience to
decide the most likely reason. If they wished to do so they asked the child
about the circumstances of any loss of permanent teeth. The four categories
concerned were unerupted, extracted due to decay, extracted for orthodontic
reasons, and missing due to trauma. In this section we are concerned only
with teeth classified as extraced due to decay.

A quarter of twelve year olds and 31% of fourteen year olds had lost some permanent
teeth due to decay (see Tables 18.22 and 18.23). Perhaps the most surprising fact,
however, is that this was so for 21% of twelve year old regular attenders and 27%
of fourteen year old regular attenders. Even among those children whose dental
background and outlook had been good over some considerable time 17% of twelve
year olds and 14% of fourteen year olds had lost some permanent teeth. However,
the children with the worst attendance patterns had much greater experience of
permanent tooth extraction; for example among those children who generally did not
go for a check-up but who had been to a dentist in the last six months, or failing
that in the last two years, the proportion who had lost some permanent teeth was 35%
and 36% for the twelve year olds and 46% and 49% for the fourteen year olds.

Earlier in Chapter II we reported the mothers' views on what treatment they would
prefer the child to have for bad back permanent teeth; a strong preference for
restoration was expressed by the mothers, and it is therefore fairly surprising
that even among the children with the best dental attendance records a considerable
proportion of children were losing permanent teeth for decay reasons.

19 Regional variations in the dental condition of children

One of the purposes of the survey was to investiage whether there are any regional variations in dental condition and, if so to establish whether such variations are accounted for by uneven distribution of dental attitudes or dental behaviour among the children (or their parents). In the first section of this chapter we examine whether or not regional variations in dental health exist, in the second section we examine whether there are any regional variations in dental behaviour and in the third section we investigate whether the latter appears to account for the former or not. Throughout the chapter we present the results for the four regions, based on grouped economic planning regions, that have been used throughout this report and the earlier report on adult dental health. In addition we show the results for Wales separately using the unweighted sample for that area.* It was requested that the sample for Wales should be increased to a size that would allow separate analysis as it was felt that grouping Wales with the South West was not a particularly happy arrangement in that the two areas had rather different levels of resources. Comparing the results which follow for Wales and the South West, and Wales separately suggests that the unease expressed about the grouping was justified. We have for the time being retained the grouping in order to make comparisons with earlier work.

19.1 Regional variations in the dental examination findings

In the Table Section at the back of the report we give in full, for each region, the number of teeth in each condition for the deciduous dentition, the permanent dentition and both together. Comparisons between regions can therefore be made in considerable detail. We have selected three factors which illustrate the regional variations that exist: the proportion of children with some extracted permanent teeᵗn, the proportion of children with some filled teeth and the proportion of children with some active decay. Since this information is derived from the dental examination it is available for children of all ages from five to fifteen.

Table 19.1 shows the proportion of children in each region who had experienced extraction of permanent teeth for decay reasons. In London and the South East the proportion ranged from zero to 19% among fifteen year olds. In Wales the

---

*A disproportionately large sample was drawn in Wales thus providing a large enough sample to analyse some Welsh results separately. The sample for Wales was downweighted for all other analyses to restore the true balance for England and Wales, see Chapter I.

proportion ranged from zero to 50% among fourteen and fifteen year olds. The
proportion in the North and in the Midlands and East Anglia were similar to each
other reaching about 40% for the oldest children. The low proportion of extractions
in London and the South East was visible even among children aged eight, and among
the children aged eleven or older London and the South East had a significantly
lower proportion having had extractions than any other region. The extraction
rate in the South West was lower than in the North or Midlands and East Anglia
for when grouped with Wales, which is shown to have a high extraction record,
the combined area of Wales and the South West maintained a lower proportion of
extractions than the North and Midlands and East Anglia.

Table 19.1

Proportion of children with some permanent teeth extracted for decay, by region

Age	Proportion of children with some permanent teeth extracted for decay in									
	The North		Midlands and East Anglia		Wales and the South West		London and the South East		Wales alone	
Five	–	323	–	200	–	158	–	271	–	172
Six	–	347	–	224	–	168	–	341	–	184
Seven	2%	390	2%	221	2%	185	1%	341	2%	191
Eight	6%	357	4%	224	3%	166	1%	344	6%	183
Nine	12%	358	5%	223	7%	169	6%	379	14%	195
Ten	17%	362	15%	213	13%	163	9%	354	22%	182
Eleven	22%	317	23%	195	19%	155	10%	319	32%	176
Twelve	26%	294	28%	182	25%	160	16%	320	38%	175
Thirteen	39%	285	34%	194	31%	146	13%	290	45%	185
Fourteen	37%	308	38%	207	34%	145	18%	263	50%	177
Fifteen	43%	218	40%	130	36%	111	19%	237	50%	120

In Table 19.2 we show the proportion of children with some filled, otherwise sound,
teeth, this excludes any teeth previously filled but now decayed. In London and
the South East there was, for each age group, except the fifteen year olds, a higher
proportion of children with some restored teeth than was the case in Wales, the
North or Midlands and East Anglia. Allowing for the inclusion of Wales in Wales and
the South West the proportion of children in the South West who had some filled
teeth was comparable with London and the South East.

Table 19.2

Proportion of children with some filled* teeth, by region

Age	Proportion of children with some filled* teeth in									
	The North		Midlands and East Anglia		Wales and the South West		London and the South East		Wales alone	
Five	24%	323	18%	200	30%	158	33%	271	22%	172
Six	30%	347	30%	224	53%	168	47%	341	33%	184
Seven	34%	390	45%	221	54%	185	58%	341	37%	191
Eight	49%	357	50%	224	65%	166	66%	344	49%	183
Nine	58%	358	55%	223	70%	169	73%	379	54%	195
Ten	59%	362	60%	213	72%	163	78%	354	57%	182
Eleven	63%	317	61%	195	77%	155	79%	319	59%	176
Twelve	69%	294	72%	182	79%	160	83%	320	72%	175
Thirteen	74%	285	66%	194	82%	146	86%	290	71%	185
Fourteen	79%	308	76%	207	84%	145	87%	263	71%	177
Fifteen	85%	218	81%	130	93%	111	90%	237	88%	120

* *Filled, otherwise sound*

In terms of the current need for treatment, expressed as the proportion of children with some active decay, Table 19.3 shows that London and the South East had less current treatment need than did Wales for children of all age groups. Again, given the situation in Wales, the South West is probably comparable to London and the South East in current treatment need for decay. The North and Midlands and East Anglia came between London and the South East and Wales.

Table 19.3

Proportion of children with some active decay, by region

Age	Proportion of children with some active decay in									
	The North		Midlands and East Anglia		Wales and the South West		London and the South East		Wales alone	
Five	63%	323	71%	200	65%	158	57%	271	71%	172
Six	67%	347	72%	224	77%	168	65%	341	75%	184
Seven	74%	390	74%	221	80%	185	66%	341	85%	191
Eight	80%	357	84%	224	80%	166	71%	344	86%	183
Nine	76%	358	79%	223	77%	169	73%	379	84%	195
Ten	72%	362	69%	213	73%	163	65%	354	76%	182
Eleven	66%	317	74%	195	64%	155	62%	319	73%	176
Twelve	60%	294	67%	182	67%	160	56%	320	70%	175
Thirteen	64%	285	66%	194	69%	146	50%	290	72%	185
Fourteen	65%	308	61%	207	68%	145	54%	263	72%	177
Fifteen	56%	218	67%	130	62%	111	50%	237	72%	120

We would therefore conclude that the survey results show significant differences in current treatment need and past treatment experience between children living in different regions.

19.2 Regional variations in dental attendance patterns

In Chapter 18 we saw that there were significant differences in treatment need and treatment experience for children in the different broad groups of attendance pattern, especially between those who were establishing a pattern of regular attendance and those who only attended when they had trouble. In this section we examine whether or not the proportion of children in those broad attendance pattern categories were similar in all the regions.

The significant variations which occurred in dental health in the different regions generally involved London and the South East and Wales at the two extremes, although in some instances it was London and the South East standing out from the rest of the regions, with the South West obviously being more similar to London and the South East than to Wales. Table 19.4 shows the proportion of children in the three main attendance pattern types by region. For all age groups except the five year olds London and the South East had significantly more children going for regular check-ups than was the case in Wales. As with earlier regional comparisons Wales would seem to be more similar to the North and Midlands and East Anglia, and the South West would appear, by deduction, to be similar to London and the South East.

The proportion of children who only go to the dentist when they have some kind of trouble was significantly lower in London and the South East compared to Wales for all age groups. Here again the most natural regional grouping would seem to be the south versus elsewhere.

Table 19.4
Dental attendance pattern by region

Region	Children aged							
	5+		8+		12+		14+	
	Proportion who go for regular check-ups							
The North	38%	312	44%	173	47%	140	43%	294
Midlands and East Anglia	32%	195	41%	109	46%	88	36%	197
Wales and the South West	43%	151	64%	80	53%	77	55%	143
London and the South East	42%	264	56%	170	61%	146	56%	252
Wales alone	34%	168	40%	90	46%	87	43%	174
	Proportion who go for occasional check-ups							
The North	8%	312	10%	173	17%	140	19%	294
Midlands and East Anglia	8%	195	10%	109	9%	88	20%	197
Wales and the South West	8%	151	9%	80	12%	77	15%	143
London and the South East	9%	264	12%	170	16%	146	22%	252
Wales alone	5%	168	9%	90	8%	87	17%	174
	Proportion who go when having trouble							
The North	54%	312	46%	173	36%	140	38%	294
Midlands and East Anglia	60%	195	49%	109	45%	88	44%	197
Wales and the South West	49%	151	27%	80	35%	77	30%	143
London and the South East	49%	264	32%	170	23%	146	22%	252
Wales alone	61%	168	51%	90	46%	87	40%	174

From the results of Table 19.4 we would conclude that there is not an even distribution of dental attendance patterns among children in different regions and therefore, since we have already seen that the different attendance patterns have different dental needs and treatment experience this must make some contribution to the regional variation in dental health.

19.3 Region, dental attendance and dental condition

We have already shown that there is a regional variation in treatment need and treatment experience and that proportionately more children with a good dental attendance pattern are to be found in some regions compared to others. In this section we look at all three factors in combination to establish whether or not the regional variation is wholly accounted for by the variation in dental attitudes and behaviour. If this were to be so we would find that regular attenders had similar dental needs and treatment experience in all regions, and that irregular dental attenders were in a similar dental condition in all regions. If this proves not to be the case then the regional variation in dental health is due to more than just the uneven distribution of children with different dental attitudes and behaviour as expressed in their dental attendance patterns.

By taking account of the child's dental attendance pattern and region simultaneously the numbers in the sub-samples become rather small. For this reason we have restricted the analysis to the age groups five and fourteen, and for the five year olds show only the two main attendance patterns.

The first section of Table 19.5 shows the proportion of children with ten or more teeth known to have been involved with decay. The results among the five year olds are difficult to interpret since any deciduous teeth extracted for decay will not be included. Among the fourteen year olds the only significant difference between London and the South East and Wales was among the regular attenders who had less decay experience in London and the South East and more decay experience in Wales.

The second section of the table gives the proportion of children with some active decay. For the five year olds this is restricted to deciduous teeth and for the fourteen year olds it refers to permanent teeth. Among neither the five year old nor fourteen year old regular attenders was there any significant difference between London and the South East and Wales in the proportion of children with active decay. Among children who do not go to the dentist for a check-up those in London and the South East were less likely to have some active decay than were those in Wales.

The regional differences in active decay are further demonstrated in the third section of the table which shows the proportion of children with some unrestorable teeth. Except among five year old regular attenders the proportion of children with some unrestorable teeth was always significantly lower in London and the South East than in Wales, whatever their attendance patterns.

Table 19.5
Decay, dental attendance pattern and region

Region	Children aged									
	5+				14+					
	Regular check-ups		Only when having trouble		Regular check-ups		Occasional check-ups		Only when having trouble	
	Proportion having ten or more teeth with decay experience									
N	8%	117	5%	167	37%	129	13%	54	22%	109
M&EA	12%	61	7%	117	31%	71	21%	38	26%	87
W&SW	7%	67	10%	73	38%	80	36%	21	30%	42
L&SE	5%	111	5%	129	25%	141	25%	56	24%	54
W	4%	57	16%	103	47%	72	26%	30	33%	70
	Proportion having some active decay *deciduous teeth* / *permanent teeth*									
N	59%	117	71%	167	54%	129	68%	54	78%	109
M&EA	61%	61	73%	117	41%	71	60%	38	75%	87
W&SW	58%	67	72%	73	63%	80	67%	21	78%	42
L&SE	53%	111	64%	129	51%	141	52%	56	65%	54
W	58%	57	82%	103	57%	72	70%	30	86%	70
	Proportion having some unrestorable teeth *deciduous teeth* / *permanent teeth*									
N	25%	117	39%	167	8%	129	22%	54	23%	109
M&EA	23%	61	38%	117	3%	71	18%	38	26%	87
W&SW	16%	67	41%	73	6%	80	16%	21	32%	42
L&SE	17%	111	33%	129	2%	141	9%	56	20%	54
W	19%	57	50%	103	8%	72	23%	30	44%	70

Table l9.6 shows the situation with respect to treatment experience. The first section shows the proportion of children who have some filled teeth. Again for the five year olds this refers to deciduous teeth and for the fourteen year olds to permanent teeth. Among regular attenders, age five or fourteen, there was no significant difference between Wales and London and the South East in the proportion of children with some filled teeth but for children who were not regular attenders the position was quite different. Among five year olds who were irregular attenders 25% of those living in London and the South East had some filled teeth compared with only 9% of those living in Wales. Among fourteen year olds who were irregular attenders 78% of those living in London and the South East had some filled teeth compared to 50% of those living in Wales. Thus the restorative treatment experience, although similar for children with a good dental attendance record whichever region they came from, was certainly different according to where they lived for children who had not established good dental behaviour.

The second section of Table l9.6 shows the proportion of children who had experienced extraction of permanent teeth for decay. Among fourteen year olds, whatever their current dental attendance pattern, the likelihood of such extractions was much lower in London and the South East than it was in Wales. Among regular attenders in London and the South East l8% had had permanent teeth extracted, the comparable proportion in Wales was 40%. Among the fourteen year olds who were irregular attenders 28% in London and the South East had had some extractions compared to 63% of fourteen year old irregular attenders in Wales.

Table 19.6

Treatment, dental attendance pattern and region

Region	Children aged				
	5+		14+		
	Regular check-ups	Only when having trouble	Regular check-ups	Occasional check-ups	Only when having trouble
	Proportion having some filled teeth				
	deciduous teeth		*permanent teeth*		
N	42% 117	16% 167	95% 129	80% 54	58% 109
M&EA	33% 61	14% 117	94% 71	82% 38	63% 87
W&SW	44% 67	22% 73	92% 80	87% 21	65% 42
L&SE	48% 111	25% 129	90% 141	88% 56	78% 54
W	51% 57	9% 103	88% 72	73% 30	50% 70
	Proportion having some permanent teeth extracted for decay				
N	–	–	36% 129	33% 54	41% 109
M&EA	–	–	31% 71	42% 38	40% 87
W&SW	–	–	26% 80	40% 21	49% 42
L&SE	–	–	18% 141	11% 56	28% 54
W	–	–	40% 72	43% 30	63% 70

During the interview we asked the mother what kind of treatment the child had received last time he went to the dentist, and to illustrate the variations in treatment shown in the previous tables we show in Table l9.7 what proportion of children were said to have had at least one filling and what proportion were said to have had at least one extraction last time they went to the dentist, according to both attendance pattern and region.

Among regular attenders in both age groups there was little regional variation in the proportion who had some fillings as a result of their last dental visit. Among the five year old irregular attenders in London and the South East 41% were said to have had some fillings last time compared to only 15% in Wales; the equivalent proportions for the fourteen year olds were 65% in London and the South East compared to 41% in Wales. Among these irregular attenders there was a considerable variation between regions as to whether or not they had any extractions; for the five year olds in London and the South East 39% had some extractions last time compared with 71% in Wales; for the fourteen year olds in London and the South East 25% had extractions, in Wales the comparable figure was 49%.

Table 19.7

Most recent treatment, dental attendance pattern and region

Region	Children who have been to the dentist, aged									
	5+				14+					
	Regular check-ups		Only when having trouble		Regular check-ups		Occasional check-ups		Only when having trouble	
	Proportion having some fillings last time									
N	33%	117	29%	74	42%	129	42%	54	34%	98
M&EA	25%	61	42%	45	33%	71	29%	38	53%	81
W&SW	37%	67	45%	39	41%	80	49%	21	58%	38
L&SE	31%	111	41%	62	44%	141	43%	56	65%	45
W	34%	57	15%	48	48%	72	33%	30	41%	65
	Proportion having some extractions last time									
N	4%	117	65%	74	8%	129	2%	54	50%	98
M&EA	5%	61	46%	45	5%	71	8%	38	41%	81
W&SW	1%	67	42%	39	3%	80	5%	21	36%	38
L&SE	1%	111	39%	62	4%	141	2%	56	25%	45
W	6%	57	71%	48	7%	72	10%	30	49%	65

The examination of attendance pattern, region and dental condition has shown that children of similar attendance patterns do not have the same treatment experience in different regions. Regular attenders do in general receive much the same opportunity for some restorative treatment but curiously they do not escape the regional disparity in extractions. The irregular attenders in London and the South East are more likely to have benefitted from the provision of some restorative work, and are less likely to have an extraction as the result of lack of dental care and attention than are their counterparts elsewhere, particularly those in Wales.

The regional variation in treatment is thus based on more than simply an uneven distribution of dental attitudes among children (and their parents). The fact that the region with the most manpower resources is the one most able to intervene and provide some dental protection for those children who have not established themselves as regular attenders is unlikely to be coincidence. Similarly the fact that the regions with the most restricted resources are the ones where such intervention is least apparent will probably be no surprise to the people operating the dental services in such areas.

20 The dental condition of individual tooth types

Chapters 18 and 19 have presented information about the dental condition of the
mouth as a whole, but different teeth have different disease risks and it is
therefore of interest to investigate the contribution to dental health that
comes from the different tooth types. In the first section of this chapter
we look in detail at the first permanent molars, the sixes, for all ages from
five to fifteen and in the second section we examine the condition of individual
permanent teeth for the fourteen year olds.

20.1 The dental condition of the sixes

The first permanent molars, the sixes, play an outstanding role in the dental
development and dental health of children. They are unique in their contribution
to the transition from deciduous to permanent teeth since they erupt when the
child is very young (about six years old), in fact at much the same time as the
first permanent incisors, but unlike the incisors, no deciduous teeth are shed
because the first permanent molars erupt in the space behind the most posterior
deciduous teeth. In Chapter 2 we showed the age at which the sixes erupt and in
Chapter 3 we showed the dental condition of the sixes for children of ages ranging
from five to fifteen. It is obvious from Figure 3.2 that the first permanent
molars bear the brunt of the disease and treatment of permanent teeth in childhood.
It is also clear that they are particularly prone to decay as compared with the
lower central permanent incisors which usually erupt at about the same time.

In Chapter 10 we showed that although mothers could give a reasonable estimate of
when a child's permanent incisors erupt, they did not know when the first permanent
molars erupt. It was felt that many mothers probably thought that the sixes were
not permanent teeth, but the last of the deciduous teeth, or perhaps they remained
unaware that the child had back teeth erupting at that age. As part of the
analysis we examined what the mother said about her child's extraction experience
for those twevle year olds who, according to the survey dental examination, had
some sixes extracted. In 45% of the cases the mother said that the child had only
ever had deciduous teeth extracted. Lack of awareness about dental development
which leads mothers to mistake permanent teeth for deciduous ones, or to be
ignorant of their presence, is particularly unfortunate as although about half of
mothers thought it was best to extract rather than fill a bad back deciduous tooth
nine out of ten said they would prefer a bad back permanent tooth to be filled.

We have seen in Chapter 19 that there is a certain amount of regional variation in
the treatment received and in the context of this regional variation and the lack
of knowledge on the part of many mothers about the child's dental development, it
is of interest to look at the dental condition of the sixes in more detail.

Figure 20.1 Conditions of UL6 for children of different ages by region

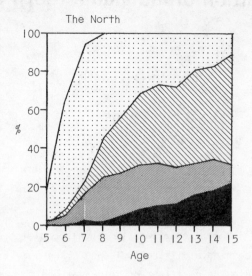

The North

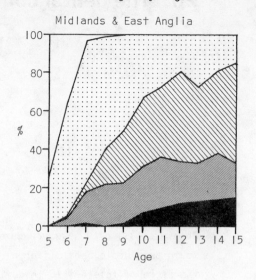

Midlands & East Anglia

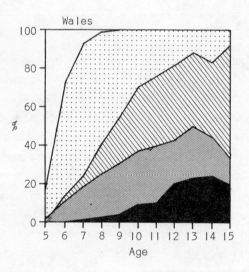

Wales

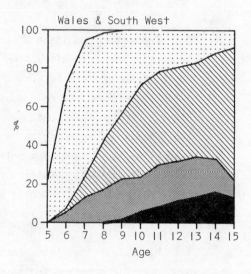

Wales & South West

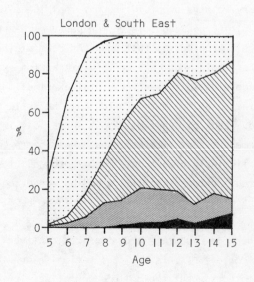

London & South East

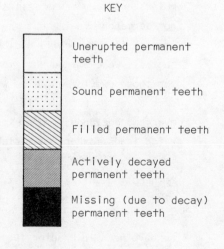

KEY

Unerupted permanent teeth

Sound permanent teeth

Filled permanent teeth

Actively decayed permanent teeth

Missing (due to decay) permanent teeth

Figure 20.2 Condition of LL6 for children of different ages by region

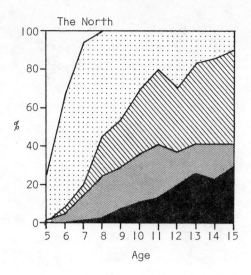

The North

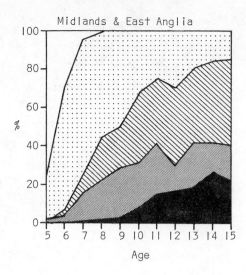

Midlands & East Anglia

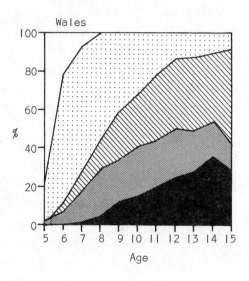

Wales

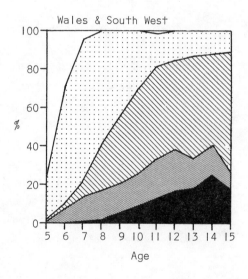

Wales & South West

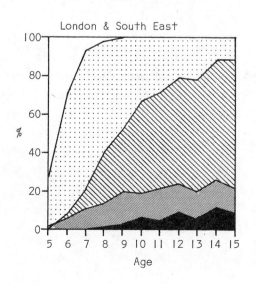

London & South East

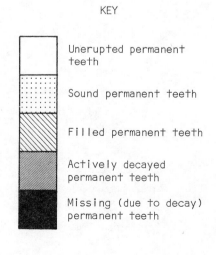

KEY

Unerupted permanent teeth

Sound permanent teeth

Filled permanent teeth

Actively decayed permanent teeth

Missing (due to decay) permanent teeth

The first permanent molars erupt at about the age of six and are intended to perform their masticatory function for the rest of the child's life. The advent of disease in the form of decay interferes with the natural state of things in so far as, left untreated, it may necessitate extraction of the tooth. Figures 20.1 and 20.2 show diagrammatically the proportion of upper left sixes and lower left sixes that have become diseased and what the treatment outcome has been for children of ages from five to fifteen. The diagrams have been drawn separately for the regions.

Both the upper left six and the lower left six have similar eruption patterns to each other and there is no appreciable difference between the regions. Although the tooth is intended to last a lifetime there are already some signs of disease among six year olds. The total disease experienced by the first permanent molar, as represented by the proportion of teeth decayed, missing and filled is very similar for the upper and lower jaw and not dissimilar between the regions. The most obvious difference between the regions is not in whether the tooth has become diseased but in how the disease has been treated.

In London and the South East the proportion of filled sixes is high and the proportion of extracted sixes is very low. This is so for both the upper left six and the lower left six. In addition, the proportion of sixes with active decay is smaller in London and the South East than elsewhere. The diagrams thus suggest that disease, although occurring to a similar extent in all regions is very much more under control with respect to treatment in London and the South East than is the case elsewhere.

Among the other regions, there is little variation between the North, the Midlands and East Anglia and Wales on its own. The region made up of Wales and the South West incorporates the Welsh figures, and since the diagrams for this region show proportionately rather more restorative work than the North, the Midlands and East Anglia and Wales alone, the South West would appear to have attained a somewhat similar pattern to London and the South East of restoration rather than extraction. For some children some sixes are being extracted within about two years of eruption. Among twelve year olds in Wales one in four lower left sixes were already extracted, not a very good record for a tooth that was intended to last a lifetime. If permanent teeth are extracted at ages such as these, it should perhaps be no surprise to find in adult dental health surveys that some people consider that all natural teeth can be dispensed with fairly early in adult life.

20.2 Dental condition of individual teeth by attendance pattern and region

In earlier chapters we have seen that even among the children who are regular dental attenders about half were likely to have some decay at the time of the examination. We have also seen that the regular attenders are at a particular advantage in terms of the number of filled teeth that they have. In addition we have established that regional variation in treatment is not wholly accounted for by an uneven distribution of dental attitudes and behaviour but that in addition it would seem that the difference between scarce and very scarce resources affect the situation.

At this point we look in detail at individual teeth among fourteen year olds to see how the impact of the dental attendance pattern of the child and the region in which he lives have affected the different teeth. The fourteen year olds in the survey were the last full year in school at the time of the inquiry and this detailed scrutiny gives some indication of their likely dental future. Figure 20.3 presents information about the teeth on the left hand side of the upper jaw. On the left of the figure is shown the situations for fourteen year olds who are regular attenders and the right hand side gives the results for irregular attenders. Each of the five small columns represents a region. The figure includes all of the teeth in the upper left quadrant except the third molar or wisdom tooth which was seldom erupted in children of this age. Each column is shaded to show the total disease experience of that particular tooth and the cross hatchings are varied so as to denote the proportion of teeth extracted due to decay, currently decayed or filled. Figure 20.4 is set out in a similar way but related to the teeth in the lower left quadrant of the mouth. Only two quadrants of the mouth have been shown since disease and treatment were symmetrical within each jaw.

The diagrams show the extent to which the first permanent molars, the sixes, dominate the situation with respect to disease and treatment of permanent teeth in children. It is of interest to note that the regional variation in extractions exists among the children who are regular attenders as well as those who are irregular attenders.

After the sixes the tooth that has the most disease experience is the second permanent molar. Among fourteen year old regular attenders about a half of second permanent molars were either decayed, missing or filled, and for this particular attendance type the large majority were filled.

Among the fourteen year old irregular attenders the disease experience of the second permanent molars, the sevens, was apparently lower than among the regular attenders, this being an illustration of how fillings can increase the apparent disease level in well cared for children as some of their fillings may well have been carried out at at stage of decay which would not have been recorded as decay using the survey definition. Although the irregular attenders would appear to be slightly less disease prone in total, their current position with respect to second permanent molars is much worse than the regular attenders since in all regions except London and the South East, a half or more of the diseased sevens are either missing or currently decayed rather than filled. It is in fact sad to see that already among the fourteen year olds in some regions a few extractions of second permanent molars are taking place

Among upper premolars the level of disease experience was not largely different for regular and irregular attenders but the amount of treatment need among the irregular attenders was again approaching half the disease experience whereas among regular attenders the fraction was much smaller.

A disappointingly high proportion of upper incisors had some decay experience even among the regular attenders. Again more of the disease had been treated among regular attenders.

Thus all the tooth types that had been involved with some decay experience contributed towards the finding that regular attenders have more filled teeth than irregular attenders, although at the age of fourteen much of this contribution comes from the first and second molars.

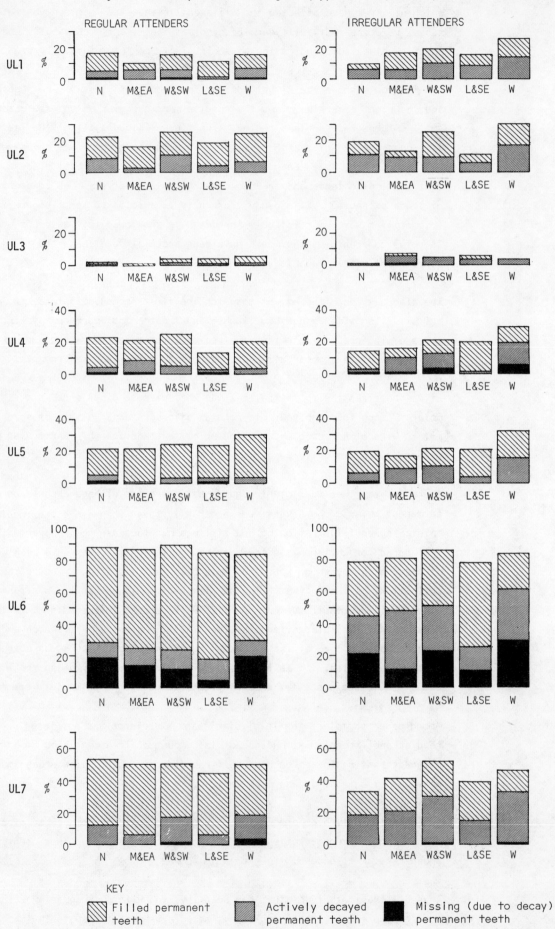

Figure 20.3 Decay and treatment experience of individual teeth in fourteen year olds by attendance pattern and region (Upper Left Quadrant)

REGULAR ATTENDERS

IRREGULAR ATTENDERS

KEY

Filled permanent teeth

Actively decayed permanent teeth

Missing (due to decay) permanent teeth

Figure 20.4 Decay and treatment experience of individual teeth in fourteen year olds by attendance pattern and region (Lower Left Quadrant)

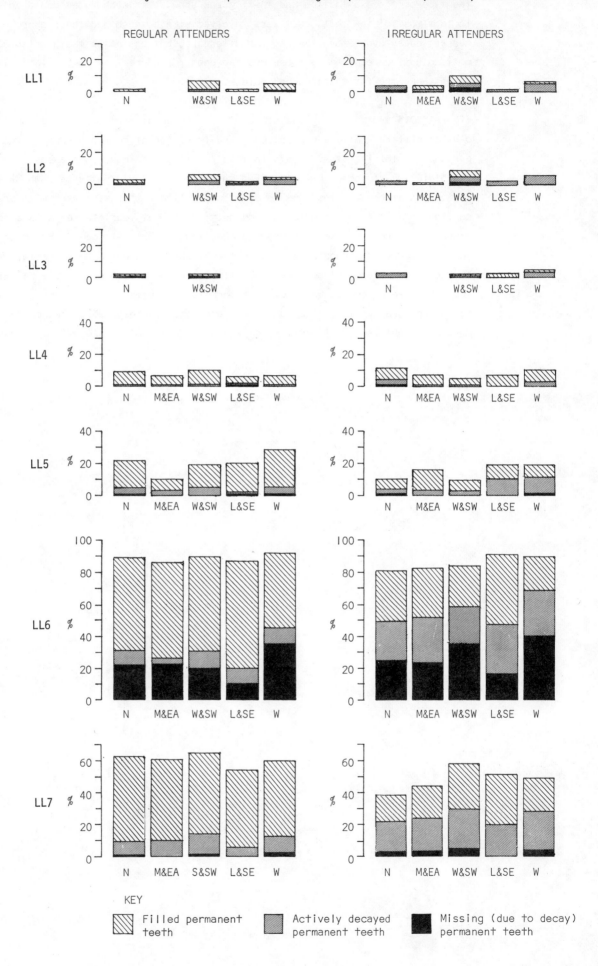

Chapter 18 showed that about half of regular attenders had some active decay at the time of the examination and the figures show where such decay could be found. In fact most of the teeth that were involved with disease had their share of current decay even among the regular attenders, but again the teeth which contributed most to active decay among those who had been for a check-up in the last six months were the first and second molars.

Figures 20.3 and 20.4 show the state of the permanent dentition among fourteen year olds of different attendance patterns and in different regions. One of the main purposes of looking at the teeth in this detail was to make some assessment of the dental future of these children. For those of the regular attenders who keep to this pattern of attendance the same level of controlled restorative work will presumably continue. Among the irregular attenders, for whom at fourteen there is a considerable amount of current treatment need, the question must be left open. For most of the fourteen year old irregular attenders the situation is not irretrievable. Very little extraction has taken place except for first permanent molars, and the majority of the teeth that were decayed were not unrestorable, but unless the current treatment need is met by restorative methods before the teeth become unrestorable then extractions of more permanent teeth will follow, and then their dental future will be bleak.

21 Disease variation among five year olds

In the fight against decay it would be of considerable interest to ascertain whether
some children are more prone to decay than others and what factors are associated
with their susceptibility. Unfortunately the measurement of susceptibility to decay
is much more difficult than the measurement of treatment experience. The survey
dental examination detected active decay at a particular level, that is when it
could be diagnosed visually*, but in the normal treatment situation decay may be
diagnosed and treated at an earlier stage. Thus to assume that fillings indicate
previous decay could lead to an overstatement of disease in survey terms as the
teeth may have been filled at a level of active decay lower than that which was
recorded in the survey dental examination. At the other end of the spectrum if
neglected disease affects other teeth in the mouth then the decay situation found
at the time of the survey examination will reflect not only how prone the child is
to decay but also, in some cases, lack of treatment experience.

For these reasons any survey measurement of the extent of decay experience among
children has many shortcomings. These can perhaps be minimised by concentrating
the analysis on the youngest age group, the five year olds, where over a quarter
have not yet experienced any decay, and where dental intervention has so far had
the least impact.

For these reasons we confine our investigation of disease variation to the five
year olds, which thereby determines that we are concerned with the disease variation
of deciduous teeth. The survey dental examination did not assess the reason for any
missing deciduous teeth but in Chapter 4 we estimated what the total deciduous decay
experience had been for the five year olds, and it is this estimated level of total
deciduous decay experience which has been used throughout the disease variation
analysis.

For the investigation we use two indicators of deciduous decay experience: the
proportion of children with no apparent decay experience and the proportion of
children with five or more teeth involved. Table 21.1 shows that 28% of five year
olds had no decay experience whereas 38% had five or more teeth that had decay
experience.

---

* See the appendix for the dental examination criteria

Table 21.1

Estimated total deciduous decay experience
of five year olds

Estimated total deciduous decay experience	Proportion of five year olds
No deciduous decay experience	28%
Five or more teeth involved	38%
Base	952

21.1 Disease variation and background characteristics

In earlier chapters we have seen that dental attitudes and the child's dental
treatment experience vary with certain characteristics of the child's mother, for
example the mother's own dental attendance pattern. We now investigate whether
the prevalence of disease is also associated with background characteristics. In
this chapter we use a greater variety of background characteristics, and for some
factors examine the father's characteristics as well as the mother's.

Table 21.2

Decay experience of five year olds according to
mother's dental attendance pattern

Mother's dental attendance pattern	Proportion of five year olds with			
	No deciduous decay experience		Five or more deciduous teeth involved	
Regular	33%	407	32%	407
Occasional	25%	101	38%	101
Irregular	26%	309	40%	309
Edentulous	13%	93	59%	93

Throughout the report one of the dominating factors has been the mother's dental
attendance pattern and we start the analysis of variation in disease by testing
whether there is any association between the two (see Table 21.2). One in three
five year olds whose mothers are regular dental attenders had no deciduous decay
experience. For the children whose mothers went for an occasional check-up, or
only when they had dental trouble, this proportion was lower but not markedly so.
However among those children whose mothers were edentulous only 13% were found to
have had no deciduous disease experience. These children also had a much greater
chance of having five or more deciduous teeth with decay experience, this being the
situation for almost two-thirds of them. The children of mothers who were irregular
and occasional attenders fared slightly better, but still over 40% of them had five
or more teeth with disease experience. Among the children of mothers who were
regular attenders, one-third were estimated to have five or more teeth with disease
experience. It is interesting to note that the mothers who are regular attenders do
not produce significantly better results than the mothers who are irregular or
occasional dental attenders in preventing disease completely, but they do perform
significantly better in the control of disease than do the other two types of mother.

We analysed various combinations of mothers' and fathers' dental attendance patterns
and found that, provided the mother was not edentulous, the dental status and
attendance pattern of the father showed no particular association with the disease
experience of the child. However, for those children with an edentulous mother, we
found a significantly lower proportion with an estimated five or more teeth diseased
where the father was a regular dental attender than in those cases where he was not.

We have also shown earlier that dental attitudes and behaviour vary with social
class, and Table 21.3 shows the relationship between dental disease among five year
olds and social class. Over a third of children whose parents are in the top social
class group have no disease experience whereas this proportion for both the lower
groups is less than a quarter. Fewer than one in three children of parents in the
top social class group had five or more teeth with disease experience while over
40% of children of parents in the lower groups had disease experience to this
extent. Thus in both the prevention of disease and the control of it, children of
parents in the top social class group do significantly better than the others.

Table 21.3

Decay experience of five year olds according to social class

Social class	Proportion of five year olds with			
	No deciduous decay experience		Five or more deciduous teeth involved	
I, II & III non-manual	38%	283	30%	283
III manual	24%	441	41%	441
IV and V	23%	158	43%	158

Social class groupings are determined by the father's occupation but it is generally
the mother who has most of the day to day responsibility for the child's upbringing
and so it is interesting to investigate the variation in dental disease with the
mother's occupation. In most cases the mother no longer worked full time and so
we classified what she considered had been her usual occupation. The mothers were
divided into three employment types; firstly those who were (had been) teachers,
nurses, social workers or other professionals, secondly those who worked in offices
or did some type of clerical job, and thirdly those who worked in factories,
hairdressers, shops and so on. Table 21.4 gives the variation in the children's
disease experience for these groups of occupations. It can be seen that the ranges
of proportions of children with no disease or with five or more teeth with disease
experience were very similar to those for social class, a result which is not
particularly surprising as the father's occupation and mother's occupation tended
to be correlated.

Table 21.4

Decay experience of five year olds according to mother's occupation

Mother's occupation	Proportion of five year olds with	
	No deciduous decay experience	Five or more deciduous teeth involved
Teacher, nurse, social worker	36% *133*	30% *133*
Office worker	31% *233*	33% *233*
Factory or shop worker	23% *515*	43% *515*

Another factor which may indicate the life style of the parents is the age at which they finished full-time education. As with occupation, we found that the educational status of the parents was correlated, so that the information about both parents in conjunction did not improve the relationship which existed with either parent alone. Table 21.5 shows the relationship which was found between the child's disease experience and the parent's education. If either or both of the parents finished their full-time education at the age of eighteen or later, then over 40% of the five year olds had no deciduous decay experience. If neither parent had been in full-time education to the age of eighteen, then only 25% of the children had no deciduous decay experience. These figures are totally reversed when one examines the proportion of children who had five or more deciduous teeth involved with decay. This proportion was between a fifth and a quarter for those children whose mother or father was educated till at least the age of eighteen, whereas 40% of children whose parents had finsished their education before eighteen had five or more deciduous teeth with decay experience.

Table 21.5

Decay experience of five year olds according to parent's education

Age of parents at end of full-time education	Proportion of five year olds with	
	No deciduous decay experience	Five or more deciduous teeth involved
Mother was under 18	26% *775*	40% *775*
Mother was 18 or more	45% *78*	21% *78*
Father was under 18	25% *757*	40% *757*
Father was 18 or more	44% *100*	25% *100*
Mother and father were under 18	25% *726*	40% *726*
Either or both were 18 or more	42% *127*	26% *127*

The variations that we have shown with the parent's dental attendance pattern, social class and full-time education are not, of course, directly related to the disease of the deciduous teeth but merely indicate that the variation in life style, behaviour and attitudes which are associated with these factors most certainly do have a bearing on the disease experience of the child. In the next section we examine whether there was any regional variation in deciduous disease experience and if so whether this was accounted for by the background characteristics being unevenly distributed between the regions or whether the variation was due to more than that.

21.2 Disease variation and region

In our investigation of regional variation in disease we are limited, of course, to the social and background factors which were covered in the survey. There are of course other factors which could affect disease which were outside the scope of this inquiry, for example, we have no information on the physical health of the child, inheritance factors, or the effects of water supply or mineral intake over the child's lifetime. Nevertheless as we have already seen that there is a significant variation in disease with broad factors such as education, it is therefore of interest to see to what extent the factors for which we do have information account for any regional differences. Initially, however, we examine whether there was in fact a regional variation in the dental disease experience of five year olds.

Table 21.6 shows the proportion of five year olds with different levels of disease experience in the different regions. Since regional variation is an issue of considerable importance we have included in this table the proportion of children who have ten or more deciduous teeth involved with decay, as this is a level often used to indicate rampant decay in young children. The region with the highest proportion of decay free five year olds was London and the South East (31%), the region with the lowest proportion of decay free children was Wales (20%). A similar situation existed in terms of the proportion of children with five or more teeth involved, the lowest proportion was in London and the South East (34%) and the highest was in Wales (48%). The proportion of children with rampant decay in deciduous teeth at the age of five was particularly high in Wales (18%) and again lowest in London and the South East (8%).

Table 21.6

Decay experience of five year olds by region

Region	Proportion of five year olds with					
	No deciduous decay experience		Five or more deciduous teeth involved		Ten or more deciduous teeth involved	
The North	28%	312	37%	312	10%	312
Midlands and East Anglia	26%	195	41%	195	13%	195
Wales and the South West	25%	151	43%	151	14%	151
London and the South East	31%	264	34%	264	8%	264
Wales alone	20%	168	48%	168	18%	168

Having established that there is a regional variation in the disease experience of five year olds, the significant difference occurring between Wales and London and the South East, we examine in Table 21.7 whether mothers of different dental attendance patterns in those regions achieve different results.

In terms of the proportion of children who were decay free there were no significant differences between children of mothers of similar attendance patterns coming from London and the South East and Wales. Neither was there any significant difference between mothers of similar attendance patterns in these two regions in terms of the proportion of children with five or more teeth involved with decay.

Table 21.7

Decay experience of five year olds by mother's dental attendance pattern and region

Region	Mother's dental attendance pattern							
	Regular		Occasional		Irregular		Edentulous	
	Proportion of five year olds with no deciduous decay experience							
The North	35%	122	24%	29	26%	108	14%	51
Midlands and East Anglia	34%	76	25%	20	22%	76	10%	20
Wales and the South West	28%	74	*	19	22%	44	*	12
London and the South East	33%	135	27%	33	32%	81	*	10
Wales alone	20%	56	*	19	21%	67	5%	22
	Proportion of five year olds with five or more deciduous teeth involved							
The North	29%	122	41%	29	36%	108	59%	51
Midlands and East Anglia	33%	76	40%	20	44%	76	60%	20
Wales and the South West	38%	74	*	19	47%	44	*	12
London and the South East	32%	135	30%	33	38%	81	*	10
Wales alone	41%	56	*	19	48%	67	73%	22

In Table 21.8 we look in a similar way at the variation in disease among children of different social class and region. For children in the social class groups IV and V there was no significant regional variation in the proportion who were disease free or who had five or more teeth involved with decay. This was true

Table 21.8

Decay experience of five year olds by social class and region

Region	Social class					
	I,II & III non-manual		III manual		IV and V	
	Proportion of five year olds with no deciduous decay experience					
The North	41%	100	21%	153	23%	44
Midlands and East Anglia	28%	40	26%	101	28%	46
Wales and the South West	27%	55	26%	66	22%	23
London and the South East	47%	88	24%	121	24%	45
Wales alone	23%	48	15%	66	23%	39
	Proportion of five year olds with five or more deciduous teeth involved					
The North	26%	100	45%	153	41%	44
Midlands and East Anglia	45%	40	40%	101	46%	46
Wales and the South West	33%	55	47%	66	46%	23
London and the South East	26%	88	35%	121	40%	45
Wales alone	40%	48	51%	66	44%	39

for the children in social class III manual in the case of decay free mouths but London and the South East had a significantly lower proportion of children with five or more teeth involved than Wales. Among the children in the top social class group there was a significantly lower proportion with no decay experience in Wales than in London and the South East although no significant variation was found between these two regions in the proportion who had five or more teeth involved.

Finally we examine the relationship between the age the parents finished full-time education and the disease experience of the five year olds in the different region The only regional variations that were significant occurred among the children of parents whose full-time education finished before the age of eighteen. In Wales there was a lower proportion of decay free children than in the other regions and in London and the South East there was a lower proportion with five or more teeth involved.

Table 21.9

Decay experience of five year olds by parent's education and region

Region	Age of parents at end of full-time education			
	Both under 18 years		One or both 18 years or over	
	Proportion of five year olds with no deciduous decay experience			
The North	23%	250	46%	41
Midlands and East Anglia	25%	169	*	13
Wales and the South West	24%	113	34%	30
London and the South East	28%	194	44%	50
Wales alone	18%	125	23%	26
	Proportion of five year olds with five or more deciduous teeth involved			
The North	41%	250	20%	41
Midlands and East Anglia	43%	169	*	13
Wales and the South West	43%	113	36%	30
London and the South East	36%	194	22%	50
Wales alone	46%	125	42%	26

Unfortunately the sample sizes were rather small for this detailed analysis and it would certainly be of interest to see whether with a bigger sample the differences which occurred but which were not significant would prove to be so.

The pattern of the differences which were significant was rather erratic and does not provide conclusive evidence that the regional variation in disease was due to more than regional variations in social and background factors.

21.3 Disease variation and early upbringing

During the interview we asked the mothers a series of questions about the child's early life, including whether he had been breast or bottle fed, whether the child had sucked a dummy, whether the mother had given him a dinky feeder and whether the child was a thumb sucker.

Table 21.10 shows the deciduous disease experience according to whether the child was breast fed, bottle fed, or both. Not many children were totally breast fed but those who were breast and bottle fed were less likely to have decayed deciduous teeth than those who were only bottle fed. It is not possible from the survey data to say whether this is a causal relationship or the result of a variable confounded with other factors which are the source of the causal relationship, for example that perhaps the mothers who breast feed give a higher priority to or are more knowledgeable about health and child development.

Table 21.10

Decay experience of breast fed and bottle fed babies

Baby feeding	Proportion of five year olds with			
	No deciduous decay experience		Five or more deciduous teeth involved	
Breast fed	30%	80	34%	80
Bottle fed	25%	605	40%	605
Both	33%	233	36%	233

We asked the mothers whether the children had ever had drinks from a bottle once they were being given solids for their main meals. We also inquired as to what age this habit continued. Table 21.11 shows that among the children who were given drinks from a bottle beyond the age of two years only 17% had no decay experience and 51% had five or more teeth involved at the age of five. It is difficult to know exactly why these children are more decay prone, whether it is because drinking from a bottle means that the teeth are washed with the liquid over a longer period than would happen when drinking from a cup, or whether it develops a desire for food and drink as a comforter which then leads to greater intake. Whatever the reason for the relationship it would appear to be an ill-advised habit from the dental health point of view.

Table 21.11

Decay experience and drinking from a bottle
once main meals are solids

Age until child drank from bottle once main meals were solids	Proportion of five year olds with			
	No deciduous decay experience		Five or more deciduous teeth involved	
Not at all	32%	301	35%	301
Under two years	28%	481	36%	481
Two years or more	17%	135	51%	135

We also asked the mothers whether the child had ever been given a dummy to suck and if so till what age the child had had a dummy. As with drinking from a bottle dummy sucking showed a relationship with deciduous decay experience. All dummy suckers were more likely to have some deciduous decay than were non dummy suckers, but those who used a dummy at the age of three or more were particularly at risk. A half of this group had five or more deciduous teeth involved with decay at the age of five. Again it is not possible to say whether this relationship exists because of the habit of dummy sucking (which might well have been accompanied by the dummy being dipped into something sweet) or whether the dummy encouraged the habit of sucking something as a comforter.

Table 21.12

Decay experience and the use of a dummy

Age until child had a dummy	Proportion of five year olds with			
	No deciduous decay experience		Five or more deciduous teeth involved	
Not at all	31%	588	36%	588
Under three years	24%	242	39%	242
Three years or more	15%	75	50%	75

Another method by which some liquid and, maybe, some comfort can be given to a baby is by the use of a dinky feeder. In the majority of cases the mothers said they had not used this method. There was hardly any difference between the dental health of children who had never had a dinky feeder and those that had, providing that they had stopped using it before the age of two. For those children who had been given a dinky feeder beyond the age of two, the likelihood of disease, and extensive disease, were both increased (see Table 21.13).

Table 21.13

Decay experience and dinky feeders

Age until child had a dinky feeder	Proportion of five year olds with			
	No deciduous decay experience		Five or more deciduous teeth involved	
Not at all	28%	661	37%	661
Under two years	30%	207	40%	207
Two years or more	18%	51	46%	51

Finally in terms of early upbringing we examine the relationship between deciduous decay experience and thumb sucking. Table 21.14 shows that from the point of view of deciduous decay, the children who sucked their thumbs till the age of three or more were much more likely to be free from decay and much less likely than other children to have five or more teeth involved with decay. Again it is not possible to detect from the survey data a causal relationship between these findings, but it is possible or indeed probable that children who suck their thumbs have not been sucking other things as comforters such as dummies, dinky feeders, drinks in bottles, sweets and so on. It is also possible that their intake of sweet things has been curbed as a result of their thumb sucking, and that their saliva flow has been increased.

Table 21.14

Decay experience and thumbsucking

Age until child sucked thumb	Proportion of five year olds with			
	No deciduous decay experience		Five or more deciduous teeth involved	
Did not suck thumb	25%	688	42%	688
Under three years	27%	23	56%	23
Three years or more	37%	205	25%	205

The survey results relating to upbringing thus suggest that there are some habits
which are associated with the disease experience of the child. Most of the factors
shown to be related to disease were matters that were largely within the discretion
of the mother, and although there was little suggestion that a single factor could
eradicate the problem of decay it would seem that the mother could, if she realised
and if she wished, choose to reduce the decay experience of her child.

21.4 Disease variation and current eating habits

In addition to the information that we obtained about early upbringing we asked a
large range of questions related to the current eating habits of the child. It is
unlikely that any individual variable is very important in relating eating habits
to dental health, but by analysing these questions we hoped to find indicators of
ranges of habits which tend either to help or hinder the cause of preventive
dentistry.

One of the biggest problems in investigating the relationship between eating habits
and dental health from survey data is that the total dental disease experience of
the five year old has been affected by eating patterns since birth. If the child
has already had dental problems, the mother may have been given advice which
resulted in a change of eating habits. Such circumstances would then abrogate the
expected relationship between eating habits and decay. In addition, of course, it
is very difficult to obtain accurate information about eating habits since some
mothers may give what they consider to be acceptable answers and mothers' views
of what is large or small will vary; furthermore, the diversity of time, place
and quantity of food consumed makes the collection of simple meaningful indicators
very difficult. We feel in retrospect that for most of the meal questions, the
information would have been better had we obtained a history of meals over a period
of time and this was considered at the planning stage, but it would have distorted
the balance of the interview to such an extent that the idea was discarded. If the
main purpose of this inquiry had been to investigate variations in disease alone
then eating habits would have justified much greater depth of study.

In terms of eating habits one of the factors of interest which emerged for the
five year olds, was whether or not the mothers said the child usually had something
to eat at break. About half of the children did. Among those who did not 32% had
no decay experience and 34% had five or more teeth involved. Among those who did
have something to eat at break 23% had no decay experience and 42% had five or more
teeth involved with decay. Perhaps this is an indication that those who had

something to eat at break were more used to having snacks between meals than the other children (see Table 21.15).

Table 21.15

Decay experience and eating at break

Whether child has anything to eat at break	Proportion of five year olds with			
	No deciduous decay experience		Five or more deciduous teeth involved	
Eats at break	23%	443	42%	443
Does not	32%	476	34%	476

We asked the mothers whether the child was used to eating a lot of cakes and biscuits, a fair number, or not many cakes and biscuits. Table 21.16 shows the relationship between this and the child's disease experience. Among the small group of children who were said to eat a lot of cakes and biscuits 21% of the children had no decay experience and 58% had five or more teeth involved. This compares with 30% decay free and 34% with five or more teeth involved among children who were said not to eat many cakes and biscuits. We also asked the mothers whether the child was allowed to help himself to biscuits or whether he had to ask first. Of the five year olds who were allowed to help themselves to biscuits only 18% had no decay experience and 50% had five or more deciduous teeth involved with decay. Thus the greater the quantity of and the more free the access to cakes and biscuits, the worse was the child's deciduous disease situation.

Table 21.16

Decay experience and consumption of cakes and biscuits

Consumption of cakes and biscuits	Proportion of five year olds with			
	No deciduous decay experience		Five or more deciduous teeth involved	
Eats a lot	21%	46	58%	46
Eats a fair number	24%	317	43%	317
Does not eat many	30%	557	34%	557
Helps himself to biscuits	18%	170	50%	170
Does not	30%	751	36%	751

Cakes and biscuits are not, of course, the only source of sweet things to eat, and we asked the mothers some similar questions about the child's fondness for sweets and how many he ate. The children said to be very fond of sweets were less likely to be decay free and more likely to have five or more teeth involved with decay than were the children who were said not to be as fond of sweets as most children (see Table 21.17). In terms of the amount consumed, the very small group of children who were said not to eat sweets at all were at a very noticeable advantage; 48% of them were decay free and only 14% had five or more teeth involved

with decay. The children who were said to eat only a small quantity of sweets
were also at an advantage. The children who were said to eat a large quantity of
sweets were at a considerable disadvantage, 42% having five or more deciduous teeth
involved with decay.

Table 21.17

Decay experience and consumption of sweets

Consumption of sweets	Proportion of five year olds with			
	No deciduous decay experience		Five or more deciduous teeth involved	
Very fond of sweets	22%	302	42%	302
About average	30%	525	38%	525
Less fond than average	31%	92	31%	92
Eats a large quantity	26%	62	42%	62
Eats a medium quantity	22%	209	38%	209
Eats a small quantity	27%	513	40%	513
Eats a very small quantity	38%	102	33%	102
Does not eat sweets	48%	21	14%	21

We have used these few illustrations of particular facets of eating to indicate
that there are relationships between eating habits and dental health and that they
can be shown from survey data. As illustrations we would not wish them to be
interpreted too narrowly. We feel that the relationship between eating habits and
dental health is based on much wider factors than sweets, biscuits and cakes and
that the survey results are merely indicative that there are certain dietary
factors, which are within the control of the mother, that do affect dental health.

In Chapter 10 we showed that mothers were aware that eating sweet things was
associated with decay. They also showed that their reaction to stopping decay
was not to restrict the intake of the sweet foods but to clean the teeth. We feel
it would be appropriate to end this section by examining whether or not the
children who were said to brush their teeth most frequently were at an advantage
with respect to total deciduous decay experience.

Table 21.18

Decay experience and frequency of toothbrushing

Frequency of toothbrushing	Proportion of five year olds with			
	No deciduous decay experience		Five or more deciduous teeth involved	
Three times a day	28%	44	36%	44
Twice a day	28%	469	37%	469
Once a day	27%	297	42%	297
Less than once a day	29%	98	35%	98

Table 21.18 shows that there was no systematic variation in disease experience
with variation in toothbrushing frequency.

22   Summary of findings and conclusions

Chapter 1   *Introduction*
The survey findings are based on the results of dental examinations conducted on
a random sample of 13,000 children aged 5-15 in maintained schools in England and
Wales, and on an interview carried out with 3,000 of the mothers of children aged
five, eight, twelve and fourteen.   Seventy dentists were seconded from their duties
in the School Dental Service to carry out the dental examinations and they all
attended a one week training course to practice using the definitions laid down for
the survey examination so as to achieve as uniform a standard of examination as
possible.

The response achieved for the survey was very high, 95% of the children who were
selected for examination were examined, and for 91% of those selected for both
parts of the inquiry we obtained both the dental examination and the interview with
the mother.

22.1   Summary of findings

Chapter 2   *Dental development*
The survey included children ranging from the age of five to fifteen, thus covering
the whole period of transition from deciduous teeth to permanent teeth.   The rate
at which this change takes place varies very much from child to child.   The first
deciduous tooth to exfoliate naturally is usually one of the lower central incisors,
a few of these teeth were already missing among children who were only just five
years old, on the other hand, a few lower central incisors were still present among
children who had recently passed their seventh birthday.

The eruption of permanent teeth occurs at different ages for different children.
In general it appeared that for boys the eruption of permanent teeth tended to
occur a little later than for girls.

Chapter 3   *Dental decay and treatment*
By far the greatest amount of contact between children and the dental profession
arises because of tooth decay.   At the time of the survey about two-thirds of
children were found to have some active decay, the proportion being lowest at 57%
among the fifteen year olds and highest at 78% among the eight year olds.   Among
the five to eight year olds more than 20% of children had five or more actively
decayed teeth, among children aged nine to fifteen more than 10% had five or more
actively decayed teeth.

The treatment available for decayed teeth is either restoration by filling or extraction. The proportion of children who had some filled teeth increased over the age groups from 26% of five year olds to 88% of fifteen year olds. The proportion of children with no filled teeth at the age of fourteen and fifteen was 19% and 12% respectively. The figure for the fourteen year olds is probably the best estimate of the proportion of children who are obtaining no restorative treatment since the fifteen year olds who are still at school do not represent the total age group because the early school leavers are excluded.

The survey only measured the extraction experience for permanent teeth since it is impossible to tell for children in the process of changing from one dentition to the other whether the missing deciduous teeth were exfoliated or extracted. Among the oldest children, the fourteen and fifteen year olds, about a third had already had some permanent teeth extracted, and at an age as early as seven, eight and nine years old some permanent teeth were being lost.

Teeth in different positions in the mouth contribute very differently to the decay experience of the child and this is so for both deciduous and permanent teeth. In both dentitions it is the molars which are most disease prone.

Chapter 4   *Total decay experience*
If one takes as an indication of total decay experience the sum of current disease and the evidence of past treatment then one can see that very few children avoid decay entirely. Seven out of ten five olds already have some evidence of decay experience, at the age of eight nine out of ten children have evidence of decay experience and among the teenagers fewer than five children in a hundred have no evidence of decay experience.

As well as knowing how many children have had some decay it is of interest to know the extent of their disease experience. For the permanent dentition this can be achieved by summing the number of teeth with current decay or evidence of past treatment but for the deciduous dentition the examination provided no estimate of the number of deciduous teeth that had been extracted for decay reasons. For the five year olds, among whom little natural exfoliation would have so far taken place we estimated the likelihood of the missing deciduous teeth being diseased. This provided an estimate of the proportion of five year olds who had ten or more teeth involved with decay, a level often used to indicate rampant decay in the deciduous dentition. By this method we estimate that 11% of five year olds had ten or more deciduous teeth, that is a half c more of the deciduous dentition, involved with decay.

Chapter 5   *Accidental damage*
In some cases children need dental attention because of damage caused to the teeth by some kind of accident. It is most likely that the front teeth are the ones to suffer in this way and the dental examiners found that about one in ten girls and one in five boys among the twelve to fourteen year olds had evidence of such damage. This relatively high involvement with accidental damage is influenced by the fact

that the criteria for the dental examination included fractures of the enamel which are fairly minor kinds of damage and would probably not require treatment and would perhaps be hardly noticeable.

Chapter 6   *Dentures*

Among all the children examined for the survey, that is about 13,000, only 46 children were found to have dentures; of these 23 had apparently suffered accidental damage to the teeth, 5 had developmental or congenital problems and 18 needed the denture because of extractions due to decay. Only one child had a full upper denture the others all had a partial denture involving one jaw.

Chapter 7   *The condition of the gums*

Another of the problems that affect dental health is the condition of the gums. The examiners recorded whether the child had any gum inflammation, debris or calculus. It is possible that the survey dental criteria for recording gum conditions were more stringent than those which are currently applied in practice. From the age of seven onwards about threequarters of children were involved with gum trouble of one or other kind. Gum inflammation and debris were found to be significantly associated.

Chapter 8   *Orthodontics*

Not all children have the good fortune to have trouble free dental development and the most common condition that arises is that of teeth crowded together. As many as 65% of eight year olds were recorded as having some crowding, and over the age range seven to fifteen the proportion was always greater than a half. Taking all the orthodontic assessments into account the dental examiners were asked to say whether, in their opinion, the child needed (or would need) orthodontic treatment. The future orthodontic need of five and six year olds was, of course, rather difficult to assess but by the age of seven about a half of the children were estimated to be in need of treatment. The proportion was highest among eight year olds where 57% were said to be in need of treatment. The need for orthodontic treatment may be apparent some considerable while before treatment is actually carried out and so the proportion in need of such treatment decreased among the older children till it reached 28% and 27% of fourteen and fifteen year olds. By that age any treatment that was going to be carried out would most likely have been started and so about a quarter of the children are likely to remain with an orthodontic treatment need that is unmet. A quarter of fourteen year olds had previously had some orthodontic treatment compared to the fact that 28% were said to be currently in need of treatment, thus about half of the estimated total orthodontic need is being met. Chapter 17 shows that mothers did not always recognise the need for orthodontic treatment which the dentists had found.

Chapter 9   *Overall dental condition*

It was of interest to assess what the total current need for dental attention was at the time of the survey and for this estimate we included the three most common sources of dental need, that is active decay, some gum trouble, or some orthodontic treatment need. By combining these three grounds for dental need we found that eight out of ten five year olds and nine out of ten children in the age range six to fifteen would benefit from dental treatment or oral hygiene instruction.

Chapter 10   *Mother's dental experience, knowledge and attitudes*

Nearly all children have their first permanent front teeth before the age of eight, many have them at the age of five or six. Similarly nearly all children have their first permanent back teeth by the age of eight and again many have them at the age of five or six. We asked the children's mothers when they thought these teeth erupted and over three-quarters said the first front teeth erupt before the age of eight but under a quarter estimated that the first permanent back teeth come through as early as that. There would thus appear to be a considerable lack of knowledge among mothers about their children's dental development. Mothers who were themselves good dental attenders were no more likely than other mothers to be aware of the pattern of permanent tooth eruption, neither were mothers in the top social class group more likely than others to know these facts. We felt that in many cases the mothers either did not know that any back teeth erupted at the age of six, or mistook them for the last of the deciduous teeth. In fact among twelve year olds who had already had some of their back permanent teeth extracted 45% of the mothers stated that all the child's extractions so far had been deciduous teeth.

In terms of knowledge about decay mothers were in no doubt that it could occur in very young children. Half of the mothers thought that such trouble could start before the age of three and three-quarters thought decay could start before the age of four. Neither were the mothers in much doubt as to what caused decay, eight out of ten blamed eating sweets and sweet things. When asked what might be done to help prevent decay the majority suggested better tooth cleaning, the minority suggested restricting the intake of sweet things.

Chapter 11   *Mother's views on the dental care of her child*

We asked the mothers whether they had any preference for different kinds of treatment for their children. Over a half said that if a bad back deciduous tooth was involved they would prefer it to be extracted. Only about one in ten said they would prefer extraction if the tooth concerned was a bad permanent tooth. In view of their different attitudes for the different dentitions it is particularly ironic that mothers are not aware which teeth are which.

The preference for different kinds of treatment reflected the mother's own attendance pattern to a considerable extent, for example a half of the mothers who were themselves regular attenders preferred fillings for deciduous teeth whereas only a quarter of mothers who were irregular attenders preferred that. Once

permanent teeth were involved, eight out of ten of even those mothers who themselves
had the worst dental attendance pattern said they would prefer their child's bad
back permanent teeth to be filled.

We asked the mothers whether they thought that their children currently needed any
dental treatment, six out of ten mothers said the child did not need any treatment.
Only about four out of ten children had in fact been classified by the dental
examination as currently free from decay.

Chapter 12   *The child's dental background*

Over the age of five very few children have not seen a dentist whether for the
relief of pain or for conservation. In fact the proportion who were said to have
never been to the dentist was 29% among the five year olds, 9% among the eight
year olds, and 3% among the twelve and fourteen year olds. Beyond the age of five
it may be that the more accurate description is that the child had seldom been to
the dentist since some of the children who were said never to have been to the
dentist had in fact had some fillings and extractions.

We asked the mothers whether the children had ever, in the past, had any extractions
either of deciduous or permanent teeth. A quarter of five year olds, two-thirds of
eight year olds and three-quarters of twelve and fourteen year olds had at some time
had at least one extraction. Having teeth extracted thus soon ceases to be a
minority experience. Even the children of mothers who were themselves regular
attenders had not noticeably escaped the experience.

The two main services through which children can obtain dental treatment are the
General Dental Service and the School Dental Service, although, in fact, the
majority of treatment is carried out through the General Dental Service. Mothers
(or children) can decide to change the service they use whenever they so wish.
Three-quarters of children had at some stage used the General Dental Service and
the proportion who had at some time used the School Dental Service reached 48%
among the fourteen year olds. Among fourteen year olds a half of the children
had always used the General Dental Service and just under a quarter had always
used the School Dental Service and just over a quarter had used both.

Children of mothers who were themselves regular attenders were much more likely to
have always used the General Dental Service, as were children in the top social
class group and children in London and the South East. Conversely children who
had always used the School Dental Service were more likely to come from less
dentally aware backgrounds. When asked the reason for using the type of dental
service the child attended the major reason for going to the General Dental Service
was that the mother took the child to her own dentist. The reasons for going to
the School Dental Service were that the mother was notified of the need to see a
dentist by the school, that the school dentist was more convenient or that the
school dentist was thought to be good with children.

Chapter 13   *Visiting the dentist*
Among those children who had been to the dentist nearly two-thirds said that the
reason for the most recent visit was for a check-up. Between a fifth and a quarter
of the different age groups said their last visit had been because of dental
trouble and about one in ten were prompted to go because of a note from school.
As might be expected the note from school was of more importance as a stimulus for
dental attendance among children who are in the habit of using the School Dental
Service. These figures reflect the fact that the majority of treatment is obtained
through the General Dental Service, and also some of the differences in the
organisation of the two services.

The treatment that was said to have been received as a result of the most recent
dental visit was highly associated with the reason for the visit. For children
whose last visit was said to have been for a check-up fewer than ten per cent had
treatment which involved extractions whereas among those whose last visit was
prompted by dental trouble over a half had some extractions.

Chapter 14   *Toothbrushing*
When asked about prevention of decay many mothers put considerable faith in toothbrushing. We asked the mothers how frequently the children brushed their teeth
and about a half said twice a day and about a third said once a day. The survey
results showed no marked variation between the frequency of toothbrushing and
decay, but there were significant differences in relation to gum inflammation and
debris.

Chapter 15   *Toothache*
We asked the mothers whether the children had ever had toothache and for a half of
them the answer was in the negative. Over a third of the children whose mothers
were regular attenders had had toothache which suggests that toothache does not
always arise in circumstances of dental neglect on the part of the parent. In
two-thirds of all cases the outcome for the tooth when a child had toothache was
extraction.

Chapter 16   *Mother's awareness of accidental damage*
We asked mothers whether the children had ever suffered any accidental damage and
compared their answers with the examination findings. Among children said by the
dentist to have traumatised incisors approximately half of the mothers said there
had been no accidental damage. We would have expected that the mothers would have
been aware of any serious accident and so we scrutinised the cases where there was
disagreement between the dentist and the mother and found that in the majority of
cases the level of trauma recorded by the dentist was very minor and could fairly
easily have escaped the notice of the mother.

Chapter 17   *Mother's views on orthodontics*

Chapter 8 has shown the level of orthodontic need as assessed by the dental examiners and this chapter discusses the mothers' attitudes to orthodontics. Mothers apparently attach considerable value to the treatment of children's teeth if they are crooked or protruding. They did not, however, have the same level of assessment as the dentists as to which conditions required orthodontic treatment. Among children aged twelve and fourteen who had previously had no orthodontic treatment but whom the dentist considered needed some, half of the mothers said the child had no orthodontic irregularity. Since the dentist's assessment for orthodontic need could arise from several sources we looked at one particular orthodontic assessment and examined whether the mother and dentist agreed about the child's teeth being crowded, but even where the dentist said there was crowding in the upper middle segment, that is among upper canines and incisors, nearly a half of the mothers said there was no irregularity.

Chapter 18   *Dental background and dental health*

Among the five year olds a considerable proportion of children had not as yet been to the dentist, but among the eight, twelve and fourteen year olds about half the children were said to have been for a check-up within the past six months. There was, on the other hand, a considerable proportion of children in the older groups who were not going to the dentist unless they had some trouble or were prompted by a note from school. This was so for about a third of children aged eight, twelve and fourteen. Among the fourteen year olds, 12% were said not to have been to the dentist at all within the previous two years.

In terms of the proportion of children who would benefit from some dental attention, that is those with some decay, some gum trouble or some orthodontic treatment need, the level was very high even among the potential regular attenders. This was also the case for the gum trouble need and the orthodontic need when examined on their own. In terms of the proportion of children with some active decay the disparity between attendance patterns was greater but the proportion of children with active decay among the potential regular attenders was disappointingly high. For fourteen year olds a half of the regular attenders had some active decay, as had two-thirds of the occasional attenders and three-quarters of the irregular attenders.

It is fairly common to find that if one calculates disease experience by adding current decay to evidence of past treatment then the most dentally well cared for children contain the highest proportion of children with extensive disease experience. This arises when the stage of decay at which some fillings are provided is earlier than the level used to detect current decay. For example, 32% of fourteen year olds who had been for a check-up in the last six months had ten or more teeth with decay experience compared to 22% of the occasional attenders and 25% of the irregular attenders.

We have already seen that the mothers' attitudes towards preferences for dental treatment vary according to whether deciduous or permanent teeth are involved. Among eight year olds 66% of potentially regular attenders had some decayed deciduous teeth, 35% having some deciduous teeth that were unrestorable. Among the eight year olds who were potential irregular attenders 76% had some decayed deciduous teeth, 43% having some that were unrestorable. The differences between the attendance patterns were thus relatively small.

The proportion of children with fillings in deciduous teeth varied between attendance patterns especially for the five year olds, being 43% for those who had been for a check-up in the last six months, 11% for those whose check-up had been longer ago than that and 18% for those who were not in the habit of going for a check-up. By the age of eight the differences were less marked being 57%, 41% and 33% for the attendance types respectively. The interesting fact here is that even among the children who have been for check-ups the proportion with deciduous filled teeth is not much greater than a half.

In terms of the filling experience of permanent teeth the advantage that the potentially regular attenders have over the children with other attendance patterns is to be seen among fourteen year olds where the regular attenders have, on average, 6.1 filled permanent teeth compared with an average of 3.3 filled permanent teeth among the irregular attenders. For the fourteen year olds who have not been to a dentist in the past two years the average number of filled teeth is as low as 1.0.

The alternative to the restoration of decayed teeth is the eventual loss of them by extraction. The proportion of children who have had some permanent teeth extracted for decay reasons by the age of fourteen varies with attendance pattern. However, even among the regular attenders a quarter have lost some permanent teeth by that age. For the irregular attenders, the proportion having lost some permanent teeth by the age of fourteen was as high as 40%.

Chapter 19   *Regional variations in the dental condition of children*
Dental attendance patterns among children were found to vary between the regions. London and the South East had a higher proportion of potential regular attenders and Wales had proportionately fewer. Conversely, Wales had considerably more irregular attenders proportionately, for example among the fourteen year olds in Wales 40% were irregular attenders compared to 22% in London and the South East.

The examination results revealed that the proportion of children with some active decay, some filled teeth and some extracted permanent teeth also varied with region, children in London and the South East being in the most advantageous position and those in Wales being in the least. For example, the proportion of fourteen year olds with some extracted permanent teeth was 50% in Wales but 18% in London and the South East.

The variation in treatment experience between the regions was not entirely accounted for by the uneven distribition of attendance pattern. In general, regular attenders had fairly similar treatment experience wherever they lived but irregular attenders were more likely to have less current decay and more restorative experience if they lived in London and the South East. For example the proportion of children aged fourteen who had some filled permanent teeth taking account of the three attendance patterns was 90%, 88% and 78% in London and the South East compared to 88%, 73% and 50% in Wales. In this respect the North, Midlands and East Anglia and Wales and the South West tended to be similar to Wales.

One factor for which regional variation affected the regular attenders as well as the irregulars was the proportion of children who had lost some permanent teeth. For fourteen year olds in the three main attendance groups the proportion who had had some permanent teeth extracted was 18%, 11% and 28% in London and the South East, but 40%, 43% and 63% in Wales.

Chapter 20   *The dental condition of individual tooth types*

When the individual tooth types are examined to see which ones are most prone to disease there is no doubt that the first permanent molars bear the brunt of both disease and treatment experience among children. It is interesting to find that there is little regional variation in the total disease experience of the first permanent molars in different regions but considerable evidence of treatment variation. Children in London and the South East retain many more of their first permanent molars, fewer of which are currently decayed, many more of which are filled, than is the case in other regions.

We looked particularly closely at the dental condition of fourteen year olds since they were the last full age group in school at the time of the survey and thus represent the best estimate we have of the dental condition of adolescents as they approach adult life. An examination of the dental condition of different tooth types for fourteen year olds of different attendance patterns from different regions revealed that those who were well cared for appeared to be more decay prone because of the variation in the level of decay at which fillings take place. The disease experienced by children who do not go for dental check-ups was more likely to be untreated than was the case for children who go for regular check-ups.

In view of the history of the first permanent molar it was of interest to investigate the condition of the tooth posterior to it, the second permanent molar. Among regular attenders aged fourteen over half of the second permanent molars already had evidence of disease experience, the great majority of which had been treated restoratively. Among irregular attenders of the same age there was less evidence of disease but, except in London and the South East, the majority of disease had not been treated restoratively. Only in a small proportion of cases had extractions of second permanent molars occurred, the majority of diseased teeth being currently decayed.

At the time that the survey dental examination was carried out the majority of decayed teeth found among fourteen year old irregular attenders were still restorable, so although the fourteen year olds who are not accustomed to going to the dentist for a check-up had considerably more current treatment need than the regular attenders the position was not for the most part irretrievable.

Chapter 21   *Disease variation among five year olds*

A detailed analysis was carried out to investigate what factors were associated with the estimated total deciduous disease experience of five year olds. It was found that social and background factors such as the mother's own dental attendance pattern, the parents' occupation and educational attainment were associated with disease experience. It was also found that disease experience was associated with region. The analysis that was carried out to see whether factors other than social and background were associated with the regional variation in disease was rather inconclusive.

Different methods of upbringing and various current eating habits showed that some patterns of behaviour were more associated with disease than others. For example, if the child had been in the habit of having drinks from a bottle beyond the age of two the likelihood was that the level of disease experience would be high. On the other hand if the child had been a thumb sucker beyond the age of three the likelihood of disease was fairly low. If the child ate something at school break-time the disease experience was higher than if he did not. If the five year old ate few or no sweets the likelihood of decay experience was lower, whereas if the child helped himself to biscuits the disease experience was higher.

None of the indicators are intended to be interpreted in isolation but they have been used to illustrate the fact that exposure to certain conditions has certain results. The results which we show may well not be direct cause and effect relationships, for example, the fact that a child of five is free to help himself to biscuits may merely reflect that he has had the opportunity to develop a liking for sweet food which could well be manifested in many different ways. Merely stopping him from helping himself to biscuits may not improve the situation.

22.2   Conclusions

One of the main purposes of the children's survey was to provide information about the dental health of children which would complement that obtained from the survey among adults, thereby showing at what stage the characteristics which so markedly distinguish adults of different attendance patterns in different regions are observable among children.

Many of the dental attitudes that people have are transmitted from parents to children very early in life. Even by the age of five many decisions have been made as to the child's dental attendance pattern and attitudes towards treatment. Some changes of attitude do take place during the child's school life and the survey results show that some children with not very good dental attendance patterns are receiving restorative treatment, but the gap between the dental condition of those who attend regularly and those who do not is apparent even among the five year olds, among whom 43% of children who have recently been for a check-up have some filled deciduous teeth compared to 18% of the children who do not go for a check-up. Although all the deciduous teeth are eventually lost the recollection of their dental treatment and the resulting expectations of dentistry remain. As the permanent dentition develops one finds that the children with the best dental background have more restorative treatment and less current decay but no less disease. However, by the age of fourteen the variation in dental condition between children of different attendance patterns and different regions has not for the most part reached irreparable dimensions (except for the state of the first permanent molars). In theory the vast majority of children at this age could be made dentally fit and have a reasonable expectation of adequate reliance on natural teeth well into adult life, provided that resources were available to carry out the backlog of treatment needed and the children were prepared to have the treatment.

However in the real world resources are limited and children's dental attitudes
have already been moulded by their experiences and expectations. The fact that at
the age of fourteen the situation would still appear to be retrievable for most
children does not mean that the future situation will in fact be saved. In the
survey of adult dental health carried out in 1968 the differences between the
treatment received by young people aged 16-34 according to their attendance pattern
and the region in which they lived were more marked than among the fourteen year
olds in 1973. The young adults had a wider range of permanent teeth extracted and
a wider range of teeth extensively filled. It is not possible to say how far the
fourteen year olds will in the next few years recreate that pattern, it is only
possible to say that at fourteen the position was still redeemable. It is hard to
say how far the attitudes of the fourteen year olds are already entrenched in terms
of the priorities attached to dental welfare but it is worrying to compare the
regional variation in loss of permanent teeth among fourteen year olds with the
regional variation in total tooth loss among adults.

Table 22.1
Tooth loss among fourteen year olds and total tooth loss among adults, by region

Region	Proportion of fourteen year olds with some permanent teeth extracted in 1973		Proportion of adults edentulous in 1968	
The North	37%	308	46%	864
Midlands and East Anglia	38%	207	34%	629
Wales and the South West	34%	145	43%	431
London and the South East	18%	263	28%	1008

The regional variations that have come to light from the analysis of the survey
results were known to exist before the survey was carried out, for the survey

Table 22.2
Regional variation in treatment carried out through the General Dental Service

Region		Ratio of conserved* to extracted deciduous teeth for children aged		Ratio of filled* to extracted permanent teeth for children aged
		0-4	5-15	5-15
North ⎤ North West ⎬ The North Yorks & Humberside ⎦		1.12 ⎤ 1.47 ⎬1.43 1.56 ⎦	0.55 ⎤ 0.88 ⎬0.78 0.79 ⎦	5.09 ⎤ 5.72 ⎬5.91 6.95 ⎦
West Midlands ⎤ Midlands and East Midlands ⎬ East Anglia East Anglia ⎦		1.95 ⎤ 2.06 ⎬2.16 3.62 ⎦	1.06 ⎤ 1.06 ⎬1.12 1.51 ⎦	6.87 ⎤ 7.38 ⎬7.21 8.05 ⎦
Wales ⎤ Wales and South West ⎦ the South West		1.58 ⎤ 3.44 ⎦2.53	0.94 ⎤ 2.11 ⎦1.54	4.25 ⎤ 8.49 ⎦6.30
G.L.C. ⎤ London and South East ⎦ the South East		10.70 ⎤ 5.55 ⎦7.04	3.40 ⎤ 2.47 ⎦2.82	17.04 ⎤ 11.38 ⎦13.40
Wales	Wales	1.58 1.58	0.94 0.94	4.25 4.25

*   Treatment carried out under the General Dental Service as reported in
    the Dental Estimates Board Annual Report for 1972

227

findings reflect the same variations as are shown by the ratios of restoration to
extraction in the dental treatment carried out within the General Dental Service
and reported in the Dental Estimates Board Annual Report 1972, and indeed in
previous annual reports. However the context in which to interpret them was not
known until background information and the overall levels of disease among children
were established. Since the survey results show no massive variation in disease
experience regionally which could have accounted for the regional variation in the
ratios these variations must be due to treatment rather than disease.

If one compares the regional variation in treatment with the regional variation
in population per dentist and pupils per school dentist then maybe one should not
be surprised to find that in the south conservative treatment has been provided
for a much larger and more varied group of children than is the case in other
regions.

Table 22.3
Regional distribution of manpower resources

Region			Persons per GDS* dentist		Pupils per school dentist†	
North		The North	5783		5633	
North West			5210	5395	6260	6189
Yorkshire and Humberside			5414		6539	
West Midlands		Midlands and East Anglia	5602		6653	
East Midlands			5765	5578	7315	6633
East Anglia			5161		5485	
Wales		Wales and the South West	5736		5093	
South West			3828	4437	4201	4552
G.L.C.		London and the South East	2682		4829	
South East			3717	3159	5511	5207
Wales		Wales	5736	5736	5093	5093

* General Dental Service
† Pupils at 1st January 1973, whole time dentist equivalents at 31st December 1972

The practising dentist sees in a clinical setting the dental situation that we have
described from the survey results. He is making his patients reasonably dentally
fit or relieving pain in situations of emergency. Since even among the children
who are regular attenders we found that nearly half had some current decay it is
not surprising that the dentist's time is fully taken up with the treatment
requirements of the children already on his books.

Without the information which a survey can provide it is very difficult to tell
what proportion of children are repeatedly dropping through the protective net of
restorative dentistry. Among fourteen year olds 12% were said not to have seen a
dentist in the previous two years and their restorative experience was very limited
compared to other groups of children. It is, on the other hand, encouraging to see
that among the 21% of fourteen year olds who have been to the dentist fairly
recently although prompted by dental trouble or a note, eight out of ten have some

filled teeth and are therefore receiving care and attention despite their attitudes
and backgrounds.

Many of the policies which have attempted to tackle the problems of scarce resources
have advocated limiting restorative dentistry to those children who demonstrate
favourable dental attitudes and behaviour. Any assessment of priorities on this
basis accentuates the marked division in dental attitudes thus perpetuating the
limited expectations that some sections of the community have of dental health.
The problem for the future, which is by no means a new one, is how to reduce disease
and how to increase treatment resources in order to provide the full amount of
restorative treatment shown to be needed among children.

Part IV

Table section

Table Section Contents

Table 1   Number of deciduous teeth present,
           for children of different ages

England and Wales

Number of deciduous teeth present	Age at 31 December 1972										
	5+	6+	7+	8+	9+	10+	11+	12+	13+	14+	15+
	%	%	%	%	%	%	%	%	%	%	%
0	-	-	-	-	6	19	46	67	85	95	97
1	-	-	-	1	2	7	11	12	7	3	2
2	-	-	-	2	5	8	10	6	4	1	1
3	-	-	-	1	4	7	6	5	2	1	-
4	-	-	1	4	6	8	6	3	1	-	-
5	-	-	1	3	6	7	5	2	1	-	-
6	-	-	2	7	8	8	4	2	-	-	-
7	-	1	3	6	9	6	3	1	-	-	-
8	-	1	6	10	11	8	4	1	-	-	-
9	-	1	6	8	9	6	2	1	-	-	-
10	1	3	8	13	9	5	1	-	-	-	-
11	-	2	8	9	8	4	1	-	-	-	-
12	1	8	24	24	15	7	1	-	-	-	-
13	1	6	8	4	2	-	-	-	-	-	-
14	3	10	11	4	-	-	-	-	-	-	-
15	3	8	6	1	-	-	-	-	-	-	-
16	4	10	6	2	-	-	-	-	-	-	-
17	6	10	3	-	-	-	-	-	-	-	-
18	15	20	5	1	-	-	-	-	-	-	-
19	11	6	1	-	-	-	-	-	-	-	-
20	55	14	1	-	-	-	-	-	-	-	-
	100	100	100	100	100	100	100	100	100	100	100
Average	18.7	15.9	12.2	9.6	7.5	5.0	2.3	0.9	0.4	0.1	0.0
Base	952	1080	1137	1091	1129	1092	986	956	915	923	696

Table 2 Number of permanent teeth erupted, for children of different ages

England and Wales

Number of permanent teeth erupted	Age at 31 December 1972										
	5+	6+	7+	8+	9+	10+	11+	12+	13+	14+	15+
	%	%	%	%	%	%	%	%	%	%	%
0	58	12	1	-	-	-	-	-	-	-	-
1	9	5	1	-	-	-	-	-	-	-	-
2	9	7	1	-	-	-	-	-	-	-	-
3	6	6	1	-	-	-	-	-	-	-	-
4	7	8	2	-	-	-	-	-	-	-	-
5	3	8	2	1	-	-	-	-	-	-	-
6	5	20	9	1	-	-	-	-	-	-	-
7	1	7	5	2	-	-	-	-	-	-	-
8	1	7	10	4	1	-	-	-	-	-	-
9	-	6	10	4	1	-	-	-	-	-	-
10	1	11	26	15	3	-	-	-	-	-	-
11	-	1	10	8	4	1	-	-	-	-	-
12	-	2	19	42	32	15	3	-	-	-	-
13	-	-	2	9	13	8	2	-	-	-	-
14	-	-	1	7	10	9	4	1	-	-	-
15	-	-	-	3	8	8	4	1	-	-	-
16	-	-	-	1	7	8	5	1	-	-	-
17	-	-	-	2	4	6	4	2	1	-	-
18	-	-	-	1	3	7	4	2	-	-	-
19	-	-	-	-	4	5	4	2	1	-	-
20	-	-	-	-	3	5	5	2	1	-	-
21	-	-	-	-	1	4	4	3	1	-	-
22	-	-	-	-	2	5	6	3	2	-	-
23	-	-	-	-	1	3	6	4	2	-	-
24	-	-	-	-	2	5	7	7	4	2	1
25	-	-	-	-	1	4	7	7	4	2	1
26	-	-	-	-	-	3	11	11	8	6	4
27	-	-	-	-	-	2	7	12	12	10	7
28	-	-	-	-	-	2	17	42	64	79	85
29	-	-	-	-	-	-	-	-	-	1	2
30	-	-	-	-	-	-	-	-	-	-	-
31	-	-	-	-	-	-	-	-	-	-	-
32	-	-	-	-	-	-	-	-	-	-	-
	100	100	100	100	100	100	100	100	100	100	100
Average	1.4	5.3	9.2	11.8	14.4	17.7	22.2	25.4	26.9	27.6	27.8
Base	952	1080	1137	1091	1129	1092	986	956	915	923	696

Table 3   Average number of teeth with known decay
experience for children of different ages,
showing type of treatment and dentition

England and Wales

Average number of teeth with known decay experience	Age at 31 December 1972										
	5+	6+	7+	8+	9+	10+	11+	12+	13+	14+	15+
Deciduous											
df	3.3	3.6	3.4	3.3	2.8	1.9	1.0	0.4	0.2	0.0	0.0
d	2.6	2.5	2.3	2.0	1.6	1.2	0.6	0.2	0.1	0.0	0.0
f	0.7	1.0	1.1	1.2	1.1	0.7	0.4	0.2	0.0	0.0	0.0
Permanent											
DMF	0.0	0.3	0.8	1.7	2.2	3.0	3.9	4.8	6.1	7.4	8.4
D	0.0	0.2	0.5	0.8	0.8	1.0	1.3	1.4	1.6	1.9	1.6
M	0.0	0.0	0.0	0.1	0.1	0.3	0.4	0.5	0.6	0.8	0.8
F	0.0	0.1	0.3	0.9	1.2	1.7	2.2	2.9	3.8	4.8	6.0
Both											
DMF + df	3.4	3.9	4.3	5.0	5.0	4.9	4.9	5.2	6.2	7.4	8.4
D+d	2.6	2.7	2.8	2.8	2.5	2.1	1.9	1.7	1.7	1.9	1.6
M	0.0	0.0	0.0	0.1	0.1	0.3	0.4	0.5	0.6	0.8	0.8
F+f	0.7	1.1	1.5	2.1	2.4	2.4	2.6	3.0	3.9	4.8	6.0
Base	*952*	*1080*	*1137*	*1091*	*1129*	*1092*	*986*	*956*	*915*	*923*	*696*

237

Table 4   Distribution of the number of teeth with known decay experience, for children of different ages (DMF + df)

Number of teeth with known decay experience	Age at 31 December 1972										
	5+	6+	7+	8+	9+	10+	11+	12+	13+	14+	15+
	%	%	%	%	%	%	%	%	%	%	%
0	29	21	14	9	7	7	5	5	5	4	3
1	12	10	10	7	6	5	5	5	4	3	3
2	11	12	8	9	9	7	7	7	7	4	3
3	8	9	10	10	11	11	10	9	8	5	4
4	9	10	12	11	13	19	21	20	14	11	7
5	8	9	12	12	12	12	14	14	12	9	8
6	7	8	10	11	12	13	13	11	12	10	9
7	4	8	8	11	9	9	8	9	10	10	9
8	4	5	6	7	8	7	8	6	6	9	9
9	2	3	4	5	6	5	4	4	6	8	9
10	2	2	3	4	4	2	2	3	3	5	7
11	1	1	1	2	2	2	1	2	4	5	6
12	1	1	1	2	1	1	1	2	2	5	7
13	-	1	1	-	-	-	1	1	3	3	4
14	1	-	-	-	-	-	-	1	1	2	3
15	-	-	-	-	-	-	-	-	2	2	2
16	⎫	-	-	-	-	-	-	-	1	2	2
17	⎬ 1	-	-	-	-	-	-	-	-	1	2
18	⎭	-	-	-	-	-	-	1	-	1	1
19	-	-	-	-	-	-	-	-	-	-	1
20	-	-	-	-	-	-	-	-	-	1	1
	100	100	100	100	100	100	100	100	100	100	100
Base	952	1080	1137	1091	1129	1092	986	956	915	923	696

Table 5 Distribution of the number of teeth in both dentitions, which are decayed, missing or filled, for children of different ages (D+d, M, F+f)

England and Wales

Number of teeth	Age at 31 December 1972										
	5+	6+	7+	8+	9+	10+	11+	12+	13+	14+	15+
Decayed (D+d)	%	%	%	%	%	%	%	%	%	%	%
0	37	31	27	22	24	31	34	39	39	38	43
1	14	16	17	18	19	19	19	22	23	20	21
2	12	13	10	14	16	16	16	14	14	14	12
3	7	9	11	13	13	11	11	9	7	8	9
4	7	8	8	10	10	9	7	6	6	6	5
5	6	6	9	7	6	6	6	4	4	5	3
6	5	5	5	6	4	3	4	2	2	3	3
7	3	4	5	3	3	2	2	2	2	1	2
8	3	3	3	2	2	1	1	1	1	2	-
9	1	2	2	2	1	1	-	-	1	1	-
10	2	1	1	1	1	1	-	1	1	1	1
11+	3	2	2	2	1	-	-	-	-	1	1
	100	100	100	100	100	100	100	100	100	100	100
Missing (M)											
0	100	100	99	96	92	87	82	77	72	69	67
1	-	-	1	2	4	5	7	8	10	10	11
2	-	-	-	2	3	4	6	7	9	9	9
3	-	-	-	-	-	1	1	2	3	3	4
4	-	-	-	-	1	3	4	6	6	7	7
5	-	-	-	-	-	-	-	-	-	1	1
6	-	-	-	-	-	-	-	-	-	-	-
7	-	-	-	-	-	-	-	-	-	1	1
8+	-	-	-	-	-	-	-	-	-	-	-
	100	100	100	100	100	100	100	100	100	100	100
Filled (F+f)											
0	74	61	53	43	36	33	30	24	23	19	13
1	10	12	13	10	13	10	12	11	8	9	6
2	6	9	10	11	11	11	11	13	11	7	6
3	4	5	7	9	12	13	11	13	11	9	6
4	3	6	6	11	10	14	14	16	12	9	9
5	2	3	5	5	6	7	9	7	9	8	8
6	-	2	3	4	4	5	5	6	8	9	8
7	1	1	1	3	4	3	3	4	4	6	9
8	-	1	1	1	2	1	2	2	3	6	9
9	-	-	1	1	1	1	1	1	3	5	7
10	-	-	-	1	1	1	1	1	3	3	5
11	-	-	-	1	-	1	-	1	2	3	4
12	-	-	-	-	-	-	1	1	1	3	3
13	-	-	-	-	-	-	-	-	-	1	2
14	-	-	-	-	-	-	-	-	1	1	1
15	-	-	-	-	-	-	-	-	-	1	2
16	-	-	-	-	-	-	-	-	1	1	1
17+	-	-	-	-	-	-	-	-	1	-	1
	100	100	100	100	100	100	100	100	100	100	100
Base	952	1080	1137	1091	1129	1092	986	956	915	923	696

Table 6   Distribution of the number of permanent teeth with decay experience, for children of different ages (DMF)

England and Wales

Number of permanent teeth that are, or have been decayed	Age at 31 December 1972										
	5+	6+	7+	8+	9+	10+	11+	12+	13+	14+	15+
	%	%	%	%	%	%	%	%	%	%	%
0	97	84	61	35	26	15	10	7	5	4	3
1	2	8	15	16	13	9	7	6	5	3	3
2	1	4	11	14	15	12	9	8	7	4	3
3	-	2	5	13	14	14	13	10	8	6	4
4	-	2	7	20	28	39	33	26	16	11	7
5	-	-	1	1	3	5	9	10	10	9	8
6	-	-	-	1	1	3	6	9	11	10	9
7	-	-	-	-	-	2	5	7	9	9	9
8	-	-	-	-	-	1	4	5	7	9	9
9	-	-	-	-	-	-	2	3	5	8	9
10	-	-	-	-	-	-	1	3	4	5	7
11	-	-	-	-	-	-	1	2	4	5	6
12	-	-	-	-	-	-	-	1	2	5	7
13	-	-	-	-	-	-	-	1	3	3	4
14	-	-	-	-	-	-	-	1	1	2	3
15	-	-	-	-	-	-	-	-	2	2	2
16	-	-	-	-	-	-	-	-	1	2	2
17	-	-	-	-	-	-	-	1	-	1	2
18	-	-	-	-	-	-	-	-	-	1	1
19	-	-	-	-	-	-	-	-	-	-	-
20	-	-	-	-	-	-	-	-	-	1	2
	100	100	100	100	100	100	100	100	100	100	100
Base	952	1080	1137	1091	1129	1092	986	956	915	923	696

Table 7 Distribution of the number of permanent teeth which are decayed, missing or filled for children of different ages (D,M,F)

England and Wales

Number of permanent teeth	Age at 31 December 1972										
	5+	6+	7+	8+	9+	10+	11+	12+	13+	14+	15+
	%	%	%	%	%	%	%	%	%	%	%
Decayed (D) 0	97	88	73	60	58	54	47	46	42	39	43
1	2	7	13	19	19	21	19	20	22	21	21
2	1	3	8	10	13	12	13	13	14	14	12
3	–	1	3	6	6	6	9	8	7	8	9
4	–	1	3	4	4	5	6	5	5	6	5
5	–	–	–	1	–	1	3	3	4	4	3
6	–	–	–	–	–	1	1	2	2	3	3
7	–	–	–	–	–	–	1	1	1	1	2
8	–	–	–	–	–	–	1	1	1	1	–
9	–	–	–	–	–	–	–	–	1	1	–
10	–	–	–	–	–	–	–	1	1	1	1
11+	–	–	–	–	–	–	–	–	–	1	1
	100	100	100	100	100	100	100	100	100	100	100
Missing (M) 0	100	100	99	96	92	87	82	77	72	69	67
1	–	–	1	2	4	5	7	8	10	10	11
2	–	–	–	2	3	4	6	7	9	9	9
3	–	–	–	–	–	1	1	2	3	3	4
4	–	–	–	–	1	3	4	6	6	7	7
5	–	–	–	–	–	–	–	–	–	1	1
6	–	–	–	–	–	–	–	–	–	} 1	} 1
7	–	–	–	–	–	–	–	–	–	}	}
8+	–	–	–	–	–	–	–	–	–	–	–
	100	100	100	100	100	100	100	100	100	100	100
Filled (F) 0	100	95	83	63	50	39	34	25	23	19	12
1	–	2	7	11	13	10	12	11	8	9	6
2	–	1	5	9	13	16	13	14	11	8	6
3	–	1	2	7	11	15	12	13	11	9	6
4	–	1	3	10	12	18	18	18	12	9	9
5	–	–	–	–	1	2	4	5	9	7	9
6	–	–	–	–	–	–	3	4	8	9	8
7	–	–	–	–	–	–	1	4	4	6	9
8	–	–	–	–	–	–	1	2	3	6	9
9	–	–	–	–	–	–	1	1	3	5	7
10	–	–	–	–	–	–	1	1	3	3	5
11	–	–	–	–	–	–	–	1	2	3	4
12	–	–	–	–	–	–	–	1	1	3	3
13	–	–	–	–	–	–	–	–	–	1	2
14	–	–	–	–	–	–	–	–	1	1	1
15	–	–	–	–	–	–	–	–	–	1	2
16	–	–	–	–	–	–	–	–	–	1	1
17+	–	–	–	–	–	–	–	–	1	–	1
	100	100	100	100	100	100	100	100	100	100	100
Base	*952*	*1080*	*1137*	*1091*	*1129*	*1092*	*986*	*956*	*915*	*923*	*696*

241

Table 8 — Distribution of the number of deciduous teeth, which are decayed or filled, for children of different ages (df, d, f)

England and Wales

Number of deciduous teeth		Age at 31 December 1972										
		5+	6+	7+	8+	9+	10+	11+	12+	13+	14+	15+
		%	%	%	%	%	%	%	%	%	%	%
Decayed or filled (df)	0	29	21	17	15	19	37	57	79	90	97	99
	1	12	11	11	12	15	14	16	11	7	2	1
	2	11	12	12	15	18	16	11	6	2	1	-
	3	8	10	14	16	12	12	7	3	1	-	-
	4	9	12	12	15	14	9	5	1	-	-	-
	5	8	10	12	9	10	6	2	-	-	-	-
	6	7	8	9	8	6	3	2	-	-	-	-
	7	4	6	6	5	4	2	-	-	-	-	-
	8	4	5	4	4	2	1	-	-	-	-	-
	9	2	2	2	1	-	-	-	-	-	-	-
	10	2	2	1	-	-	-	-	-	-	-	-
	11	1	1	-	-	-	-	-	-	-	-	-
	12	1	-	-	-	-	-	-	-	-	-	-
	13	-	-	-	-	-	-	-	-	-	-	-
	14	1	-	-	-	-	-	-	-	-	-	-
	15+	1	-	-	-	-	-	-	-	-	-	-
		100	100	100	100	100	100	100	100	100	100	100
Decayed (d)	0	37	32	32	28	34	49	68	85	93	98	99
	1	14	16	17	23	24	19	17	10	5	2	1
	2	12	13	11	15	18	14	8	4	2	-	-
	3	7	9	12	15	10	9	4	1	-	-	-
	4	7	8	8	8	6	5	2	-	-	-	-
	5	6	6	8	4	4	3	1	-	-	-	-
	6	5	5	5	4	2	1	-	-	-	-	-
	7	3	4	3	2	1	-	-	-	-	-	-
	8	3	3	2	1	1	-	-	-	-	-	-
	9	1	1	1	-	-	-	-	-	-	-	-
	10	2	1	1	-	-	-	-	-	-	-	-
	11	1	1	-	-	-	-	-	-	-	-	-
	12	1	1	-	-	-	-	-	-	-	-	-
	13	1	-	-	-	-	-	-	-	-	-	-
		100	100	100	100	100	100	100	100	100	100	100
Filled (f)	0	74	62	58	55	56	67	79	90	96	99	99
	1	10	13	13	14	15	13	10	6	3	1	1
	2	6	9	11	11	11	10	6	3	1	-	-
	3	4	5	7	8	7	5	3	1	-	-	-
	4	3	6	5	5	5	2	1	-	-	-	-
	5	2	2	4	3	3	1	1	-	-	-	-
	6	-	1	1	2	2	1	-	-	-	-	-
	7	1	1	1	1	1	1	-	-	-	-	-
	8	-	1	-	1	-	-	-	-	-	-	-
		100	100	100	100	100	100	100	100	100	100	100
Base		952	1080	1137	1091	1129	1092	986	956	915	923	696

Table 9   Average number of teeth with known decay
            experience, for children of different ages,
            showing type of treatment and dentition.

Average number of teeth with known decay experience	Age at 31 December 1972										
	5+	6+	7+	8+	9+	10+	11+	12+	13+	14+	15+
Deciduous											
df	3.2	3.4	3.1	3.0	2.4	1.8	0.9	0.3	0.1	0.0	0.0
d	2.6	2.6	2.4	2.1	1.6	1.2	0.6	0.2	0.1	0.0	0.0
f	0.6	0.8	0.8	0.9	0.8	0.6	0.3	0.1	0.0	0.0	0.0
Permanent											
DMF	0.0	0.3	0.9	1.9	2.3	3.0	3.9	4.6	6.4	7.3	8.6
D	0.0	0.2	0.5	0.9	0.9	1.1	1.5	1.5	1.7	1.9	1.6
M	0.0	0.0	0.0	0.1	0.2	0.4	0.5	0.7	1.0	0.9	1.2
F	0.0	0.1	0.3	0.9	1.1	1.5	2.0	2.5	3.7	4.5	5.8
Both											
DMF + df	3.2	3.7	4.0	4.8	4.7	4.7	4.9	4.9	6.5	7.4	8.6
D+d	2.6	2.8	2.9	3.0	2.5	2.3	2.1	1.6	1.8	2.0	1.6
M	0.0	0.0	0.0	0.1	0.2	0.4	0.5	0.7	1.0	0.9	1.2
F+f	0.6	0.8	1.1	1.7	2.0	2.1	2.3	2.6	3.7	4.5	5.8
Base	*323*	*347*	*390*	*357*	*358*	*362*	*317*	*294*	*285*	*308*	*218*

Table 10   Distribution of the number of teeth with known decay experience, for children of different ages   (DMF + df)

Number of teeth with known decay experience	Age at 31 December 1972										
	5+	6+	7+	8+	9+	10+	11+	12+	13+	14+	15+
	%	%	%	%	%	%	%	%	%	%	%
0	28	25	14	9	6	7	5	6	4	4	3
1	13	9	11	7	6	5	5	5	4	4	2
2	11	10	9	9	10	8	7	9	8	5	3
3	8	9	13	10	13	10	7	10	8	6	5
4	11	8	12	13	15	19	24	22	13	11	8
5	7	8	13	10	13	16	17	13	11	12	6
6	5	9	9	13	12	12	13	8	13	8	7
7	3	8	7	11	9	7	8	11	10	8	8
8	6	6	5	7	6	7	7	5	7	8	10
9	3	4	3	4	4	4	2	3	5	8	10
10	2	1	2	2	3	2	1	3	2	5	6
11	2	1	1	3	1	2	1	2	4	4	6
12	-	1	1	1	1	1	1	1	2	5	6
13	-	-	-	1	-	-	1	1	3	3	5
14	1	1	-	-	1	-	1	-	2	1	4
15	-	-	-	-	-	-	-	-	2	3	3
16	-	-	-	-	-	-	-	-	-	3	2
17	-	-	-	-	-	-	-	1	-	1	2
18	-	-	-	-	-	-	-	-	1	1	1
19	-	-	-	-	-	-	-	-	1	-	1
20	-	-	-	-	-	-	-	-	1	-	-
21	-	-	-	-	-	-	-	-	-	-	-
22	-	-	-	-	-	-	-	-	-	-	1
23+	-	-	-	-	-	-	-	-	-	-	1
	100	100	100	100	100	100	100	100	100	100	100
Base	*323*	*347*	*390*	*357*	*358*	*362*	*317*	*294*	*285*	*308*	*218*

Table 11 Distribution of the number of teeth in both
dentitions, which are decayed, missing or filled,
for children of different ages (D+d, M, F+f)

North

Number of teeth	Age at 31 December 1972										
	5+	6+	7+	8+	9+	10+	11+	12+	13+	14+	15+
	%	%	%	%	%	%	%	%	%	%	%
Decayed (D+d) 0	37	33	26	20	24	28	34	40	36	35	44
1	14	13	16	19	18	17	18	21	23	19	19
2	10	12	12	13	16	18	14	14	14	16	14
3	8	7	11	12	13	12	10	7	9	11	7
4	8	8	8	10	12	9	9	7	8	6	7
5	5	6	10	7	7	6	8	6	4	5	3
6	5	7	7	8	4	2	3	1	2	3	1
7	3	5	4	4	2	3	3	2	2	2	4
8	4	4	3	3	2	3	1	1	-	2	1
9	2	1	1	2	1	1	-	1	1	-	-
10	1	1	1	-	1	1	-	-	-	-	-
11+	3	3	1	2	-	-	-	-	1	1	-
	100	100	100	100	100	100	100	100	100	100	100
Missing (M) 0	100	100	98	94	88	83	78	74	61	63	57
1	-	-	2	4	5	6	9	8	11	12	13
2	-	-	-	2	5	7	7	8	13	11	9
3	-	-	-	-	1	-	1	3	4	2	6
4	-	-	-	-	1	4	5	7	9	11	11
5	-	-	-	-	-	-	-	-	-	1	2
6	-	-	-	-	-	-	-	-	1	-	1
7	-	-	-	-	-	-	-	-	-	-	1
8+	-	-	-	-	-	-	-	-	1	-	-
	100	100	100	100	100	100	100	100	100	100	100
Filled (F+f) 0	76	70	66	51	42	41	37	31	26	21	15
1	12	11	11	10	13	9	11	11	7	11	6
2	4	6	6	10	10	12	12	14	12	9	8
3	3	4	5	7	12	13	9	10	10	10	7
4	2	3	5	9	10	12	14	14	11	7	7
5	1	2	3	4	4	5	8	5	9	6	7
6	-	2	2	3	4	3	4	5	7	7	6
7	1	-	2	3	2	2	2	4	5	3	8
8	1	1	-	1	1	1	2	3	2	8	8
9	-	1	-	1	1	-	1	1	2	5	8
10	-	-	-	-	1	1	-	1	2	3	6
11	-	-	-	1	-	1	-	-	3	3	3
12	-	-	-	-	-	-	-	1	1	4	3
13	-	-	-	-	-	-	-	-	1	1	3
14	-	-	-	-	-	-	-	-	1	-	2
15	-	-	-	-	-	-	-	-	-	1	2
16	-	-	-	-	-	-	-	-	-	1	-
17+	-	-	-	-	-	-	-	-	1	-	1
	100	100	100	100	100	100	100	100	100	100	100
Base	*323*	*347*	*390*	*357*	*358*	*362*	*317*	*294*	*285*	*308*	*218*

Table 12   Distribution of the number of permanent
            teeth with decay experience for children
            of different ages   (DMF)

North

Number of permanent teeth that are, or have been decayed	Age at 31 December 1972										
	5+	6+	7+	8+	9+	10+	11+	12+	13+	14+	15+
	%	%	%	%	%	%	%	%	%	%	%
0	96	84	60	33	25	16	8	8	4	4	3
1	3	8	16	16	11	9	8	7	3	4	2
2	1	4	11	13	16	11	9	8	8	5	4
3	-	3	6	12	15	14	13	9	8	6	4
4	-	1	7	24	28	40	35	26	16	12	8
5	-	-	-	2	3	5	10	11	10	10	6
6	-	-	-	-	2	2	6	9	12	8	7
7	-	-	-	-	-	1	5	8	9	8	9
8	-	-	-	-	-	1	4	4	7	9	10
9	-	-	-	-	-	1	2	3	5	7	10
10	-	-	-	-	-	-	-	2	3	5	6
11	-	-	-	-	-	-	-	3	3	4	6
12	-	-	-	-	-	-	-	-	2	5	6
13	-	-	-	-	-	-	-	1	3	3	5
14	-	-	-	-	-	-	-	-	2	1	4
15	-	-	-	-	-	-	-	-	2	3	3
16	-	-	-	-	-	-	-	-	-	3	2
17	-	-	-	-	-	-	-	1	-	1	2
18	-	-	-	-	-	-	-	-	1	1	1
19	-	-	-	-	-	-	-	-	1	-	1
20	-	-	-	-	-	-	-	-	-	1	-
21	-	-	-	-	-	-	-	-	-	-	-
22	-	-	-	-	-	-	-	-	-	-	1
23+	-	-	-	-	-	-	-	-	1	-	-
	100	100	100	100	100	100	100	100	100	100	100
Base	*323*	*347*	*390*	*357*	*358*	*362*	*317*	*294*	*285*	*308*	*218*

Table 13 — Distribution of the number of permanent teeth which are decayed, missing or filled for children of different ages (D, M, F)

Number of permanent teeth	Age at 31 December 1972										
	5+	6+	7+	8+	9+	10+	11+	12+	13+	14+	15+
	%	%	%	%	%	%	%	%	%	%	%
Decayed (D) 0	96	88	70	55	55	48	44	45	38	35	44
1	3	8	14	20	18	23	21	20	22	20	19
2	1	2	10	12	14	14	13	13	13	16	14
3	-	1	3	6	9	7	8	7	10	10	6
4	-	1	3	6	4	6	8	6	7	6	7
5	-	-	-	1	-	1	3	5	3	4	3
6	-	-	-	-	-	1	1	1	2	3	1
7	-	-	-	-	-	-	2	1	1	2	4
8	-	-	-	-	-	-	-	-	1	2	1
9	-	-	-	-	-	-	-	1	1	-	1
10	-	-	-	-	-	-	-	-	-	-	-
11+	-	-	-	-	-	-	-	-	2	2	-
	100	100	100	100	100	100	100	100	100	100	100
Missing (M) 0	100	100	98	94	88	83	78	74	61	63	57
1	-	-	2	4	5	6	9	8	11	12	13
2	-	-	-	2	5	7	7	8	13	11	9
3	-	-	-	-	1	-	1	3	4	2	6
4	-	-	-	-	1	4	5	7	9	11	11
5	-	-	-	-	-	-	-	-	-	1	2
6	-	-	-	-	-	-	-	-	1	-	1
7	-	-	-	-	-	-	-	-	-	-	1
8+	-	-	-	-	-	-	-	-	1	-	-
	100	100	100	100	100	100	100	100	100	100	100
Filled (F) 0	100	95	87	65	56	47	39	32	27	21	15
1	-	2	6	10	10	8	11	11	7	11	6
2	-	2	3	10	11	14	14	15	12	9	8
3	-	1	1	6	12	13	10	10	10	10	7
4	-	-	3	9	10	17	16	15	10	7	7
5	-	-	-	-	1	1	5	4	9	6	7
6	-	-	-	-	-	-	3	4	7	7	6
7	-	-	-	-	-	-	1	3	5	3	8
8	-	-	-	-	-	-	1	3	2	8	8
9	-	-	-	-	-	-	-	1	2	5	8
10	-	-	-	-	-	-	-	1	2	3	6
11	-	-	-	-	-	-	-	-	3	3	3
12	-	-	-	-	-	-	-	1	1	4	3
13	-	-	-	-	-	-	-	-	1	1	3
14	-	-	-	-	-	-	-	-	1	-	2
15	-	-	-	-	-	-	-	-	-	1	2
16	-	-	-	-	-	-	-	-	-	1	-
17+	-	-	-	-	-	-	-	-	1	-	1
	100	100	100	100	100	100	100	100	100	100	100
Base	323	347	390	357	358	362	317	294	285	308	218

247

Table 14 Distribution of the number of deciduous teeth, which are decayed or filled, for children of different ages (df,d,f)

North

Number of deciduous teeth	Age at 31 December 1972										
	5+	6+	7+	8+	9+	10+	11+	12+	13+	14+	15+
	%	%	%	%	%	%	%	%	%	%	%
Decayed or filled (df) 0	29	26	16	16	21	39	60	84	93	97	99
1	13	11	14	10	19	15	15	9	5	2	1
2	11	10	13	16	17	15	12	3	2	1	-
3	8	9	17	21	13	13	5	3	-	-	-
4	11	9	12	16	14	9	3	1	-	-	-
5	7	11	12	8	9	4	2	-	-	-	-
6	6	8	7	6	3	2	2	-	-	-	-
7	3	6	3	4	2	2	-	-	-	-	-
8	5	4	4	2	1	1	1	-	-	-	-
9	2	3	1	1	-	-	-	-	-	-	-
10	2	2	1	-	1	-	-	-	-	-	-
11	1	1	-	-	-	-	-	-	-	-	-
12	-	-	-	-	-	-	-	-	-	-	-
13	-	-	-	-	-	-	-	-	-	-	-
14	1	-	-	-	-	-	-	-	-	-	-
15+	1	-	-	-	-	-	-	-	-	-	-
	100	100	100	100	100	100	100	100	100	100	100
Decayed (d) 0	38	35	30	27	34	49	70	88	92	98	99
1	14	14	16	20	26	18	14	9	5	2	1
2	10	12	13	17	18	14	9	2	2	-	-
3	8	6	14	15	9	9	2	1	1	-	-
4	8	8	7	10	6	5	2	-	-	-	-
5	5	8	8	4	4	2	2	-	-	-	-
6	5	6	6	4	1	1	1	-	-	-	-
7	3	4	2	2	-	1	-	-	-	-	-
8	3	3	3	1	1	1	-	-	-	-	-
9	1	1	-	-	-	-	-	-	-	-	-
10	1	2	1	-	1	-	-	-	-	-	-
11	1	1	-	-	-	-	-	-	-	-	-
12	1	-	-	-	-	-	-	-	-	-	-
13	2	-	-	-	-	-	-	-	-	-	-
	100	100	100	100	100	100	100	100	100	100	100
Filled (f) 0	76	71	70	65	65	75	84	92	99	99	100
1	12	12	10	11	13	11	9	5	1	1	-
2	4	6	7	10	10	6	4	2	-	-	-
3	4	3	6	6	6	3	1	1	-	-	-
4	2	4	3	4	3	1	1	-	-	-	-
5	1	2	4	1	1	1	1	-	-	-	-
6	-	1	-	2	2	1	-	-	-	-	-
7	1	-	-	1	-	1	-	-	-	-	-
8	-	1	-	-	-	1	-	-	-	-	-
	100	100	100	100	100	100	100	100	100	100	100
Base	323	347	390	357	358	362	317	294	285	308	218

Table 15   Average number of teeth with known decay
experience, for children of different ages,
showing type of treatment and dentition

Midlands and East Anglia

Average number of teeth with known decay experience	Age at 31 December 1972										
	5+	6+	7+	8+	9+	10+	11+	12+	13+	14+	15+
Deciduous											
df	3.5	3.1	3.5	3.0	2.5	1.5	1.0	0.5	0.2	0.1	0.0
d	3.1	2.5	2.5	2.1	1.7	1.1	0.6	0.3	0.1	0.0	0.0
f	0.4	0.6	1.0	0.9	0.8	0.4	0.3	0.2	0.0	0.0	0.0
Permanent											
DMF	0.0	0.3	0.9	1.7	2.1	3.0	3.7	4.9	5.7	6.9	8.4
D	0.0	0.2	0.6	1.0	1.0	1.1	1.5	1.6	1.9	2.1	1.9
M	0.0	0.0	0.0	0.0	0.1	0.3	0.5	0.6	0.7	0.9	1.1
F	0.0	0.1	0.3	0.8	1.0	1.6	1.7	2.6	3.1	3.9	5.4
Both											
DMF + df	3.5	3.4	4.4	4.8	4.6	4.5	4.7	5.4	5.9	7.0	8.4
D+d	3.1	2.7	3.1	3.1	2.7	2.2	2.1	2.0	2.0	2.1	1.9
M	0.0	0.0	0.0	0.0	0.1	0.3	0.5	0.6	0.7	0.9	1.1
F+f	0.4	0.7	1.2	1.7	1.8	2.0	2.1	2.8	3.1	4.0	5.4
Base	200	224	221	224	223	213	195	182	194	207	130

Table 16   Distribution of the number of teeth with known decay experience for children of different ages   (DMF + df)

Midlands and East Anglia

Number of teeth with known decay experience	Age at 31 December 1972										
	5+	6+	7+	8+	9+	10+	11+	12+	13+	14+	15+
	%	%	%	%	%	%	%	%	%	%	%
0	26	20	14	8	11	8	5	4	3	5	5
1	12	11	12	5	8	6	6	6	7	4	2
2	12	14	6	13	11	7	8	8	8	5	5
3	8	12	11	12	9	14	15	12	8	6	3
4	9	11	11	9	11	21	18	19	12	11	5
5	4	12	10	17	12	9	14	17	16	9	5
6	10	6	8	9	11	12	11	6	10	11	10
7	6	5	10	9	5	11	5	6	7	9	6
8	2	3	5	7	9	6	10	7	8	7	11
9	1	2	5	4	7	3	3	3	7	7	10
10	4	1	3	3	2	1	1	3	3	7	5
11	1	2	2	1	3	1	2	3	6	5	8
12	1	1	1	2	1	1	2	3	1	5	9
13	2	-	1	-	-	-	-	1	2	2	2
14	1	-	1	-	-	-	-	1	2	2	1
15	1	-	-	1	-	-	-	-	-	1	2
16	-	-	-	-	-	-	-	-	-	-	4
17	-	-	-	-	-	-	-	1	-	1	2
18	-	-	-	-	-	-	-	-	-	1	1
19	-	-	-	-	-	-	-	-	-	-	1
20	-	-	-	-	-	-	-	-	-	-	-
21	-	-	-	-	-	-	-	-	-	-	1
22	-	-	-	-	-	-	-	-	-	-	-
23+	-	-	-	-	-	-	-	-	-	-	2
	100	100	100	100	100	100	100	100	100	100	100
Base	200	224	221	224	223	213	195	182	194	207	130

Table 17   Distribution of the number of teeth in both
            dentitions, which are decayed, missing or filled,
            for children of different ages (D+d,M,F+f)

Midlands and East Anglia

Number of teeth	Age at 31 December 1972										
	5+	6+	7+	8+	9+	10+	11+	12+	13+	14+	15+
	%	%	%	%	%	%	%	%	%	%	%
Decayed (D+d) 0	29	28	26	16	21	31	26	33	34	39	33
1	16	17	15	17	17	18	24	25	22	23	25
2	14	11	9	16	18	15	16	15	16	11	15
3	8	10	12	15	15	12	10	12	10	6	8
4	6	11	9	12	10	9	9	5	3	4	5
5	6	7	9	9	7	6	8	1	5	6	4
6	10	4	3	5	3	5	3	2	4	3	5
7	4	6	7	4	4	2	2	3	2	1	2
8	2	2	4	2	2	1	2	1	1	1	1
9	1	1	2	2	1	1	-	-	1	3	-
10	3	1	1	2	1	-	-	2	2	1	1
11+	1	2	3	-	1	-	-	1	-	2	1
	100	100	100	100	100	100	100	100	100	100	100
Missing (M) 0	100	100	98	96	95	85	77	72	66	62	60
1	-	-	1	3	2	6	8	10	15	13	11
2	-	-	1	1	2	4	8	10	8	11	11
3	-	-	-	-	1	-	2	2	4	4	7
4	-	-	-	-	-	5	5	6	6	8	8
5	-	-	-	-	-	-	-	-	1	1	1
6	-	-	-	-	-	-	-	-	-	1	1
7	-	-	-	-	-	-	-	-	-	-	-
8+	-	-	-	-	-	-	-	-	-	-	1
	100	100	100	100	100	100	100	100	100	100	100
Filled (F+f) 0	82	70	55	50	45	40	39	28	34	29	19
1	7	13	19	10	12	11	13	15	7	9	7
2	4	8	9	10	12	13	13	9	12	9	5
3	2	4	6	10	11	12	11	14	9	10	5
4	2	3	4	9	8	12	8	14	9	10	9
5	1	1	2	5	5	5	6	6	8	6	6
6	1	-	2	2	1	3	6	4	5	9	9
7	-	1	1	2	3	2	2	4	4	6	12
8	1	-	-	-	3	1	1	3	4	5	7
9	-	-	-	-	-	-	1	2	4	4	7
10	-	-	1	1	-	-	-	-	2	2	3
11	-	-	1	1	-	-	-	1	2	2	4
12	-	-	-	-	-	-	-	-	-	2	2
13	-	-	-	-	-	-	-	-	-	1	-
14	-	-	-	-	-	-	-	-	-	1	1
15	-	-	-	-	-	-	-	-	-	-	2
16	-	-	-	-	-	-	-	-	-	-	2
17+	-	-	-	-	-	-	-	-	-	-	-
	100	100	100	100	100	100	100	100	100	100	100
Base	*200*	*224*	*221*	*224*	*223*	*213*	*195*	*182*	*194*	*207*	*130*

Table 18   Distribution of the number of permanent teeth with decay experience for children of different ages (DMF)

Midlands and East Anglia

Number of permanent teeth that are, or have been decayed	Age at 31 December 1972										
	5+	6+	7+	8+	9+	10+	11+	12+	13+	14+	15+
	%	%	%	%	%	%	%	%	%	%	%
0	99	81	59	33	27	16	13	9	4	5	5
1	1	13	15	16	16	10	6	6	7	4	2
2	-	4	13	15	16	12	10	7	9	5	5
3	-	1	5	17	12	10	18	14	7	7	3
4	-	1	8	18	22	39	29	26	14	11	5
5	-	-	-	1	4	5	6	9	14	9	5
6	-	-	-	-	1	4	6	5	9	11	10
7	-	-	-	-	1	3	4	4	8	9	6
8	-	-	-	-	1	1	5	6	9	7	11
9	-	-	-	-	-	-	1	2	5	7	10
10	-	-	-	-	-	-	-	3	3	7	6
11	-	-	-	-	-	-	1	3	5	5	8
12	-	-	-	-	-	-	1	3	2	5	8
13	-	-	-	-	-	-	-	1	2	2	2
14	-	-	-	-	-	-	-	1	2	2	1
15	-	-	-	-	-	-	-	-	-	1	2
16	-	-	-	-	-	-	-	-	-	1	4
17	-	-	-	-	-	-	-	1	-	1	2
18	-	-	-	-	-	-	-	-	-	1	1
19	-	-	-	-	-	-	-	-	-	-	1
20	-	-	-	-	-	-	-	-	-	-	-
21	-	-	-	-	-	-	-	-	-	-	1
22	-	-	-	-	-	-	-	-	-	-	-
23+	-	-	-	-	-	-	-	-	-	-	2
	100	100	100	100	100	100	100	100	100	100	100
Base	*200*	*224*	*221*	*224*	*223*	*213*	*195*	*182*	*194*	*207*	*130*

Table 19   Distribution of the number of permanent
teeth which are decayed, missing or filled
for children of different ages   (D,M,F)

Midlands and East Anglia

Number of permanent teeth	Age at 31 December 1972										
	5+	6+	7+	8+	9+	10+	11+	12+	13+	14+	15+
	%	%	%	%	%	%	%	%	%	%	%
Decayed (D) 0	99	84	68	52	50	52	41	46	36	40	33
1	1	12	15	22	22	18	22	20	22	22	25
2	–	4	9	13	16	13	14	11	17	11	15
3	–	–	5	7	7	7	9	10	7	6	8
4	–	–	3	5	3	6	8	4	2	4	5
5	–	–	–	1	1	2	4	1	5	5	4
6	–	–	–	–	–	1	–	1	5	4	4
7	–	–	–	–	1	–	1	3	2	1	3
8	–	–	–	–	–	1	1	1	2	1	–
9	–	–	–	–	–	–	–	–	1	3	1
10	–	–	–	–	–	–	–	2	1	1	1
11+	–	–	–	–	–	–	–	1	–	2	1
	100	100	100	100	100	100	100	100	100	100	100
Missing (M) 0	100	100	98	96	95	85	77	72	66	62	60
1	–	–	1	3	2	6	8	10	15	13	11
2	–	–	1	1	2	4	8	10	8	11	11
3	–	–	–	–	1	–	2	2	4	4	7
4	–	–	–	–	–	5	5	6	6	8	8
5	–	–	–	–	–	–	–	–	1	1	1
6	–	–	–	–	–	–	–	–	–	1	1
7	–	–	–	–	–	–	–	–	–	–	–
8+	–	–	–	–	–	–	–	–	–	–	1
	100	100	100	100	100	100	100	100	100	100	100
Filled (F) 0	100	96	86	68	57	43	43	30	34	24	19
1	–	2	7	11	13	13	14	13	8	9	7
2	–	–	5	6	11	13	12	10	11	9	5
3	–	1	1	7	9	13	12	14	9	11	5
4	–	1	1	8	8	15	9	17	9	10	9
5	–	–	–	–	1	2	4	3	9	5	6
6	–	–	–	–	1	–	3	3	5	9	9
7	–	–	–	–	–	1	1	3	4	6	12
8	–	–	–	–	–	–	1	2	4	5	7
9	–	–	–	–	–	1	1	2	4	4	7
10	–	–	–	–	–	–	–	1	1	2	3
11	–	–	–	–	–	–	–	1	2	2	4
12	–	–	–	–	–	–	–	1	–	2	2
13	–	–	–	–	–	–	–	–	–	1	–
14	–	–	–	–	–	–	–	–	–	1	1
15	–	–	–	–	–	–	–	–	–	–	2
16	–	–	–	–	–	–	–	–	–	–	2
17+	–	–	–	–	–	–	–	–	–	–	–
	100	100	100	100	100	100	100	100	100	100	100
Base	*200*	*224*	*221*	*224*	*223*	*213*	*195*	*182*	*194*	*207*	*130*

Table 20　　Distribution of the number of deciduous teeth which are decayed or filled, for children of different ages　(df,d,f)

Midlands and East Anglia

Number of deciduous teeth	Age at 31 December 1972										
	5+	6+	7+	8+	9+	10+	11+	12+	13+	14+	15+
	%	%	%	%	%	%	%	%	%	%	%
Decayed or filled (df)											
0	26	21	21	14	24	43	57	75	91	96	99
1	13	13	11	15	17	17	17	14	5	3	1
2	12	14	10	18	18	16	10	6	3	-	-
3	8	12	12	16	11	9	6	3	1	1	-
4	9	13	10	11	12	8	8	1	-	-	-
5	5	11	12	9	9	4	1	1	-	-	-
6	10	5	9	8	3	2	1	-	-	-	-
7	6	5	8	5	4	1	-	-	-	-	-
8	2	1	3	3	2	-	-	-	-	-	-
9	1	2	3	-	-	-	-	-	-	-	-
10	5	1	1	-	-	-	-	-	-	-	-
11	1	2	-	1	-	-	-	-	-	-	-
12	1	-	-	-	-	-	-	-	-	-	-
13	1	-	-	-	-	-	-	-	-	-	-
14	-	-	-	-	-	-	-	-	-	-	-
15+	-	-	-	-	-	-	-	-	-	-	-
	100	100	100	100	100	100	100	100	100	100	100
Decayed (d)											
0	29	30	33	24	33	53	65	80	92	97	99
1	16	18	15	24	25	18	21	14	6	2	1
2	14	10	9	17	18	12	7	5	2	-	-
3	8	12	12	15	9	7	4	1	-	1	-
4	6	11	8	9	6	7	3	-	-	-	-
5	7	6	9	4	4	2	-	-	-	-	-
6	9	4	4	5	2	1	-	-	-	-	-
7	4	5	5	1	1	-	-	-	-	-	-
8	2	2	2	1	1	-	-	-	-	-	-
9	1	1	2	-	-	-	-	-	-	-	-
10	3	-	1	-	1	-	-	-	-	-	-
11	-	1	-	-	-	-	-	-	-	-	-
12	-	-	-	-	-	-	-	-	-	-	-
13+	1	-	-	-	-	-	-	-	-	-	-
	100	100	100	100	100	100	100	100	100	100	100
Filled (f)											
0	82	71	60	62	63	76	83	90	97	98	100
1	7	13	17	14	17	14	8	5	2	1	-
2	5	8	10	10	8	5	5	3	1	1	-
3	2	4	4	8	6	3	3	1	-	-	-
4	2	3	4	3	3	1	1	1	-	-	-
5	2	1	1	1	2	1	-	-	-	-	-
6	-	-	1	1	1	-	-	-	-	-	-
7	-	-	2	-	-	-	-	-	-	-	-
8+	-	-	1	1	-	-	-	-	-	-	-
	100	100	100	100	100	100	100	100	100	100	100
Base	*200*	*224*	*221*	*224*	*223*	*213*	*195*	*182*	*194*	*207*	*130*

Table 21   Average number of teeth with known decay
            experience, for children of different ages,
            showing type of treatment and dentition

Average number of teeth with known decay experience	Age at 31 December 1972										
	5+	6+	7+	8+	9+	10+	11+	12+	13+	14+	15+
Deciduous											
df	3.7	4.1	4.0	3.8	3.2	2.3	0.9	0.6	0.1	0.0	0.0
d	2.8	2.7	2.7	2.2	1.9	1.4	0.6	0.3	0.1	0.0	0.0
f	0.9	1.4	1.3	1.6	1.4	0.9	0.4	0.2	0.0	0.0	0.0
Permanent											
DMF	0.0	0.3	1.0	1.7	2.4	3.1	4.4	5.0	6.7	8.5	8.8
D	0.0	0.3	0.6	0.7	0.9	1.0	1.4	1.7	2.2	2.4	1.8
M	0.0	0.0	0.0	0.1	0.2	0.3	0.4	0.6	0.7	1.0	0.8
F	0.0	0.1	0.4	1.0	1.4	1.9	2.5	2.7	3.7	5.2	6.2
Both											
DMF + df	3.8	4.5	5.0	5.5	5.6	5.3	5.3	5.6	6.8	8.5	8.8
D+d	2.9	3.0	3.3	2.9	2.7	2.3	2.0	2.0	2.3	2.4	1.8
M	0.0	0.0	0.0	0.1	0.2	0.3	0.4	0.6	0.7	1.0	0.8
F+f	0.9	1.5	1.7	2.6	2.8	2.8	2.9	3.0	3.8	5.2	6.2
Base	*158*	*168*	*185*	*166*	*169*	*163*	*155*	*160*	*146*	*145*	*111*

Table 22   Distribution of the number of teeth with
known decay experience for children of
different ages   (DMF + df)

Wales and South West

Number of teeth with known decay experience	Age at 31 December 1972										
	5+	6+	7+	8+	9+	10+	11+	12+	13+	14+	15+
	%	%	%	%	%	%	%	%	%	%	%
0	26	12	8	9	7	4	3	3	3	2	2
1	12	10	10	5	6	5	4	4	4	1	3
2	10	11	9	5	7	7	7	5	5	2	2
3	6	8	8	7	6	9	10	8	5	5	3
4	9	13	11	11	12	16	21	18	13	8	8
5	9	8	11	12	10	12	14	15	8	6	8
6	6	8	13	11	11	15	13	12	11	11	6
7	6	11	10	11	10	8	9	12	14	9	8
8	5	9	8	10	13	8	7	6	7	12	10
9	3	3	4	7	8	8	6	7	8	8	8
10	4	3	4	6	6	4	3	4	6	8	11
11	-	2	1	3	2	4	1	3	5	8	5
12	2	1	2	3	2	-	1	1	2	2	9
13	-	1	1	-	-	-	-	1	3	3	4
14	1	-	-	-	-	-	1	-	1	2	4
15	1	-	-	-	-	-	-	-	2	3	-
16	-	-	-	-	-	-	-	-	1	3	2
17	-	-	-	-	-	-	-	1	-	2	2
18	-	-	-	-	-	-	-	-	1	2	1
19	-	-	-	-	-	-	-	-	1	-	2
20	-	-	-	-	-	-	-	-	-	1	1
21	-	-	-	-	-	-	-	-	-	1	1
22	-	-	-	-	-	-	-	-	-	1	-
23+	-	-	-	-	-	-	-	-	-	-	-
	100	100	100	100	100	100	100	100	100	100	100
Base	*158*	*168*	*185*	*166*	*169*	*163*	*155*	*160*	*146*	*145*	*111*

Table 23   Distribution of the number of teeth in both dentitions, which are decayed, missing or filled, for children of different ages (D+d,M,F+f)

Wales and South West

Number of teeth	Age at 31 December 1972										
	5+	6+	7+	8+	9+	10+	11+	12+	13+	14+	15+
	%	%	%	%	%	%	%	%	%	%	%
Decayed (D+d) 0	35	23	20	20	23	27	36	33	31	32	38
1	13	18	17	18	20	17	14	21	22	16	23
2	13	17	9	16	15	17	15	14	14	16	14
3	5	9	14	12	11	13	15	11	10	11	11
4	9	8	8	10	14	10	7	8	8	11	3
5	9	6	8	8	4	9	5	5	6	5	1
6	2	4	8	6	4	4	4	5	3	3	5
7	3	5	6	3	3	2	1	2	1	2	3
8	4	4	3	3	3	1	2	1	1	1	–
9	2	2	2	2	1	–	–	–	1	1	1
10	2	1	1	2	1	–	1	–	1	2	1
11+	3	3	4	–	1	–	–	–	2	–	–
	100	100	100	100	100	100	100	100	100	100	100
Missing (M) 0	100	100	98	97	93	87	81	75	69	66	64
1	–	–	1	1	3	5	7	7	11	8	17
2	–	–	1	2	2	5	6	7	8	11	10
3	–	–	–	–	–	–	1	2	3	4	2
4	–	–	–	–	2	3	5	9	8	7	5
5	–	–	–	–	–	–	–	–	1	2	1
6	–	–	–	–	–	–	–	–	–	–	–
7	–	–	–	–	–	–	–	–	–	1	1
8+	–	–	–	–	–	–	–	–	–	1	–
	100	100	100	100	100	100	100	100	100	100	100
Filled (F+f) 0	70	47	46	35	30	28	23	21	18	16	7
1	9	15	14	10	12	10	12	12	8	8	8
2	6	14	14	12	11	11	13	12	14	8	7
3	5	8	8	7	9	10	9	18	13	7	5
4	4	7	6	15	12	17	18	15	12	6	9
5	2	4	6	4	8	6	11	7	8	12	8
6	1	2	2	7	7	8	6	5	11	10	8
7	1	2	2	3	6	5	5	5	2	8	13
8	1	–	1	2	3	4	1	1	5	5	8
9	1	–	1	2	1	1	1	3	5	3	5
10	–	1	–	2	1	–	1	1	2	3	3
11	–	–	–	1	–	–	–	–	–	1	2
12	–	–	–	–	–	–	–	–	2	2	2
13	–	–	–	–	–	–	–	–	–	2	2
14	–	–	–	–	–	–	–	–	–	2	1
15	–	–	–	–	–	–	–	–	–	1	1
16	–	–	–	–	–	–	–	–	–	2	–
17+	–	–	–	–	–	–	–	–	–	–	2
	100	100	100	100	100	100	100	100	100	100	100
Base	*158*	*168*	*185*	*166*	*169*	*163*	*155*	*160*	*146*	*145*	*111*

Table 24   Distribution of the number of permanent
            teeth with decay experience for children
            of different ages   (DMF)

Number of permanent teeth that are, or have been decayed	Age at 31 December 1972										
	5+	6+	7+	8+	9+	10+	11+	12+	13+	14+	15+
	%	%	%	%	%	%	%	%	%	%	%
0	96	82	52	35	24	13	6	4	3	2	2
1	2	7	20	18	13	10	5	6	5	1	3
2	2	7	16	14	11	12	9	8	5	3	2
3	-	2	4	12	16	13	10	9	4	4	3
4	-	2	8	19	30	39	34	25	15	9	8
5	-	-	-	1	4	6	14	12	7	6	8
6	-	-	-	1	2	5	6	9	14	11	7
7	-	-	-	-	-	1	6	10	11	10	7
8	-	-	-	-	-	1	4	5	6	11	10
9	-	-	-	-	-	-	4	5	8	8	8
10	-	-	-	-	-	-	-	4	7	8	11
11	-	-	-	-	-	-	1	1	5	8	5
12	-	-	-	-	-	-	-	1	2	2	9
13	-	-	-	-	-	-	-	1	3	3	4
14	-	-	-	-	-	-	1	-	1	3	4
15	-	-	-	-	-	-	-	-	1	3	-
16	-	-	-	-	-	-	-	-	1	3	2
17	-	-	-	-	-	-	-	-	-	2	2
18	-	-	-	-	-	-	-	-	1	2	1
19	-	-	-	-	-	-	-	-	1	-	2
20	-	-	-	-	-	-	-	-	-	1	1
21	-	-	-	-	-	-	-	-	-	-	1
22	-	-	-	-	-	-	-	-	-	-	-
23+	-	-	-	-	-	-	-	-	-	-	-
	100	100	100	100	100	100	100	100	100	100	100
Base	*158*	*168*	*185*	*166*	*169*	*163*	*155*	*160*	*146*	*145*	*111*

Table 25   Distribution of the number of permanent
teeth which are decayed, missing or filled,
for children of different ages   (D,M,F)

Wales and South West

Number of permanent teeth	Age at 31 December 1972										
	5+	6+	7+	8+	9+	10+	11+	12+	13+	14+	15+
	%	%	%	%	%	%	%	%	%	%	%
Decayed (D) 0	96	85	67	62	62	54	47	38	33	32	38
1	3	6	18	22	13	21	14	21	22	16	23
2	1	6	9	9	12	13	15	14	15	16	13
3	-	2	2	3	7	7	13	11	7	11	11
4	-	1	4	3	5	4	6	6	7	11	3
5	-	-	-	1	-	1	2	5	7	5	2
6	-	-	-	-	1	-	2	3	2	3	5
7	-	-	-	-	-	-	-	1	1	2	3
8	-	-	-	-	-	-	1	1	1	2	-
9	-	-	-	-	-	-	-	-	1	1	1
10	-	-	-	-	-	-	-	-	1	1	1
11+	-	-	-	-	-	-	-	-	3	-	-
	100	100	100	100	100	100	100	100	100	100	100
Missing (M) 0	100	100	98	97	93	87	81	75	69	66	64
1	-	-	1	1	3	4	7	7	11	8	17
2	-	-	1	2	2	5	6	7	8	11	10
3	-	-	-	-	-	-	1	2	3	4	2
4	-	-	-	-	2	4	5	9	8	7	5
5	-	-	-	-	-	-	-	-	1	2	1
6	-	-	-	-	-	-	-	-	-	-	-
7	-	-	-	-	-	-	-	-	-	1	1
8+	-	-	-	-	-	-	-	-	-	1	-
	100	100	100	100	100	100	100	100	100	100	100
Filled (F) 0	99	95	81	58	45	34	27	22	18	16	7
1	1	3	9	14	16	11	11	13	8	8	8
2	-	2	5	12	13	16	12	15	15	8	7
3	-	-	2	5	11	16	13	16	12	7	6
4	-	-	2	11	14	21	24	18	13	7	8
5	-	-	1	-	1	2	5	5	8	11	8
6	-	-	-	-	-	-	4	3	11	10	8
7	-	-	-	-	-	-	2	4	2	8	10
8	-	-	-	-	-	-	-	1	5	6	13
9	-	-	-	-	-	-	1	2	5	5	8
10	-	-	-	-	-	-	1	1	1	3	5
11	-	-	-	-	-	-	-	-	-	3	3
12	-	-	-	-	-	-	-	-	2	1	2
13	-	-	-	-	-	-	-	-	-	2	2
14	-	-	-	-	-	-	-	-	-	2	2
15	-	-	-	-	-	-	-	-	-	1	1
16	-	-	-	-	-	-	-	-	-	2	-
17+	-	-	-	-	-	-	-	-	-	-	2
	100	100	100	100	100	100	100	100	100	100	100
Base	*158*	*168*	*185*	*166*	*169*	*163*	*155*	*160*	*146*	*145*	*111*

Table 26   Distribution of the number of deciduous teeth, which are decayed or filled, for children of different ages   (df,d,f)

Wales and South West

Number of deciduous teeth	Age at 31 December 1972										
	5+	6+	7+	8+	9+	10+	11+	12+	13+	14+	15+
	%	%	%	%	%	%	%	%	%	%	%
Decayed or filled (df) 0	26	13	11	11	16	31	61	73	90	99	99
1	12	10	9	11	10	13	15	10	8	1	1
2	10	13	13	10	17	16	10	7	1	-	-
3	6	7	13	12	12	11	5	5	-	-	-
4	9	15	13	16	14	8	5	3	1	-	-
5	8	8	13	15	11	12	1	1	-	-	-
6	7	9	10	10	11	6	3	-	-	-	-
7	6	10	8	6	3	2	-	1	-	-	-
8	4	9	4	7	3	-	-	-	-	-	-
9	3	1	2	2	1	1	-	-	-	-	-
10	4	2	3	-	1	-	-	-	-	-	-
11	-	2	1	-	-	-	-	-	-	-	-
12	2	-	-	-	1	-	-	-	-	-	-
13	1	1	-	-	-	-	-	-	-	-	-
14	1	-	-	-	-	-	-	-	-	-	-
15+	1	-	-	-	-	-	-	-	-	-	-
	100	100	100	100	100	100	100	100	100	100	100
Decayed (d) 0	36	26	25	25	32	46	72	83	92	100	99
1	13	18	17	23	21	15	15	8	6	-	1
2	12	17	12	15	18	17	5	5	2	-	-
3	6	9	14	15	11	9	5	3	-	-	-
4	10	8	10	6	8	8	1	1	-	-	-
5	7	6	8	4	2	3	1	-	-	-	-
6	2	5	5	7	3	1	1	-	-	-	-
7	3	4	5	2	2	-	-	-	-	-	-
8	4	3	2	2	1	1	-	-	-	-	-
9	2	1	1	1	1	-	-	-	-	-	-
10	2	1	1	-	-	-	-	-	-	-	-
11	1	1	-	-	1	-	-	-	-	-	-
12	1	1	-	-	-	-	-	-	-	-	-
13+	1	-	-	-	-	-	-	-	-	-	-
	100	100	100	100	100	100	100	100	100	100	100
Filled (f) 0	70	49	51	47	48	61	79	84	97	99	99
1	9	15	15	11	15	12	11	10	2	1	1
2	7	13	14	14	16	12	5	4	1	-	-
3	5	8	7	10	8	5	3	1	-	-	-
4	4	7	4	7	4	8	1	1	-	-	-
5	2	3	7	6	4	1	1	-	-	-	-
6	1	2	-	3	4	-	-	-	-	-	-
7	1	2	2	1	1	-	-	-	-	-	-
8+	1	1	-	1	-	1	-	-	-	-	-
	100	100	100	100	100	100	100	100	100	100	100
Base	*158*	*168*	*185*	*166*	*169*	*163*	*155*	*160*	*146*	*145*	*111*

Table 27   Average number of teeth with known decay
experience, for children of different ages,
showing type of treatment and dentition.

London and South East

Average number of teeth with known decay experience		Age at 31 December 1972										
		5+	6+	7+	8+	9+	10+	11+	12+	13+	14+	15+
Deciduous df		3.1	3.8	3.4	3.5	3.0	2.1	1.2	0.4	0.2	0.0	0.0
	d	2.2	2.4	1.9	1.8	1.6	1.1	0.6	0.2	0.1	0.0	0.0
	f	0.9	1.5	1.5	1.7	1.5	1.0	0.6	0.2	0.1	0.0	0.0
Permanent DMF		0.0	0.3	0.8	1.6	2.2	2.9	3.8	4.8	5.8	7.2	8.1
	D	0.0	0.2	0.3	0.5	0.7	0.7	1.0	1.2	1.0	1.3	1.3
	M	0.0	0.0	0.0	0.0	0.1	0.2	0.2	0.3	0.3	0.4	0.4
	F	0.0	0.1	0.4	1.0	1.4	2.0	2.7	3.4	4.5	5.5	6.4
Both DMF + df		3.2	4.1	4.2	5.0	5.2	5.0	5.0	5.2	6.0	7.3	8.1
	D+d	2.3	2.5	2.2	2.3	2.2	1.9	1.6	1.4	1.1	1.4	1.3
	M	0.0	0.0	0.0	0.0	0.1	0.2	0.2	0.3	0.3	0.4	0.4
	F+f	0.9	1.6	1.9	2.7	2.9	3.0	3.2	3.5	4.6	5.5	6.4
Base		*271*	*341*	*341*	*344*	*379*	*354*	*319*	*320*	*290*	*263*	*237*

Table 28 Distribution of the number of teeth with known decay experience for children of different ages (DMF+df)

Number of teeth with known decay experience	Age at 31 December 1972										
	5+	6+	7+	8+	9+	10+	11+	12+	13+	14+	15+
	%	%	%	%	%	%	%	%	%	%	%
0	32	20	18	10	6	8	7	6	8	5	3
1	10	8	9	8	6	5	6	4	3	3	4
2	11	11	7	7	6	6	7	7	6	3	2
3	8	9	8	10	13	9	8	8	8	5	4
4	7	11	12	8	12	18	20	20	15	11	6
5	10	9	13	12	12	12	11	11	11	8	10
6	6	9	10	11	13	15	14	17	12	10	10
7	4	7	7	12	10	9	10	8	10	13	11
8	3	5	7	7	7	6	7	7	5	8	8
9	2	4	4	6	5	5	4	4	5	9	8
10	1	4	2	4	5	2	2	2	3	3	6
11	1	2	1	2	3	2	1	2	3	4	6
12	1	1	1	2	2	2	1	2	2	6	5
13	1	-	1	-	-	1	1	1	2	3	3
14	1	-	-	1	-	-	-	1	1	3	4
15	1	-	-	-	-	-	1	-	3	2	2
16	1	-	-	-	-	-	-	-	1	2	2
17	-	-	-	-	-	-	-	-	1	1	2
18	-	-	-	-	-	-	-	-	1	1	-
19	-	-	-	-	-	-	-	-	-	-	1
20	-	-	-	-	-	-	-	-	-	-	2
21	-	-	-	-	-	-	-	-	-	-	-
22	-	-	-	-	-	-	-	-	-	-	1
23+	-	-	-	-	-	-	-	-	-	-	-
	100	100	100	100	100	100	100	100	100	100	100
Base	*172*	*184*	*191*	*183*	*195*	*182*	*176*	*175*	*185*	*177*	*120*

Table 29   Distribution of the number of teeth in both dentitions, which are decayed, missing or filled, for children of different ages   (D+d,M,F+f)

London and South East

Number of teeth	Age at 31 December 1972										
	5+	6+	7+	8+	9+	10+	11+	12+	13+	14+	15+
	%	%	%	%	%	%	%	%	%	%	%
Decayed (D+d) 0	43	35	34	29	27	35	38	44	50	46	50
1	14	16	21	20	20	21	21	21	23	23	19
2	13	12	10	12	17	15	17	15	13	13	10
3	6	10	9	14	13	10	10	8	3	7	9
4	6	6	7	9	8	7	5	4	5	4	5
5	6	5	8	4	6	4	3	4	2	3	3
6	4	4	3	6	3	4	4	2	2	1	3
7	1	3	3	3	3	2	2	1	2	-	1
8	3	2	2	1	2	-	-	1	-	1	-
9	1	3	1	1	1	1	-	-	-	-	-
10	1	2	1	-	-	1	-	-	-	1	-
11+	2	2	1	1	-	-	-	-	-	1	-
	100	100	100	100	100	100	100	100	100	100	100
Missing (M) 0	100	100	99	99	94	91	90	84	87	82	81
1	-	-	1	-	4	4	6	8	5	8	7
2	-	-	-	1	1	2	3	5	5	4	8
3	-	-	-	-	1	1	-	1	1	2	1
4	-	-	-	-	-	2	1	2	2	3	3
5	-	-	-	-	-	-	-	-	-	-	-
6	-	-	-	-	-	-	-	-	-	-	-
7	-	-	-	-	-	-	-	-	-	1	-
8+	-	-	-	-	-	-	-	-	-	-	-
	100	100	100	100	100	100	100	100	100	100	100
Filled (F+f) 0	67	53	42	34	27	22	21	17	14	13	10
1	9	12	12	10	13	12	12	8	9	8	4
2	9	9	13	12	11	11	10	16	8	5	5
3	4	6	11	10	13	16	12	11	12	8	6
4	5	8	8	12	11	17	16	20	14	11	11
5	4	4	7	7	7	9	10	8	10	9	11
6	-	3	4	5	4	6	5	8	10	10	9
7	1	2	1	3	6	2	5	5	5	7	7
8	1	2	1	3	3	1	4	3	3	5	8
9	-	-	-	2	2	2	1	-	3	6	7
10	-	-	1	1	2	1	1	1	4	3	5
11	-	-	-	1	1	1	1	1	1	4	4
12	-	1	-	-	-	-	-	-	2	4	4
13	-	-	-	-	-	-	1	1	-	2	3
14	-	-	-	-	-	-	1	-	2	2	-
15	-	-	-	-	-	-	-	1	2	1	1
16	-	-	-	-	-	-	-	-	-	1	3
17+	-	-	-	-	-	-	-	-	1	1	2
	100	100	100	100	100	100	100	100	100	100	100
Base	271	341	341	344	379	354	319	320	290	263	237

Table 30 — Distribution of the number of permanent teeth with decay experience for children of different ages (DMF)

London and South East

Number of permanent teeth that are, or have been decayed	Age at 31 December 1972										
	5+	6+	7+	8+	9+	10+	11+	12+	13+	14+	15+
	%	%	%	%	%	%	%	%	%	%	%
0	97	87	67	39	26	17	11	8	9	5	3
1	2	6	11	15	12	8	9	5	4	3	4
2	1	3	10	16	16	14	9	9	7	3	2
3	-	2	5	13	12	16	11	8	9	5	4
4	-	2	6	16	31	38	33	26	18	12	6
5	-	-	1	1	3	2	7	9	8	8	11
6	-	-	-	-	-	2	7	13	12	10	11
7	-	-	-	-	-	2	3	7	8	12	11
8	-	-	-	-	-	-	4	5	5	8	8
9	-	-	-	-	-	-	2	3	4	8	8
10	-	-	-	-	-	1	1	2	3	3	6
11	-	-	-	-	-	-	1	1	3	4	5
12	-	-	-	-	-	-	1	2	2	6	5
13	-	-	-	-	-	-	-	1	2	3	3
14	-	-	-	-	-	-	-	1	1	2	4
15	-	-	-	-	-	-	1	-	3	2	2
16	-	-	-	-	-	-	-	-	1	3	2
17	-	-	-	-	-	-	-	-	1	1	2
18	-	-	-	-	-	-	-	-	-	1	-
19	-	-	-	-	-	-	-	-	-	-	1
20	-	-	-	-	-	-	-	-	-	-	2
21	-	-	-	-	-	-	-	-	-	-	-
22	-	-	-	-	-	-	-	-	-	-	-
23+	-	-	-	-	-	-	-	-	-	1	-
	100	100	100	100	100	100	100	100	100	100	100
Base	271	341	341	344	379	354	319	320	290	263	237

Table 31   Distribution of the number of permanent teeth which are decayed, missing or filled for children of different ages   (D,M,F)

London and South East

Number of permanent teeth	Age at 31 December 1972										
	5+	6+	7+	8+	9+	10+	11+	12+	13+	14+	15+
	%	%	%	%	%	%	%	%	%	%	%
Decayed (D) 0	98	92	82	71	64	62	55	51	54	47	51
1	2	4	10	14	19	20	18	21	23	24	19
2	-	2	6	8	9	9	12	12	12	12	9
3	-	1	1	5	4	5	7	7	2	6	9
4	-	1	1	2	4	4	4	3	5	4	5
5	-	-	-	-	-	-	3	3	2	3	3
6	-	-	-	-	-	-	1	1	1	1	3
7	-	-	-	-	-	-	-	1	1	-	-
8	-	-	-	-	-	-	-	1	-	1	-
9	-	-	-	-	-	-	-	-	-	1	-
10	-	-	-	-	-	-	-	-	-	-	1
11+	-	-	-	-	-	-	-	-	-	1	-
	100	100	100	100	100	100	100	100	100	100	100
Missing (M) 0	100	100	99	99	94	91	90	84	87	82	81
1	-	-	1	-	4	4	6	8	5	8	7
2	-	-	-	1	1	2	3	5	5	4	8
3	-	-	-	1	1	1	1	1	1	2	1
4	-	-	-	-	-	2	-	2	2	3	3
5	-	-	-	-	-	-	-	-	-	-	-
6	-	-	-	-	-	-	-	-	-	-	-
7	-	-	-	-	-	-	-	-	-	1	-
8+	-	-	-	-	-	-	-	-	-	-	-
	100	100	100	100	100	100	100	100	100	100	100
Filled (F) 0	99	95	79	59	44	31	27	18	15	13	10
1	1	3	8	12	14	10	10	8	9	8	4
2	-	1	8	10	16	19	12	16	9	5	5
3	-	1	2	9	10	16	14	14	13	8	6
4	-	-	3	10	15	22	23	21	15	11	12
5	-	-	-	-	1	1	4	6	9	9	12
6	-	-	-	-	-	-	3	6	9	10	9
7	-	-	-	-	-	-	2	4	5	7	7
8	-	-	-	-	-	-	2	3	3	5	8
9	-	-	-	-	-	1	1	-	3	6	7
10	-	-	-	-	-	-	1	1	4	4	4
11	-	-	-	-	-	-	1	1	1	4	4
12	-	-	-	-	-	-	-	-	2	4	4
13	-	-	-	-	-	-	-	1	-	2	3
14	-	-	-	-	-	-	-	-	1	2	-
15	-	-	-	-	-	-	-	1	1	1	1
16	-	-	-	-	-	-	-	-	-	1	3
17+	-	-	-	-	-	-	-	-	1	-	1
	100	100	100	100	100	100	100	100	100	100	100
Base	*271*	*341*	*341*	*344*	*379*	*354*	*319*	*320*	*290*	*263*	*237*

Table 32   Distribution of the number of deciduous teeth which are decayed or filled for children of different ages (df,d,f)

London and South East

Number of deciduous teeth		Age at 31 December 1972										
		5+	6+	7+	8+	9+	10+	11+	12+	13+	14+	15+
		%	%	%	%	%	%	%	%	%	%	%
Decayed or filled (df)	0	33	20	20	16	16	34	51	79	87	97	97
	1	10	9	11	12	12	12	16	10	9	2	2
	2	11	11	10	12	19	16	13	7	3	1	1
	3	8	9	11	13	13	14	10	3	-	-	-
	4	8	12	14	15	14	9	5	-	1	-	-
	5	10	9	11	10	10	8	3	-	-	-	-
	6	6	10	10	10	6	3	1	-	-	-	-
	7	4	7	7	5	6	2	1	1	-	-	-
	8	3	6	4	5	3	2	-	-	-	-	-
	9	2	3	2	1	1	-	-	-	-	-	-
	10	1	2	-	1	-	-	-	-	-	-	-
	11	1	1	-	-	-	-	-	-	-	-	-
	12	1	1	-	-	-	-	-	-	-	-	-
	13	-	-	-	-	-	-	-	-	-	-	-
	14	1	-	-	-	-	-	-	-	-	-	-
	15+	1	-	-	-	-	-	-	-	-	-	-
		100	100	100	100	100	100	100	100	100	100	100
Decayed (d)	0	43	36	38	34	36	50	66	86	93	97	99
	1	14	16	21	24	22	20	18	8	5	2	1
	2	12	13	9	12	18	13	9	5	2	1	-
	3	6	10	10	14	11	9	5	1	-	-	-
	4	7	6	7	7	5	3	2	-	-	-	-
	5	6	5	6	3	3	3	-	-	-	-	-
	6	4	5	3	3	2	2	-	-	-	-	-
	7	1	3	3	1	1	-	-	-	-	-	-
	8	3	3	2	1	2	-	-	-	-	-	-
	9	1	1	-	1	-	-	-	-	-	-	-
	10	1	1	1	-	-	-	-	-	-	-	-
	11	1	1	-	-	-	-	-	-	-	-	-
	12	-	-	-	-	-	-	-	-	-	-	-
	13+	1	-	-	-	-	-	-	-	-	-	-
		100	100	100	100	100	100	100	100	100	100	100
Filled (f)	0	68	54	48	43	47	56	73	91	93	99	99
	1	10	11	13	17	16	17	10	5	6	1	1
	2	8	10	13	12	1	14	8	3	1	-	-
	3	4	7	11	8	7	7	6	1	-	-	-
	4	5	9	6	8	7	3	1	-	-	-	-
	5	3	3	5	5	4	1	1	-	-	-	-
	6	-	2	2	4	3	1	1	-	-	-	-
	7	1	2	1	2	2	1	-	-	-	-	-
	8	1	2	1	1	-	-	-	-	-	-	-
		100	100	100	100	100	100	100	100	100	100	100
Base		271	341	341	344	379	354	319	320	290	263	237

Table 33   Average number of teeth with known decay
            experience, for children of different ages,
            showing type of treatment and dentition   *Wales*

Average number of teeth with known decay experience	Age at 31 December 1972										
	5+	6+	7+	8+	9+	10+	11+	12+	13+	14+	15+
Deciduous											
df	4.0	4.2	4.0	3.5	3.2	1.7	0.8	0.4	0.1	0.0	0.0
d	3.5	3.4	3.2	2.6	2.3	1.3	0.6	0.3	0.1	0.0	0.0
f	0.5	0.8	0.8	0.9	0.8	0.4	0.2	0.1	0.0	0.0	0.0
Permanent											
DMF	0.0	0.5	1.0	1.7	2.4	3.3	4.1	5.5	6.9	8.6	10.1
D	0.0	0.4	0.7	1.0	1.2	1.4	1.9	2.0	2.6	2.9	2.6
M	0.0	0.0	0.0	0.1	0.3	0.5	0.6	1.0	1.1	1.4	1.5
F	0.0	0.1	0.3	0.6	1.0	1.4	1.5	2.5	3.1	4.3	5.9
Both											
DMF + df	4.1	4.7	5.0	5.2	5.6	5.0	4.9	5.9	7.0	8.6	10.1
D+d	3.5	3.7	3.9	3.6	3.5	2.7	2.6	2.3	2.7	2.9	2.6
M	0.0	0.0	0.0	0.1	0.3	0.5	0.6	1.0	1.1	1.4	1.5
F+f	0.5	1.0	1.1	1.6	1.8	1.8	1.7	2.6	3.1	4.3	5.9
Base	*172*	*184*	*191*	*183*	*195*	*182*	*176*	*175*	*185*	*177*	*120*

Table 34   Distribution of the number of teeth with
            known decay experience for children of
            different ages (DMF+df)

Wales

Number of teeth with known decay experience	Age at 31 December 1972										
	5+	6+	7+	8+	9+	10+	11+	12+	13+	14+	15+
	%	%	%	%	%	%	%	%	%	%	%
0	21	15	8	6	6	5	5	2	2	2	1
1	14	7	8	4	4	5	5	3	6	2	3
2	9	11	8	8	5	9	8	5	2	6	2
3	7	8	8	9	8	12	11	10	4	3	2
4	9	9	14	13	17	17	22	13	14	11	4
5	9	10	12	15	12	16	19	17	11	6	7
6	6	7	13	14	10	11	10	18	8	8	5
7	6	11	8	8	13	5	9	6	12	7	8
8	5	7	8	9	10	11	3	6	11	7	6
9	2	4	3	7	5	6	2	7	9	9	11
10	6	5	4	5	4	1	1	6	4	9	8
11	1	4	4	2	3	1	1	1	5	6	4
12	3	1	2	-	1	1	1	1	2	4	9
13	1	1	-	-	-	-	-	2	3	4	9
14	1	-	-	-	2	-	1	1	2	1	6
15	-	-	-	-	-	-	-	-	2	4	1
16	-	-	-	-	-	-	1	-	-	4	3
17	-	-	-	-	-	-	1	1	-	2	2
18	-	-	-	-	-	-	-	-	-	1	2
19	-	-	-	-	-	-	-	-	1	-	2
20	-	-	-	-	-	-	-	-	1	1	2
21	-	-	-	-	-	-	-	-	1	1	2
22	-	-	-	-	-	-	-	1	-	1	-
23+	-	-	-	-	-	-	-	-	-	1	1
	100	100	100	100	100	100	100	100	100	100	100
Base	*172*	*184*	*191*	*183*	*195*	*182*	*176*	*175*	*185*	*177*	*120*

Table 35 Distribution of the number of teeth in both dentitions, which are decayed, missing or filled, for children of different ages (D+d,M,F+f)

Wales

Number of teeth	Age at 31 December 1972										
	5+	6+	7+	8+	9+	10+	11+	12+	13+	14+	15+
	%	%	%	%	%	%	%	%	%	%	%
Decayed (D+d) 0	29	25	15	14	16	24	27	30	28	28	28
1	16	10	10	14	14	13	11	18	16	15	23
2	11	13	15	15	13	18	20	16	15	13	10
3	3	8	13	10	12	13	14	10	10	8	9
4	6	7	9	14	14	13	10	11	7	14	5
5	10	7	11	10	8	7	8	5	11	6	4
6	3	5	8	8	7	4	3	6	3	6	7
7	5	8	6	3	5	3	2	2	2	2	7
8	5	5	4	6	6	3	1	–	2	2	1
9	2	4	1	3	1	1	1	1	2	2	2
10	5	3	2	3	2	–	1	1	2	2	2
11+	5	5	6	–	2	1	2	–	2	2	2
	100	100	100	100	100	100	100	100	100	100	100
Missing (M) 0	100	100	98	94	86	78	68	62	55	50	50
1	–	–	1	2	5	7	12	11	14	11	17
2	–	–	1	3	6	8	13	8	10	16	10
3	–	–	–	1	–	1	2	5	8	7	5
4	–	–	–	–	3	6	5	13	12	9	12
5	–	–	–	–	–	–	–	1	1	4	2
6	–	–	–	–	–	–	–	–	–	1	–
7	–	–	–	–	–	–	–	–	–	2	2
8+	–	–	–	–	–	–	–	–	–	–	2
	100	100	100	100	100	100	100	100	100	100	100
Filled (F+f) 0	78	67	63	51	46	43	41	28	29	29	12
1	11	9	11	11	13	12	14	12	9	9	8
2	3	9	11	11	10	16	14	14	10	9	9
3	1	3	5	8	9	8	6	14	10	5	8
4	5	7	3	10	8	13	15	10	13	5	7
5	1	2	2	3	5	3	6	10	8	8	8
6	1	1	2	3	5	3	2	3	8	7	5
7	–	1	3	2	2	1	1	3	4	6	9
8	–	1	–	1	1	1	1	2	5	4	7
9	–	–	–	–	1	–	–	2	2	4	7
10	–	–	–	–	–	–	–	1	1	3	4
11	–	–	–	–	–	–	–	–	–	3	3
12	–	–	–	–	–	–	–	–	1	2	3
13	–	–	–	–	–	–	–	1	–	2	4
14	–	–	–	–	–	–	–	–	–	1	2
15	–	–	–	–	–	–	–	–	–	1	2
16	–	–	–	–	–	–	–	–	–	1	1
17+	–	–	–	–	–	–	–	–	–	1	1
	100	100	100	100	100	100	100	100	100	100	100
Base	*172*	*184*	*191*	*183*	*135*	*182*	*176*	*175*	*185*	*177*	*120*

Table 36   Distribution of the number of permanent teeth with decay experience for children of different ages   (DMF)

Number of permanent teeth that are, or have been decayed	Age at 31 December 1972										
	5+	6+	7+	8+	9+	10+	11+	12+	13+	14+	15+
	%	%	%	%	%	%	%	%	%	%	%
0	97	76	57	33	25	13	9	2	3	2	1
1	2	8	15	19	14	11	5	5	6	2	3
2	1	10	9	16	13	14	11	9	2	6	2
3	-	3	7	11	14	11	12	10	5	2	2
4	-	3	12	17	24	32	31	15	14	12	4
5	-	-	-	2	5	9	14	14	10	5	7
6	-	-	-	2	3	4	6	17	9	8	5
7	-	-	-	-	1	1	4	5	11	7	8
8	-	-	-	-	1	3	3	6	10	7	6
9	-	-	-	-	-	1	1	6	9	9	11
10	-	-	-	-	-	1	1	5	4	9	8
11	-	-	-	-	-	-	-	1	5	6	4
12	-	-	-	-	-	-	-	1	2	5	9
13	-	-	-	-	-	-	-	2	3	4	9
14	-	-	-	-	-	-	1	1	2	1	6
15	-	-	-	-	-	-	-	-	2	4	1
16	-	-	-	-	-	-	1	-	-	4	3
17	-	-	-	-	-	-	1	1	-	2	2
18	-	-	-	-	-	-	-	-	-	1	2
19	-	-	-	-	-	-	-	-	1	-	2
20	-	-	-	-	-	-	-	-	1	1	2
21	-	-	-	-	-	-	-	-	1	1	2
22	-	-	-	-	-	-	-	-	-	1	-
23+	-	-	-	-	-	-	-	-	-	1	I
	100	100	100	100	100	100	100	100	100	100	100
Base	*172*	*184*	*191*	*183*	*195*	*182*	*176*	*175*	*185*	*177*	*120*

Table 37 — Distribution of the number of permanent teeth which are decayed, missing or filled for children of different ages (D,M,F)

Wales

Number of permanent teeth	Age at 31 December 1972										
	5+	6+	7+	8+	9+	10+	11+	12+	13+	14+	15+
	%	%	%	%	%	%	%	%	%	%	%
Decayed (D) 0	97	81	67	50	51	41	37	32	30	29	29
1	2	6	14	25	15	22	12	21	17	14	22
2	1	8	7	12	16	14	19	16	13	13	10
3	-	2	5	6	8	11	15	12	8	8	9
4	-	3	7	5	7	7	10	7	7	14	5
5	-	-	-	2	2	2	2	3	12	6	4
6	-	-	-	-	1	1	2	6	3	6	7
7	-	-	-	-	-	1	-	2	2	2	7
8	-	-	-	-	-	1	1	-	2	2	1
9	-	-	-	-	-	-	1	-	2	2	2
10	-	-	-	-	-	-	-	-	2	2	2
11+	-	-	-	-	-	-	1	1	2	2	2
	100	100	100	100	100	100	100	100	100	100	100
Missing (M) 0	100	100	98	94	86	78	68	62	55	50	50
1	-	-	1	2	5	7	12	11	14	11	17
2	-	-	1	3	6	8	13	8	10	16	10
3	-	-	-	1	-	1	2	5	8	7	5
4	-	-	-	-	3	6	5	13	12	9	12
5	-	-	-	-	-	-	-	1	1	4	2
6	-	-	-	-	-	-	-	-	-	1	-
7	-	-	-	-	-	-	-	-	-	2	2
8+	-	-	-	-	-	-	-	-	-	-	2
	100	100	100	100	100	100	100	100	100	100	100
Filled (F) 0	100	93	86	72	59	48	45	29	29	30	12
1	-	2	6	9	14	12	12	14	9	8	8
2	-	4	3	10	13	18	14	14	10	8	9
3	-	1	3	4	7	8	9	14	10	5	8
4	-	-	2	4	5	10	17	10	14	6	7
5	-	-	-	1	1	2	2	8	8	7	8
6	-	-	-	-	1	1	-	3	8	7	5
7	-	-	-	-	-	-	1	3	4	6	9
8	-	-	-	-	-	-	-	2	5	5	7
9	-	-	-	-	-	-	-	2	2	4	7
10	-	-	-	-	-	-	-	1	-	3	4
11	-	-	-	-	-	-	-	-	-	3	3
12	-	-	-	-	-	-	-	-	1	2	3
13	-	-	-	-	-	-	-	-	-	2	4
14	-	-	-	-	-	-	-	-	-	1	2
15	-	-	-	-	-	-	-	-	-	1	2
16	-	-	-	-	-	-	-	-	-	1	1
17+	-	-	-	-	-	1	-	-	-	1	1
	100	100	100	100	100	100	100	100	100	100	100
Base	172	184	191	183	195	182	176	175	185	177	120

Table 38   Distribution of the number of deciduous teeth which are decayed or filled, for children of different ages   (df,d,f)

Wales

Number of deciduous teeth		Age at 31 December 1972										
		5+	6+	7+	8+	9+	10+	11+	12+	13+	14+	15+
		%	%	%	%	%	%	%	%	%	%	%
Decayed or filled (df)	0	22	17	14	12	16	43	62	80	94	98	99
	1	15	7	7	11	9	17	18	8	4	2	-
	2	9	11	12	14	17	12	8	8	1	-	1
	3	6	9	10	13	18	7	7	3	1	-	-
	4	9	10	14	19	15	8	2	1	-	-	-
	5	9	10	14	14	10	8	1	-	-	-	-
	6	6	10	12	6	7	3	1	-	-	-	-
	7	5	11	8	5	4	1	1	-	-	-	-
	8	5	6	4	5	2	1	-	-	-	-	-
	9	2	2	2	1	1	-	-	-	-	-	-
	10	5	3	3	-	1	-	-	-	-	-	-
	11	1	2	-	-	-	-	-	-	-	-	-
	12	3	1	-	-	-	-	-	-	-	-	-
	13	1	-	-	-	-	-	-	-	-	-	-
	14	1	-	-	-	-	-	-	-	-	-	-
	15+	1	1	-	-	-	-	-	-	-	-	-
		100	100	100	100	100	100	100	100	100	100	100
Decayed (d)	0	29	26	21	21	26	50	68	86	95	99	99
	1	17	11	10	18	15	18	15	5	3	1	1
	2	10	12	14	19	18	9	8	6	1	-	-
	3	4	7	14	11	17	9	5	2	1	-	-
	4	6	10	9	11	10	9	2	1	-	-	-
	5	9	8	12	7	4	2	-	-	-	-	-
	6	3	9	6	7	4	2	1	-	-	-	-
	7	5	8	7	2	3	-	1	-	-	-	-
	8	5	3	2	4	1	1	-	-	-	-	-
	9	2	2	1	-	1	-	-	-	-	-	-
	10	5	2	3	-	1	-	-	-	-	-	-
	11	1	2	1	-	-	-	-	-	-	-	-
	12	2	-	-	-	-	-	-	-	-	-	-
	13+	2	-	-	-	-	-	-	-	-	-	-
		100	100	100	100	100	100	100	100	100	100	100
Filled (f)	0	78	70	67	62	66	81	88	92	99	99	99
	1	11	9	15	13	11	7	9	6	1	1	1
	2	3	8	7	9	10	8	2	2	-	-	-
	3	1	2	6	6	7	2	1	-	-	-	-
	4	5	7	2	7	3	2	-	-	-	-	-
	5	1	1	2	1	1	-	-	-	-	-	-
	6	1	2	-	2	2	-	-	-	-	-	-
	7	-	1	1	-	-	-	-	-	-	-	-
	8	-	-	-	-	-	-	-	-	-	-	-
		100	100	100	100	100	100	100	100	100	100	100
Base		*172*	*184*	*191*	*183*	*195*	*182*	*176*	*175*	*185*	*177*	*120*

Table 39   Average number of teeth with known decay
experience, for children of different ages,
showing type of treatment and dentition

Male

Average number of teeth with known decay experience	Age at 31 December 1972										
	5+	6+	7+	8+	9+	10+	11+	12+	13+	14+	15+
Deciduous											
df	3.3	3.5	3.5	3.2	3.1	2.1	1.2	0.5	0.2	–	–
d	2.7	2.5	2.3	2.0	1.8	1.3	0.7	0.3	0.1	–	–
f	0.7	1.0	1.2	1.3	1.2	0.8	0.5	0.2	0.0	–	–
Permanent											
DMF	0.0	0.3	0.8	1.6	2.1	2.8	3.7	4.8	5.7	7.0	8.1
D	0.0	0.2	0.4	0.7	0.8	0.9	1.2	1.5	1.7	2.1	1.7
M	0.0	0.0	0.0	0.1	0.1	0.3	0.3	0.6	0.6	0.8	0.8
F	0.0	0.1	0.3	0.8	1.2	1.7	2.1	2.7	3.4	4.2	5.6
Both											
DMF + df	3.3	3.8	4.2	4.8	5.2	5.0	4.8	5.2	5.9	7.1	8.1
D+d	2.7	2.7	2.7	2.7	2.6	2.3	1.9	1.8	1.8	2.1	1.7
M	0.0	0.0	0.0	0.1	0.1	0.3	0.3	0.6	0.6	0.8	0.8
F+f	0.7	1.1	1.5	2.1	2.4	2.5	2.6	2.9	3.4	4.2	5.6
Base	*482*	*554*	*587*	*556*	*576*	*556*	*495*	*477*	*461*	*457*	*328*

Table 40   Distribution of the number of teeth with
            known decay experience for children of
            different ages (DMF+df)

Male

Number of teeth with known decay experience	Age at 31 December 1972										
	5+	6+	7+	8+	9+	10+	11+	12+	13+	14+	15+
	%	%	%	%	%	%	%	%	%	%	%
0	29	21	15	9	8	6	5	5	6	5	3
1	12	10	11	7	6	5	6	5	4	4	4
2	10	11	8	9	9	7	7	8	9	6	4
3	9	8	11	11	11	11	11	11	9	6	4
4	8	11	11	12	11	16	23	20	14	10	7
5	8	10	11	12	10	14	14	12	10	10	8
6	7	8	10	9	12	13	12	10	12	11	10
7	5	8	7	11	10	10	8	10	10	9	9
8	3	6	7	7	8	6	6	7	6	7	10
9	3	3	4	5	6	5	3	3	5	6	7
10	2	1	2	4	5	2	2	2	2	6	8
11	1	2	1	2	3	3	1	2	4	4	5
12	1	1	1	2	1	1	1	2	1	3	5
13	1	-	1	-	-	1	-	1	3	2	4
14	1	-	-	-	-	-	1	1	1	2	2
15	-	-	-	-	-	-	-	-	1	2	2
16	-	-	-	-	-	-	-	-	1	3	3
17	-	-	-	-	-	-	-	1	-	1	3
18	-	-	-	-	-	-	-	-	1	2	1
19	-	-	-	-	-	-	-	-	1	-	-
20+	-	-	-	-	-	-	-	-	-	1	1
	100	100	100	100	100	100	100	100	100	100	100
Base	*482*	*554*	*587*	*556*	*576*	*556*	*495*	*477*	*461*	*457*	*328*

Table 41   Distribution of the number of teeth in both
            dentitions, which are decayed, missing or filled,
            for children of different ages   (D+d,M,F+f)

Male

Age at 31 December 1972

Number of teeth	5+	6+	7+	8+	9+	10+	11+	12+	13+	14+	15+
	%	%	%	%	%	%	%	%	%	%	%
Decayed (D+d) 0	37	32	29	22	24	27	34	36	37	36	41
1	14	15	18	19	16	19	18	22	21	19	21
2	10	13	10	15	16	19	17	17	15	14	12
3	9	9	12	14	14	11	11	9	9	8	11
4	7	8	8	10	10	9	7	7	6	8	6
5	6	6	7	6	6	6	6	4	4	5	3
6	5	5	5	6	5	3	4	2	3	4	2
7	3	4	4	3	4	3	2	1	1	1	3
8	3	3	3	2	2	1	1	1	1	2	1
9	2	2	2	1	1	1	-	-	1	1	-
10	1	1	1	1	-	1	-	1	1	1	-
11+	3	2	1	1	2	-	-	-	1	1	-
	100	100	100	100	100	100	100	100	100	100	100
Missing (M) 0	100	100	98	97	93	89	83	76	72	72	69
1	-	-	2	1	3	3	8	8	11	9	10
2	-	-	-	1	2	4	4	7	9	7	7
3	-	-	-	-	1	1	1	2	3	3	5
4	-	-	-	1	1	3	4	7	5	8	7
5	-	-	-	-	-	-	-	-	-	1	1
6	-	-	-	-	-	-	-	-	-	-	1
7	-	-	-	-	-	-	-	-	-	-	-
8+	-	-	-	-	-	-	-	-	-	-	-
	100	100	100	100	100	100	100	100	100	100	100
Filled (F+f) 0	75	62	53	43	37	34	31	25	28	23	12
1	9	12	12	11	12	11	12	11	9	12	8
2	6	9	11	9	11	11	12	15	12	9	9
3	4	5	7	10	11	11	10	13	10	11	6
4	4	6	5	11	10	15	15	16	10	7	8
5	2	3	5	5	5	6	8	5	8	6	8
6	-	1	3	3	4	5	6	6	8	6	9
7	-	1	2	3	5	3	3	4	3	5	8
8	-	1	1	2	2	1	2	3	2	4	8
9	-	-	1	1	2	1	1	1	3	4	7
10	-	-	-	1	1	1	-	1	3	2	5
11	-	-	-	1	-	1	-	-	2	3	4
12	-	-	-	-	-	-	-	-	1	3	2
13	-	-	-	-	-	-	-	-	-	1	2
14	-	-	-	-	-	-	-	-	-	1	-
15	-	-	-	-	-	-	-	-	1	2	1
16	-	-	-	-	-	-	-	-	-	1	2
17+	-	-	-	-	-	-	-	-	-	-	1
	100	100	100	100	100	100	100	100	100	100	100
Base	482	554	587	556	576	556	495	477	461	457	328

Table 42　　Distribution of the number of permanent
　　　　　　teeth with decay experience for children
　　　　　　of different ages　　(DMF)

Male

Number of permanent teeth that are, or have been decayed	Age at 31 December 1972										
	5+	6+	7+	8+	9+	10+	11+	12+	13+	14+	15+
	%	%	%	%	%	%	%	%	%	%	%
0	98	84	64	40	29	16	11	7	7	4	3
1	2	8	14	16	14	10	8	7	5	4	4
2	-	4	10	13	14	13	10	8	9	5	4
3	-	3	5	13	12	14	14	11	9	6	4
4	-	1	7	17	27	39	34	27	16	11	7
5	-	-	-	1	2	4	8	8	8	10	8
6	-	-	-	-	1	2	5	8	12	11	10
7	-	-	-	-	-	1	4	8	9	8	9
8	-	-	-	-	1	1	3	5	6	8	10
9	-	-	-	-	-	-	1	3	4	6	7
10	-	-	-	-	-	-	-	2	2	6	8
11	-	-	-	-	-	-	1	2	4	4	5
12	-	-	-	-	-	-	-	1	1	4	5
13	-	-	-	-	-	-	-	1	3	2	4
14	-	-	-	-	-	-	-	1	1	2	2
15	-	-	-	-	-	-	1	-	1	2	2
16	-	-	-	-	-	-	-	-	1	3	3
17	-	-	-	-	-	-	-	1	-	1	3
18	-	-	-	-	-	-	-	-	1	2	1
19	-	-	-	-	-	-	-	-	1	-	-
20	-	-	-	-	-	-	-	-	-	1	1
21	-	-	-	-	-	-	-	-	-	-	-
22	-	-	-	-	-	-	-	-	-	-	-
23+	-	-	-	-	-	-	-	-	-	-	-
	100	100	100	100	100	100	100	100	100	100	100
Base	482	554	587	556	576	556	495	477	461	457	328

Table 43   Distribution of the number of permanent teeth which are decayed, missing or filled for children of different ages (D,M,F)   *Male*

Number of permanent teeth.	Age at 31 December 1972										
	5+	6+	7+	8+	9+	10+	11+	12+	13+	14+	15+
	%	%	%	%	%	%	%	%	%	%	%
Decayed (D) 0	98	88	77	63	61	55	50	45	40	36	41
1	2	7	11	19	16	20	17	20	22	20	21
2	-	3	7	9	12	12	13	14	14	13	12
3	-	1	2	5	6	7	9	8	7	8	11
4	-	1	3	3	5	4	6	5	6	8	6
5	-	-	-	1	-	1	3	3	4	5	3
6	-	-	-	-	-	1	1	2	3	4	2
7	-	-	-	-	-	-	1	-	1	1	3
8	-	-	-	-	-	-	-	1	1	2	1
9	-	-	-	-	-	-	-	-	1	1	-
10	-	-	-	-	-	-	-	1	1	1	-
11+	-	-	-	-	-	-	-	1	-	1	-
	100	100	100	100	100	100	100	100	100	100	100
Missing (M) 0	100	100	98	97	93	89	83	76	72	72	69
1	-	-	2	1	3	3	8	8	11	9	10
2	-	-	-	1	2	4	4	7	9	7	7
3	-	-	-	-	1	1	1	2	3	3	5
4	-	-	-	1	1	3	4	7	5	8	7
5	-	-	-	-	-	-	-	-	-	1	1
6	-	-	-	-	-	-	-	-	-	-	1
7	-	-	-	-	-	-	-	-	-	-	-
8+	-	-	-	-	-	-	-	-	-	-	-
	100	100	100	100	100	100	100	100	100	100	100
Filled (F) 0	100	96	83	66	53	40	35	26	29	23	12
1	-	2	8	10	13	11	12	12	8	12	8
2	-	1	5	10	13	16	13	15	12	9	9
3	-	1	2	7	9	12	12	14	10	11	7
4	-	-	2	7	11	19	20	17	10	8	8
5	-	-	-	-	1	1	3	4	8	6	8
6	-	-	-	-	-	1	3	4	8	6	9
7	-	-	-	-	-	-	1	3	3	5	8
8	-	-	-	-	-	-	1	2	2	4	8
9	-	-	-	-	-	-	-	1	3	4	7
10	-	-	-	-	-	-	-	1	2	2	5
11	-	-	-	-	-	-	-	1	2	3	4
12	-	-	-	-	-	-	-	-	1	2	2
13	-	-	-	-	-	-	-	-	-	1	2
14	-	-	-	-	-	-	-	-	-	1	-
15	-	-	-	-	-	-	-	-	1	2	1
16	-	-	-	-	-	-	-	-	-	1	2
17+	-	-	-	-	-	-	-	-	1	-	-
	100	100	100	100	100	100	100	100	100	100	100
Base	*482*	*554*	*587*	*556*	*576*	*556*	*495*	*477*	*461*	*457*	*328*

Table 44　Distribution of the number of deciduous teeth which are decayed or filled for children of different ages　(df,d,f)

Male

Number of deciduous teeth		Age at 31 December 1972										
		5+	6+	7+	8+	9+	10+	11+	12+	13+	14+	15+
		%	%	%	%	%	%	%	%	%	%	%
Decayed or filled (df)	0	30	22	17	15	16	32	52	74	90	97	99
	1	12	11	12	12	12	14	17	13	7	2	1
	2	10	11	11	14	18	15	12	8	2	1	-
	3	9	8	13	16	13	15	8	4	1	-	-
	4	8	14	14	15	14	9	6	1	-	-	-
	5	7	9	11	9	10	7	2	-	-	-	-
	6	7	8	8	8	7	4	2	-	-	-	-
	7	5	6	7	7	5	2	1	-	-	-	-
	8	3	5	5	3	3	2	-	-	-	-	-
	9	3	2	1	1	1	-	-	-	-	-	-
	10	2	2	1	-	1	-	-	-	-	-	-
	11	1	2	-	-	-	-	-	-	-	-	-
	12	1	-	-	-	-	-	-	-	-	-	-
	13	1	-	-	-	-	-	-	-	-	-	-
	14	1	-	-	-	-	-	-	-	-	-	-
	15+	-	-	-	-	-	-	-	-	-	-	-
		100	100	100	100	100	100	100	100	100	100	100
Decayed (d)	0	38	33	32	28	31	43	64	81	93	98	99
	1	14	16	18	23	21	22	18	12	5	2	1
	2	10	12	11	16	18	14	9	6	1	-	-
	3	8	9	12	14	12	10	5	1	1	-	-
	4	7	8	9	8	8	6	3	-	-	-	-
	5	6	6	6	4	4	3	1	-	-	-	-
	6	5	5	4	4	3	1	-	-	-	-	-
	7	3	4	3	1	1	-	-	-	-	-	-
	8	2	3	3	1	1	1	-	-	-	-	-
	9	2	1	1	1	-	-	-	-	-	-	-
	10	2	2	1	-	1	-	-	-	-	-	-
	11	1	1	-	-	-	-	-	-	-	-	-
	12	1	-	-	-	-	-	-	-	-	-	-
	13	1	-	-	-	-	-	-	-	-	-	-
		100	100	100	100	100	100	100	100	100	100	100
Filled (f)	0	75	63	59	54	53	65	77	89	96	98	99
	1	9	12	11	15	17	14	10	6	3	1	1
	2	6	9	11	10	12	11	7	4	1	1	-
	3	4	5	7	7	6	5	4	1	-	-	-
	4	4	6	5	7	4	2	1	-	-	-	-
	5	2	2	4	3	4	1	1	-	-	-	-
	6	-	1	1	3	3	1	-	-	-	-	-
	7	-	1	2	1	1	1	-	-	-	-	-
	8	-	1	-	-	-	-	-	-	-	-	-
		100	100	100	100	100	100	100	100	100	100	100
Base		*482*	*554*	*587*	*556*	*576*	*556*	*495*	*477*	*461*	*457*	*328*

Table 45   Average number of teeth with known decay
            experience, for children of different ages,
            showing type of treatment and dentition

Average number of teeth with known decay experience	Age at 31 December 1972										
	5+	6+	7+	8+	9+	10+	11+	12+	13+	14+	15+
Deciduous											
df	3.3	3.6	3.4	3.3	2.5	1.7	0.9	0.3	0.1	-	-
d	2.6	2.5	2.3	2.1	1.4	1.0	0.5	0.2	0.1	-	-
f	0.7	1.1	1.1	1.2	1.0	0.7	0.3	0.1	0.1	-	-
Permanent											
DMF	0.1	0.3	1.0	1.9	2.4	3.1	4.2	4.9	6.5	7.8	8.7
D	0.0	0.2	0.6	0.8	0.9	1.0	1.4	1.4	1.5	1.6	1.5
M	0.0	0.0	0.0	0.1	0.2	0.3	0.4	0.5	0.7	0.8	0.8
F	0.0	0.1	0.4	1.0	1.3	1.8	2.4	3.0	4.3	5.4	6.3
Both											
DMF + df	3.4	4.0	4.3	5.2	4.9	4.8	5.1	5.2	6.6	7.8	8.8
D+d	2.6	2.7	2.9	2.9	2.3	2.0	1.9	1.6	1.6	1.7	1.5
M	0.0	0.0	0.0	0.1	0.2	0.3	0.4	0.5	0.7	0.8	0.8
F+f	0.7	1.2	1.4	2.2	2.4	2.4	2.7	3.1	4.3	5.4	6.4
Base	*470*	*526*	*549*	*534*	*553*	*535*	*490*	*479*	*453*	*466*	*368*

Table 46   Distribution of the number of teeth with
            known decay experience for children of
            different ages   (DMF + df)

Female

Number of teeth with known decay experience	Age at 31 December 1972										
	5+	6+	7+	8+	9+	10+	11+	12+	13+	14+	15+
	%	%	%	%	%	%	%	%	%	%	%
0	28	20	13	9	6	8	6	6	3	4	3
1	11	9	10	6	7	5	5	5	4	2	1
2	12	12	8	8	8	7	7	7	5	3	2
3	6	10	9	9	12	10	9	7	6	5	4
4	10	9	12	9	15	21	19	20	14	10	7
5	8	9	14	13	14	11	15	15	14	8	8
6	7	9	9	14	12	13	13	13	11	9	8
7	5	7	10	11	8	8	8	8	10	11	8
8	5	5	5	8	8	7	9	5	7	9	9
9	2	4	4	5	5	5	4	5	7	10	11
10	3	4	3	4	3	2	2	3	5	5	6
11	1	1	1	2	1	2	1	3	4	5	7
12	1	1	2	2	1	1	1	2	3	6	8
13	-	-	-	-	-	-	1	1	3	4	4
14	1	-	-	-	-	-	-	-	2	2	5
15	-	-	-	-	-	-	-	-	2	2	2
16	-	-	-	-	-	-	-	-	-	2	2
17	-	-	-	-	-	-	-	-	-	1	2
18	-	-	-	-	-	-	-	-	-	1	1
19	-	-	-	-	-	-	-	-	-	-	1
20	-	-	-	-	-	-	-	-	-	1	1
	100	100	100	100	100	100	100	100	100	100	100
Base	*470*	*526*	*549*	*534*	*553*	*535*	*490*	*479*	*453*	*466*	*368*

Table 47   Distribution of the number of teeth in both
            dentitions, which are decayed, missing or filled,
            for children of different ages   (D+d,M,F+f)

Female

Number of teeth	Age at 31 December 1972										
	5+	6+	7+	8+	9+	10+	11+	12+	13+	14+	15+
	%	%	%	%	%	%	%	%	%	%	%
Decayed (D+d) 0	36	31	26	22	24	34	34	42	41	41	45
1	14	16	17	18	22	19	21	22	24	22	21
2	14	12	11	12	16	14	15	12	14	14	13
3	5	9	10	12	12	11	10	8	6	9	7
4	8	8	7	10	11	8	7	5	5	4	5
5	6	6	11	7	7	6	6	6	3	4	3
6	5	5	6	8	2	3	3	1	2	1	4
7	3	4	5	4	2	2	2	2	2	2	1
8	3	3	3	3	2	1	2	1	1	1	-
9	1	2	1	3	1	1	-	1	1	1	-
10	2	2	1	1	1	1	-	-	-	-	1
11+	3	2	2	-	-	-	-	-	1	1	-
	100	100	100	100	100	100	100	100	100	100	100
Missing (M) 0	100	100	98	96	91	85	81	78	72	66	65
1	-	-	1	2	4	6	7	8	9	12	12
2	-	-	1	2	3	5	7	7	9	11	11
3	-	-	-	-	1	-	1	2	3	3	3
4	-	-	-	-	1	4	4	4	7	7	7
5	-	-	-	-	-	-	-	-	-	1	1
6	-	-	-	-	-	-	-	-	-	-	1
7	-	-	-	-	-	-	-	-	-	-	-
8+	-	-	-	-	-	-	-	1	-	-	-
	100	100	100	100	100	100	100	100	100	100	100
Filled (F+f) 0	72	60	53	42	35	31	29	23	17	14	13
1	10	12	14	9	13	10	12	11	7	7	4
2	6	9	9	13	10	11	11	13	10	6	4
3	4	5	7	7	12	16	12	12	12	7	6
4	3	5	7	11	11	14	13	16	13	10	10
5	2	3	4	5	6	7	9	8	10	9	9
6	1	2	3	5	4	4	5	6	9	12	7
7	1	1	1	3	4	3	4	4	5	6	9
8	1	1	1	1	2	1	3	2	5	8	9
9	-	1	1	1	1	1	1	2	3	6	8
10	-	1	-	1	2	1	1	1	3	4	4
11	-	-	-	1	-	1	-	-	2	3	4
12	-	-	-	1	-	-	-	1	2	3	4
13	-	-	-	-	-	-	-	1	1	2	2
14	-	-	-	-	-	-	-	-	1	1	2
15	-	-	-	-	-	-	-	-	-	-	2
16	-	-	-	-	-	-	-	-	-	1	1
17+	-	-	-	-	-	-	-	-	-	1	2
	100	100	100	100	100	100	100	100	100	100	100
Base	*470*	*526*	*549*	*534*	*553*	*535*	*490*	*479*	*453*	*466*	*368*

Table 48   Distribution of the number of permanent
            teeth with decay experience for children
            of different ages   (DMF)

Female

Number of permanent teeth that are, or have been decayed	Age at 31 December 1972										
	5+	6+	7+	8+	9+	10+	11+	12+	13+	14+	15+
	%	%	%	%	%	%	%	%	%	%	%
0	96	84	57	30	23	15	9	8	3	4	3
1	2	8	15	16	11	7	7	5	5	2	1
2	1	4	14	16	16	12	9	8	5	3	2
3	1	2	6	13	15	13	11	9	6	5	4
4	-	2	8	23	29	39	31	25	16	11	7
5	-	-	-	1	4	5	9	12	12	8	8
6	-	-	-	1	1	4	8	10	11	9	8
7	-	-	-	-	1	2	5	6	9	11	9
8	-	-	-	-	-	1	5	5	7	9	9
9	-	-	-	-	-	1	2	4	6	9	11
10	-	-	-	-	-	1	1	3	5	5	6
11	-	-	-	-	-	-	1	2	4	6	7
12	-	-	-	-	-	-	1	1	3	6	8
13	-	-	-	-	-	-	1	1	3	4	4
14	-	-	-	-	-	-	-	-	2	2	5
15	-	-	-	-	-	-	-	1	2	2	2
16	-	-	-	-	-	-	-	-	-	2	2
17	-	-	-	-	-	-	-	-	-	1	2
18	-	-	-	-	-	-	-	-	-	1	1
19	-	-	-	-	-	-	-	-	1	-	1
20	-	-	-	-	-	-	-	-	-	-	-
21	-	-	-	-	-	-	-	-	-	-	-
22	-	-	-	-	-	-	-	-	-	-	-
23+	-	-	-	-	-	-	-	-	-	-	-
	100	100	100	100	100	100	100	100	100	100	100
Base	*470*	*526*	*549*	*534*	*553*	*535*	*490*	*479*	*453*	*466*	*368*

Table 49   Distribution of the number of permanent teeth which are decayed, missing or filled for children of different ages (D,M,F)

Female

Number of permanent teeth	Age at 31 December 1972										
	5+	6+	7+	8+	9+	10+	11+	12+	13+	14+	15+
	%	%	%	%	%	%	%	%	%	%	%
Decayed (D)											
0	97	87	68	58	55	53	44	46	44	42	45
1	2	7	16	19	20	22	22	21	23	22	21
2	1	4	10	12	13	12	13	12	13	14	12
3	-	1	3	7	7	6	8	8	6	8	7
4	-	1	3	4	3	5	6	5	5	4	5
5	-	-	-	-	1	1	3	4	3	4	3
6	-	-	-	-	1	1	1	1	2	2	4
7	-	-	-	-	-	-	2	2	1	1	1
8	-	-	-	-	-	-	1	1	1	1	-
9	-	-	-	-	-	-	-	-	1	1	1
10	-	-	-	-	-	-	-	-	-	-	1
11+	-	-	-	-	-	-	-	-	1	1	-
	100	100	100	100	100	100	100	100	100	100	100
Missing (M)											
0	100	100	98	96	91	85	81	78	72	66	65
1	-	-	1	2	4	6	7	8	9	12	12
2	-	-	1	2	3	5	7	7	9	11	11
3	-	-	-	-	1	-	1	2	3	3	3
4	-	-	-	-	1	4	4	4	7	7	7
5	-	-	-	-	-	-	-	-	-	1	1
6	-	-	-	-	-	-	-	-	-	-	1
7	-	-	-	-	-	-	-	-	-	-	-
8+	-	-	-	-	-	-	-	1	-	-	-
	100	100	100	100	100	100	100	100	100	100	100
Filled (F)											
0	99	95	83	59	48	38	32	25	17	15	12
1	1	3	6	13	13	9	11	10	7	7	4
2	-	1	6	9	13	15	13	14	10	6	4
3	-	-	2	7	12	17	12	12	13	7	6
4	-	1	3	12	13	18	17	18	14	10	10
5	-	-	-	-	1	2	6	5	9	9	9
6	-	-	-	-	-	-	3	5	8	11	7
7	-	-	-	-	-	1	2	4	5	6	9
8	-	-	-	-	-	-	2	2	5	8	10
9	-	-	-	-	-	-	1	2	3	6	8
10	-	-	-	-	-	-	1	1	3	4	4
11	-	-	-	-	-	-	-	-	2	3	4
12	-	-	-	-	-	-	-	1	2	3	4
13	-	-	-	-	-	-	-	1	1	2	2
14	-	-	-	-	-	-	-	-	1	1	2
15	-	-	-	-	-	-	-	-	-	-	2
16	-	-	-	-	-	-	-	-	-	1	1
17+	-	-	-	-	-	-	-	-	-	1	2
	100	100	100	100	100	100	100	100	100	100	100
Base	*470*	*526*	*549*	*534*	*553*	*535*	*490*	*479*	*453*	*466*	*368*

Table 50   Distribution of the number of deciduous
            teeth which are decayed or filled for
            children of different ages (df,d,f)   *Female*

Number of deciduous teeth		Age at 31 December 1972										
		5+	6+	7+	8+	9+	10+	11+	12+	13+	14+	15+
		%	%	%	%	%	%	%	%	%	%	%
Decayed or filled df	0	28	20	17	14	23	42	62	84	91	97	98
	1	11	10	12	11	17	14	15	8	6	2	1
	2	13	13	12	15	18	16	11	4	3	1	1
	3	7	11	14	16	12	10	5	3	-	-	-
	4	10	9	11	15	13	8	4	1	-	-	-
	5	8	10	13	10	8	6	2	-	-	-	-
	6	7	8	10	9	4	2	1	-	-	-	-
	7	4	7	5	3	3	2	-	-	-	-	-
	8	5	5	3	5	2	-	-	-	-	-	-
	9	1	3	2	2	-	-	-	-	-	-	-
	10	3	2	1	-	-	-	-	-	-	-	-
	11	1	1	-	-	-	-	-	-	-	-	-
	12	-	1	-	-	-	-	-	-	-	-	-
	13	-	-	-	-	-	-	-	-	-	-	-
	14	1	-	-	-	-	-	-	-	-	-	-
	15+	1	-	-	-	-	-	-	-	-	-	-
		100	100	100	100	100	100	100	100	100	100	100
Decayed (d)	0	36	32	32	29	37	56	72	89	94	97	99
	1	15	16	17	21	26	15	15	7	4	2	1
	2	13	13	12	14	17	14	6	2	2	1	-
	3	6	9	12	15	9	7	3	2	-	-	-
	4	9	8	7	8	4	4	2	-	-	-	-
	5	6	7	9	4	3	3	1	-	-	-	-
	6	4	5	5	5	1	1	1	-	-	-	-
	7	2	4	3	2	2	-	-	-	-	-	-
	8	4	2	1	2	1	-	-	-	-	-	-
	9	1	2	1	-	-	-	-	-	-	-	-
	10	2	1	1	-	-	-	-	-	-	-	-
	11	1	1	-	-	-	-	-	-	-	-	-
	12	-	-	-	-	-	-	-	-	-	-	-
	13+	1	-	-	-	-	-	-	-	-	-	-
		100	100	100	100	100	100	100	100	100	100	100
Filled (f)	0	73	61	57	55	59	70	82	91	96	99	100
	1	10	13	15	13	14	14	10	5	3	1	-
	2	6	8	11	13	11	8	4	2	1	-	-
	3	3	6	7	9	7	4	3	2	-	-	-
	4	3	5	4	4	5	2	1	-	-	-	-
	5	2	3	4	2	1	1	-	-	-	-	-
	6	1	2	1	2	2	-	-	-	-	-	-
	7	1	1	-	1	1	1	-	-	-	-	-
	8+	1	1	1	1	-	-	-	-	-	-	-
		100	100	100	100	100	100	100	100	100	100	100
Base		*470*	*526*	*549*	*534*	*553*	*535*	*490*	*479*	*453*	*466*	*368*

Table 51   Average number of teeth with known decay
            experience, for children of different ages,
            showing type of treatement and dentition

Average number of teeth decay experience	Age at 31 December 1972										
	5+	6+	7+	8+	9+	10+	11+	12+	13+	14+	15+
Deciduous											
df	3.3	3.6	3.5	3.3	2.8	1.9	1.0	0.4	0.2	0.0	0.0
d	2.6	2.5	2.3	2.1	1.6	1.2	0.6	0.2	0.1	0.0	0.0
f	0.7	1.1	1.1	1.2	1.2	0.7	0.4	0.2	0.1	0.0	0.0
Permanent											
DMF	0.0	0.3	0.9	1.8	2.3	3.0	4.0	4.9	6.2	7.5	8.6
D	0.0	0.2	0.5	0.8	0.9	1.0	1.3	1.4	1.6	1.9	1.6
M	0.0	0.0	0.0	0.1	0.1	0.3	0.4	0.5	0.9	0.8	0.9
F	0.0	0.1	0.3	0.9	1.3	1.7	2.3	2.9	3.9	4.8	6.2
Both											
DMF + df	3.4	3.9	4.3	5.0	5.1	4.9	5.0	5.3	6.3	7.5	8.6
D+d	2.7	2.7	2.8	2.8	2.5	2.2	2.0	1.7	1.7	1.9	1.6
M	0.0	0.0	0.0	0.1	0.1	0.3	0.4	0.5	0.9	0.8	0.9
F+f	0.7	1.2	1.5	2.2	2.4	2.5	2.7	3.1	4.0	4.9	6.2
Base	*895*	*1005*	*1080*	*1032*	*1068*	*1033*	*923*	*917*	*872*	*887*	*651*

Table 52   Distribution of the number of teeth with
            known decay experience for children of
            different ages   (DMF + df)

Racial Origin: White

Number of teeth with known decay experience	Age at 31 December 1972										
	5+	6+	7+	8+	9+	10+	11+	12+	13+	14+	15+
	%	%	%	%	%	%	%	%	%	%	%
0	28	20	14	9	7	7	5	5	4	4	2
1	12	10	10	6	6	5	5	5	4	3	3
2	11	11	8	8	8	7	7	7	7	4	3
3	8	10	10	10	11	11	10	9	8	6	4
4	9	10	12	11	13	18	21	20	14	11	7
5	8	9	12	13	12	13	14	14	12	9	8
6	7	9	10	12	13	14	13	11	12	10	9
7	5	8	9	11	9	8	8	10	10	10	9
8	4	5	6	7	8	7	8	6	7	8	9
9	2	3	4	5	5	5	4	4	6	8	9
10	2	3	3	4	4	2	2	3	3	6	7
11	1	1	1	2	2	2	1	2	4	5	6
12	1	1	1	2	1	1	1	2	2	5	7
13	1	-	-	-	-	-	1	1	3	3	4
14	1	-	-	-	1	-	-	1	1	2	4
15	-	-	-	-	-	-	-	-	2	2	2
16	-	-	-	-	-	-	-	-	1	2	2
17	-	-	-	-	-	-	-	-	-	1	2
18	-	-	-	-	-	-	-	-	-	1	1
19	-	-	-	-	-	-	-	-	-	-	1
20+	-	-	-	-	-	-	-	-	-	-	1
	100	100	100	100	100	100	100	100	100	100	100
Base	*895*	*1005*	*1080*	*1032*	*1068*	*1033*	*923*	*917*	*872*	*887*	*651*

Table 53   Distribution of the numbers of teeth, in both
            dentitions, which are decayed, missing or filled,
            for children of different ages   (D+d,M,F+f)

Racial Origin: White

Number of teeth		5+	6+	7+	8+	9+	10+	11+	12+	13+	14+	15+
		%	%	%	%	%	%	%	%	%	%	%
Decayed (D+d)	0	37	31	27	22	24	30	34	39	39	38	43
	1	14	16	17	18	19	19	19	23	23	21	21
	2	12	13	10	14	16	16	16	14	14	14	12
	3	7	9	12	13	13	12	11	9	8	9	8
	4	7	8	7	10	11	9	7	6	6	6	5
	5	6	6	9	6	6	6	6	4	4	5	3
	6	5	5	6	7	4	3	4	2	3	2	3
	7	3	4	5	3	3	2	2	1	1	1	2
	8	3	3	3	2	2	1	1	1	1	2	1
	9	2	2	2	2	1	1	-	-	1	1	-
	10	2	1	1	1	1	1	-	1	-	1	1
	11	1	1	1	1	-	-	-	-	-	-	-
	12	1	1	-	1	-	-	-	-	-	-	1
	13+	-	-	-	-	-	-	-	-	-	-	-
		100	100	100	100	100	100	100	100	100	100	100
Missing (M)	0	100	100	98	97	92	87	82	77	72	69	66
	1	-	-	2	2	4	5	7	8	10	11	12
	2	-	-	-	1	3	5	6	8	9	9	9
	3	-	-	-	-	1	-	1	2	3	3	4
	4	-	-	-	-	-	3	4	5	6	7	8
	5	-	-	-	-	-	-	-	-	-	1	1
	6	-	-	-	-	-	-	-	-	-	-	-
	7	-	-	-	-	-	-	-	-	-	-	-
	8+	-	-	-	-	-	-	-	-	-	-	-
		100	100	100	100	100	100	100	100	100	100	100
Filled (F+f)	0	73	60	53	42	35	32	29	23	21	18	10
	1	10	13	13	11	13	10	12	11	8	9	6
	2	6	9	10	11	11	11	12	14	11	7	6
	3	4	5	8	9	12	14	11	13	11	9	6
	4	3	6	6	11	11	15	15	16	12	9	9
	5	2	3	5	5	6	7	9	7	9	8	9
	6	-	2	3	4	4	5	5	6	9	9	8
	7	1	1	1	3	4	3	3	4	4	6	9
	8	1	1	1	1	2	1	2	3	3	6	9
	9	-	-	-	1	1	1	1	1	3	5	8
	10	-	-	-	1	1	1	1	1	3	3	5
	11	-	-	-	1	-	-	-	1	2	3	4
	12	-	-	-	-	-	-	-	-	2	3	3
	13	-	-	-	-	-	-	-	-	1	2	3
	14	-	-	-	-	-	-	-	-	1	1	1
	15	-	-	-	-	-	-	-	-	-	1	2
	16	-	-	-	-	-	-	-	-	-	1	1
	17+	-	-	-	-	-	-	-	-	-	-	1
		100	100	100	100	100	100	100	100	100	100	100
Base		*895*	*1005*	*1080*	*1032*	*1068*	*1033*	*923*	*917*	*872*	*887*	*651*

Table 54　Distribution of the number of permanent teeth with decay experience for children of different ages　(DMF)

Racial Origin: White

Number of permanent teeth that are, or have been decayed	Age at 31 December 1972										
	5+	6+	7+	8+	9+	10+	11+	12+	13+	14+	15+
	%	%	%	%	%	%	%	%	%	%	%
0	97	84	60	35	25	15	9	7	4	4	2
1	2	8	15	16	13	9	7	6	4	3	3
2	1	4	12	14	15	12	9	8	7	4	3
3	-	2	5	13	14	14	13	9	8	6	3
4	-	2	7	20	28	39	34	26	16	12	7
5	-	-	1	1	3	5	9	11	10	9	8
6	-	-	-	1	1	3	6	10	12	10	9
7	-	-	-	-	-	2	5	7	9	9	9
8	-	-	-	-	1	1	4.	5	7	8	10
9	-	-	-	-	-	-	2	3	5	8	9
10	-	-	-	-	-	-	1	3	4	5	7
11	-	-	-	-	-	-	1	2	4	5	6
12	-	-	-	-	-	-	-	1	2	5	7
13	-	-	-	-	-	-	-	1	3	3	4
14	-	-	-	-	-	-	-	1	1	2	4
15	-	-	-	-	-	-	-	-	2	2	2
16	-	-	-	-	-	-	-	-	1	3	2
17	-	-	-	-	-	-	-	-	1	1	2
18	-	-	-	-	-	-	-	-	-	1	1
19	-	-	-	-	-	-	-	-	-	-	1
20+	-	-	-	-	-	-	-	-	-	-	1
	100	100	100	100	100	100	100	100	100	100	100
Base	895	1005	1080	1032	1068	1033	923	917	872	887	651

Table 55 Distribution of the number of permanent teeth which are decayed, missing or filled for children of different ages (D,M,F)

Racial Origin: White

Number of permanent teeth	Age at 31 December 1972										
	5+	6+	7+	8+	9+	10+	11+	12+	13+	14+	15+
	%	%	%	%	%	%	%	%	%	%	%
Decayed (D)											
0	98	88	73	60	57	53	47	46	42	39	43
1	2	7	14	19	19	22	19	21	23	21	22
2	-	3	8	11	13	12	13	13	14	14	12
3	-	1	2	5	6	6	9	8	7	8	8
4	-	1	3	4	4	5	6	5	5	6	5
5	-	-	-	1	1	1	3	3	4	4	3
6	-	-	-	-	-	1	1	2	2	2	3
7	-	-	-	-	-	-	1	1	1	1	2
8	-	-	-	-	-	-	1	1	1	2	-
9	-	-	-	-	-	-	-	-	1	1	-
10	-	-	-	-	-	-	-	-	-	1	1
11+	-	-	-	-	-	-	-	-	-	1	1
	100	100	100	100	100	100	100	100	100	100	100
Missing (M)											
0	100	100	98	97	92	87	82	77	72	69	66
1	-	-	2	2	4	5	7	8	10	11	12
2	-	-	-	1	3	5	6	8	9	9	9
3	-	-	-	-	1	-	1	2	3	3	4
4	-	-	-	-	-	3	4	5	6	7	8
5	-	-	-	-	-	-	-	-	-	1	1
6	-	-	-	-	-	-	-	-	-	-	-
7	-	-	-	-	-	-	-	-	-	-	-
8+	-	-	-	-	-	-	-	-	-	-	-
	100	100	100	100	100	100	100	100	100	100	100
Filled (F)											
0	100	95	83	62	50	38	32	24	21	18	10
1	-	3	7	12	13	11	12	11	8	9	6
2	-	1	5	9	13	16	14	15	11	8	6
3	-	1	2	7	11	15	12	13	12	9	7
4	-	-	3	10	12	18	18	18	12	9	9
5	-	-	-	-	1	2	5	5	9	7	9
6	-	-	-	-	-	-	3	4	8	9	8
7	-	-	-	-	-	-	1	4	4	6	9
8	-	-	-	-	-	-	1	2	3	6	9
9	-	-	-	-	-	-	1	1	3	5	8
10	-	-	-	-	-	-	1	1	3	3	5
11	-	-	-	-	-	-	-	1	2	3	4
12	-	-	-	-	-	-	-	1	2	3	3
13	-	-	-	-	-	-	-	-	1	2	3
14	-	-	-	-	-	-	-	-	1	1	1
15	-	-	-	-	-	-	-	-	-	1	2
16	-	-	-	-	-	-	-	-	-	1	1
17+	-	-	-	-	-	-	-	-	-	-	-
	100	100	100	100	100	100	100	100	100	100	100
Base	*895*	*1005*	*1080*	*1032*	*1068*	*1033*	*923*	*917*	*872*	*887*	*651*

Table 56   Distribution of the number of deciduous teeth which are decayed or filled, for children of different ages   (df,d,f)

Racial Origin: White

Number of deciduous teeth	Age at 31 December 1972										
	5+	6+	7+	8+	9+	10+	11+	12+	13+	14+	15+
	%	%	%	%	%	%	%	%	%	%	%
Decayed or filled (df) 0	28	21	17	15	19	36	57	79	90	97	99
1	11	11	11	12	15	14	16	10	7	2	1
2	11	12	11	14	18	16	12	6	2	1	-
3	8	10	14	16	13	12	6	4	1	-	-
4	10	12	13	15	14	9	5	1	-	-	-
5	8	10	12	10	9	7	2	-	-	-	-
6	7	8	9	8	5	3	2	-	-	-	-
7	4	6	6	5	4	2	-	-	-	-	-
8	4	5	4	4	2	1	-	-	-	-	-
9	2	2	2	1	-	-	-	-	-	-	-
10	3	2	1	-	1	-	-	-	-	-	-
11	1	1	-	-	-	-	-	-	-	-	-
12	1	-	-	-	-	-	-	-	-	-	-
13	1	-	-	-	-	-	-	-	-	-	-
14	1	-	-	-	-	-	-	-	-	-	-
15+	-	-	-	-	-	-	-	-	-	-	-
	100	100	100	100	100	100	100	100	100	100	100
Decayed (D) 0	37	32	32	28	34	49	67	85	93	98	99
1	14	16	17	22	24	18	17	10	5	2	1
2	12	13	11	15	18	14	8	4	2	-	-
3	7	9	12	15	10	9	4	1	-	-	-
4	7	8	8	8	7	5	2	-	-	-	-
5	6	7	8	4	3	3	1	-	-	-	-
6	5	5	5	4	2	1	1	-	-	-	-
7	3	4	3	2	1	-	-	-	-	-	-
8	3	3	2	1	1	1	-	-	-	-	-
9	2	1	1	1	-	-	-	-	-	-	-
10	2	1	1	-	-	-	-	-	-	-	-
11	1	1	-	-	-	-	-	-	-	-	-
12	1	-	-	-	-	-	-	-	-	-	-
13	-	-	-	-	-	-	-	-	-	-	-
	100	100	100	100	100	100	100	100	100	100	100
Filled (f) 0	73	61	58	54	55	67	79	90	96	99	100
1	10	13	13	14	15	14	10	6	3	1	-
2	6	9	11	12	12	10	6	3	1	-	-
3	4	5	7	8	7	4	3	1	-	-	-
4	3	6	5	5	5	2	1	-	-	-	-
5	2	3	4	3	3	1	1	-	-	-	-
6	-	1	1	2	2	1	-	-	-	-	-
7	1	1	1	1	1	1	-	-	-	-	-
8+	1	1	-	1	-	-	-	-	-	-	-
	100	100	100	100	100	100	100	100	100	100	100
Base	*895*	*1005*	*1080*	*1032*	*1068*	*1033*	*923*	*917*	*872*	*887*	*651*

Table 57   Average number of teeth with known decay
            experience, for children of different ages,
            showing type of treatement and dentition

Racial Origin: Non-white

Average number of teeth with known decay experience	Age at 31 December 1972										
	5+	6+	7+	8+	9+	10+	11+	12+	13+	14+	15+
Deciduous df	3.1	3.6	2.8	2.8	2.2	1.5	0.7	0.2	0.0	0.1	0.1
d	2.7	2.7	1.8	1.7	1.6	0.7	0.6	0.1	0.0	0.1	0.1
f	0.4	0.9	1.0	1.1	0.6	0.8	0.2	0.1	0.0	0.1	0.0
Permanent DMF	0.1	0.2	0.7	1.2	1.6	2.2	3.0	3.8	4.3	5.1	5.2
D	0.1	0.1	0.4	0.7	0.6	0.7	0.9	1.5	1.9	1.6	1.6
M	0.0	0.0	0.0	0.1	0.1	0.2	0.3	0.5	0.5	0.6	0.5
F	0.1	0.1	0.3	0.4	0.9	1.3	1.8	1.8	1.9	2.9	3.2
Both DMF + df	3.2	3.8	3.5	4.0	3.8	3.6	3.7	4.0	4.4	5.2	5.3
D+d	2.8	2.9	2.3	2.4	2.2	1.5	1.4	1.7	2.1	1.7	1.6
M	0.0	0.0	0.0	0.1	0.1	0.2	0.3	0.5	0.5	0.6	0.5
F+f	0.4	0.9	1.2	1.5	1.5	2.0	2.0	1.9	1.9	3.0	3.2
Base	*57*	*75*	*52*	*57*	*60*	*58*	*60*	*39*	*42*	*34*	*44*

Table 58   Distribution of the number of teeth with
           known decay experience for children of
           different ages   (DMF + df)

Racial Origin: Non-white

Number of teeth with known decay experience	Age at 31 December 1972										
	5+	6+	7+	8+	9+	10+	11+	12+	13+	14+	15+
	%	%	%	%	%	%	%	%	%	%	%
0	34	24	23	16	19	17	14	18	22	11	20
1	18	6	18	7	8	10	13	8	10	14	5
2	7	15	9	13	15	12	9	8	12	9	5
3	5	9	2	17	17	5	11	16	2	3	9
4	5	11	10	9	8	23	15	21	12	4	7
5	3	8	14	5	10	7	11	5	10	9	4
6	7	4	5	5	3	8	10	3	10	11	9
7	9	7	3	12	2	9	10	-	5	11	9
8	2	8	2	7	2	6	3	5	2	8	11
9	2	4	9	5	8	-	-	8	2	8	7
10	2	1	-	-	5	-	2	4	5	3	2
11	-	1	2	-	-	3	1	2	2	3	4
12	2	1	-	2	3	-	-	-	2	-	4
13	-	1	3	-	-	-	-	2	-	3	-
14	2	-	-	2	-	-	1	-	2	3	2
15	-	-	-	-	-	-	-	-	-	-	-
16	2	-	-	-	-	-	-	-	2	-	-
17	-	-	-	-	-	-	-	-	-	-	-
18	-	-	-	-	-	-	-	-	-	-	-
19	-	-	-	-	-	-	-	-	-	-	2
20	-	-	-	-	-	-	-	-	-	-	-
	100	100	100	100	100	100	100	100	100	100	100
Base	57	75	52	57	60	58	60	39	42	34	44

Table 59   Distribution of the number of teeth, in both dentitions, which are decayed, missing or filled, for children of different ages   (D+d,M,F+f)

Racial Origin: Non-white

Number of teeth	Age at 31 December 1972										
	5+	6+	7+	8+	9+	10+	11+	12+	13+	14+	15+
	%	%	%	%	%	%	%	%	%	%	%
Decayed (D+d) 0	39	35	36	25	32	43	41	45	43	39	42
1	16	13	25	18	13	18	19	10	14	20	13
2	7	12	7	14	23	18	14	17	19	17	16
3	3	9	2	17	17	7	13	10	3	4	13
4	9	6	10	5	3	7	5	8	3	6	7
5	5	4	9	10	3	3	6	5	5	3	5
6	6	7	–	2	2	3	2	–	2	11	2
7	3	4	3	7	–	–	–	5	7	–	2
8	2	4	3	2	2	1	–	–	–	–	–
9	2	3	–	–	2	–	–	–	2	–	–
10	2	–	–	–	–	–	–	–	–	–	–
11	2	1	3	–	–	–	–	–	2	–	–
12	2	1	–	–	3	–	–	–	–	–	–
13+	2	1	2	–	–	–	–	–	–	–	–
	100	100	100	100	100	100	100	100	100	100	100
Missing (M) 0	100	100	100	93	95	94	85	75	76	74	82
1	–	–	–	5	2	2	6	15	7	9	2
2	–	–	–	2	2	1	2	5	14	9	9
3	–	–	–	–	–	–	2	–	3	–	5
4	–	–	–	–	1	3	5	5	–	8	–
5	–	–	–	–	–	–	–	–	–	–	–
6	–	–	–	–	–	–	–	–	–	–	2
7	–	–	–	–	–	–	–	–	–	–	–
8+	–	–	–	–	–	–	–	–	–	–	–
	100	100	100	100	100	100	100	100	100	100	100
Filled (F+f) 0	80	72	66	58	57	42	43	46	60	40	40
1	9	6	12	5	8	16	13	14	7	12	7
2	3	5	4	10	10	11	10	13	5	6	9
3	5	3	2	9	5	8	11	5	5	6	–
4	2	7	5	2	7	7	6	8	5	3	9
5	–	3	2	5	5	7	6	–	5	8	7
6	1	–	2	3	1	3	3	5	7	11	7
7	–	3	2	6	7	3	2	5	2	–	7
8	–	1	2	2	–	–	2	–	–	3	4
9	–	–	3	–	–	–	–	–	–	8	4
10	–	–	–	–	–	–	–	1	2	–	4
11	–	–	–	–	–	3	2	3	–	–	–
12	–	–	–	–	–	–	–	–	–	3	–
13	–	–	–	–	–	–	2	–	–	–	–
14	–	–	–	–	–	–	–	–	2	–	–
15	–	–	–	–	–	–	–	–	–	–	–
16	–	–	–	–	–	–	–	–	–	–	–
17+	–	–	–	–	–	–	–	–	–	–	2
	100	100	100	100	100	100	100	100	100	100	100
Base	*57*	*75*	*52*	*57*	*60*	*58*	*60*	*39*	*42*	*34*	*44*

Table 60   Distribution of the number of permanent
            teeth with decay experience for children
            of different ages   (DMF)

Racial Origin: Non-white

Number of permanent teeth that are, or have been decayed	Age at 31 December 1972										
	5+	6+	7+	8+	9+	10+	11+	12+	13+	14+	15+
	%	%	%	%	%	%	%	%	%	%	%
0	95	86	68	46	42	27	23	18	21	11	20
1	2	13	9	17	14	10	15	10	12	14	5
2	2	-	11	12	10	18	9	5	10	9	5
3	1	-	5	14	10	9	8	19	5	6	9
4	-	1	7	10	22	34	23	24	12	1	7
5	-	-	-	1	2	2	6	3	7	8	7
6	-	-	-	-	-	-	5	-	10	11	9
7	-	-	-	-	-	-	5	-	5	11	9
8	-	-	-	-	-	-	2	10	5	11	11
9	-	-	-	-	-	-	-	3	-	6	4
10	-	-	-	-	-	-	2	4	5	3	2
11	-	-	-	-	-	-	1	2	2	3	4
12	-	-	-	-	-	-	-	-	2	3	4
13	-	-	-	-	-	-	-	2	-	3	-
14	-	-	-	-	-	-	1	-	2	-	2
15	-	-	-	-	-	-	-	-	-	-	-
16	-	-	-	-	-	-	-	-	2	-	-
17	-	-	-	-	-	-	-	-	-	-	-
18	-	-	-	-	-	-	-	-	-	-	-
19	-	-	-	-	-	-	-	-	-	-	2
20	-	-	-	-	-	-	-	-	-	-	-
	100	100	100	100	100	100	100	100	100	100	100
Base	57	75	52	57	60	58	60	39	42	34	44

Table 61 Distribution of the number of permanent teeth which are decayed, missing or filled for children of different ages   (D,M,F)

Racial Origin: Non-white

Number of permanent teeth	Age at 31 December 1972										
	5+	6+	7+	8+	9+	10+	11+	12+	13+	14+	15+
	%	%	%	%	%	%	%	%	%	%	%
Decayed (D)											
0	96	88	79	63	69	65	54	45	43	43	44
1	2	12	7	18	14	11	19	15	17	17	11
2	2	-	7	7	11	16	15	14	17	17	16
3	-	-	4	9	3	2	5	10	5	6	13
4	-	-	3	3	3	6	5	8	2	3	7
5	-	-	-	-	-	-	2	3	2	3	7
6	-	-	-	-	-	-	-	-	5	11	2
7	-	-	-	-	-	-	-	5	5	-	-
8	-	-	-	-	-	-	-	-	-	-	-
9	-	-	-	-	-	-	-	-	2	-	-
10	-	-	-	-	-	-	-	-	-	-	-
11+	-	-	-	-	-	-	-	-	2	-	-
	100	100	100	100	100	100	100	100	100	100	100
Missing (M)											
0	100	100	100	93	95	94	85	75	76	74	82
1	-	-	-	5	2	2	6	15	7	9	2
2	-	-	-	2	2	1	2	5	14	9	9
3	-	-	-	-	-	-	2	-	3	-	5
4	-	-	-	-	1	3	5	5	-	8	-
5	-	-	-	-	-	-	-	-	-	-	-
6	-	-	-	-	-	-	-	-	-	-	2
7	-	-	-	-	-	-	-	-	-	-	-
8+	-	-	-	-	-	-	-	-	-	-	-
	100	100	100	100	100	100	100	100	100	100	100
Filled (F)											
0	96	98	86	79	67	56	54	46	60	40	40
1	2	1	5	6	10	5	6	14	7	12	7
2	2	1	5	7	3	13	6	14	5	6	9
3	-	-	2	3	7	7	10	5	5	6	-
4	-	-	2	3	13	17	10	10	5	3	11
5	-	-	-	2	-	2	3	-	5	8	5
6	-	-	-	-	-	-	3	3	7	11	7
7	-	-	-	-	-	-	2	5	2	-	7
8	-	-	-	-	-	-	2	-	-	3	4
9	-	-	-	-	-	-	-	-	-	8	4
10	-	-	-	-	-	-	-	1	2	3	4
11	-	-	-	-	-	-	2	2	-	-	-
12	-	-	-	-	-	-	-	-	-	-	-
13	-	-	-	-	-	-	2	-	-	-	-
14	-	-	-	-	-	-	-	-	2	-	-
15	-	-	-	-	-	-	-	-	-	-	-
16	-	-	-	-	-	-	-	-	-	-	-
17+	-	-	-	-	-	-	-	-	-	-	2
	100	100	100	100	100	100	100	100	100	100	100
Base	*57*	*75*	*52*	*57*	*60*	*58*	*60*	*39*	*42*	*34*	*44*

Table 62   Distribution of the number of deciduous teeth which are decayed or filled for children of different ages (df,d,f)

Racial Origin: Non-white

Number of deciduous teeth		5+	6+	7+	8+	9+	10+	11+	12+	13+	14+	15+
		%	%	%	%	%	%	%	%	%	%	%
Decayed or filled (df)	0	36	26	23	23	31	50	67	84	90	91	93
	1	16	5	20	9	17	15	11	13	10	6	5
	2	7	15	12	21	19	9	7	3	-	3	2
	3	5	10	9	14	9	12	10	-	-	-	-
	4	9	13	9	12	5	4	2	-	-	-	-
	5	3	4	9	5	8	3	3	-	-	-	-
	6	5	4	4	9	6	4	-	-	-	-	-
	7	7	8	7	2	-	3	-	-	-	-	-
	8	2	6	3	3	5	-	-	-	-	-	-
	9	2	4	2	-	-	-	-	-	-	-	-
	10	2	3	-	2	-	-	-	-	-	-	-
	11	-	-	-	-	-	-	-	-	-	-	-
	12	2	1	-	-	-	-	-	-	-	-	-
	13	-	1	2	-	-	-	-	-	-	-	-
	14	2	-	-	-	-	-	-	-	-	-	-
	15+	2	-	-	-	-	-	-	-	-	-	-
		100	100	100	100	100	100	100	100	100	100	100
Decayed (d)	0	41	38	39	31	39	62	76	87	90	94	96
	1	14	10	25	25	23	22	8	13	10	6	2
	2	7	14	5	19	14	7	6	-	-	-	-
	3	3	7	9	12	12	3	6	-	-	-	-
	4	11	8	10	3	2	2	2	-	-	-	-
	5	5	3	2	3	3	3	2	-	-	-	-
	6	4	7	-	7	2	1	-	-	-	-	-
	7	3	4	7	-	-	-	-	-	-	-	-
	8	2	3	2	-	5	-	-	-	-	-	-
	9	2	3	-	-	-	-	-	-	-	-	-
	10	2	1	-	-	-	-	-	-	-	-	-
	11	2	-	-	-	-	-	-	-	-	-	-
	12	2	1	-	-	-	-	-	-	-	-	-
	13+	2	1	1	-	-	-	-	-	-	-	-
		100	100	100	100	100	100	100	100	100	100	100
Filled (f)	0	84	73	68	59	73	69	85	97	100	97	98
	1	7	7	12	12	13	16	10	3	-	-	2
	2	2	6	5	12	5	3	3	-	-	3	-
	3	5	4	2	5	5	7	2	-	-	-	-
	4	2	5	2	6	3	2	-	-	-	-	-
	5	-	1	7	2	-	-	-	-	-	-	-
	6	-	-	-	2	1	-	-	-	-	-	-
	7	-	3	4	2	-	3	-	-	-	-	-
	8+	-	1	-	-	-	-	-	-	-	-	-
		100	100	100	100	100	100	100	100	100	100	100
Base		*57*	*75*	*52*	*57*	*60*	*58*	*60*	*39*	*42*	*34*	*44*

Table 63
Known disease experience of individual teeth for children aged five

(a) Upper jaw

Condition of teeth	Left 8	7	6	e 5	d 4	c 3	b 2	a 1	a 1	b 2	c 3	d 4	e 5	6	7	Right 8
	%	%	%	%	%	%	%	%	%	%	%	%	%	%	%	%
Deciduous																
Sound				60	74	95	90	78	78	90	94	76	59			
Filled				10	6	–	–	–	–	–	–	5	11			
Decayed				26	16	5	7	14	15	7	6	15	26			
Unerupted	100	100	77	4	4	–	3	6	5	3	–	4	4	78	100	100
Permanent																
Sound	–	–	22	–	–	–	–	2	2	–	–	–	–	21	–	–
Filled	–	–	–	–	–	–	–	–	–	–	–	–	–	–	–	–
Decayed	–	–	1	–	–	–	–	–	–	–	–	–	–	1	–	–
Missing, decayed	–	–	–	–	–	–	–	–	–	–	–	–	–	–	–	–
" trauma	–	–	–	–	–	–	–	–	–	–	–	–	–	–	–	–
" ortho	–	–	–	–	–	–	–	–	–	–	–	–	–	–	–	–
Decay categories																
Deciduous																
Decayed				17	10	4	5	11	12	5	5	9	17			
Unrestorable				7	5	1	2	3	3	2	1	5	7			
Filled & decayed				2	1	–	–	–	–	–	–	1	2			
Permanent																
Decayed	–	–	1	–	–	–	–	–	–	–	–	–	–	1	–	–
Unrestorable	–	–	–	–	–	–	–	–	–	–	–	–	–	–	–	–
Filled & decayed	–	–	–	–	–	–	–	–	–	–	–	–	–	–	–	–

(b) Lower jaw

Condition of teeth	Right 8	7	6	e 5	d 4	c 3	b 2	a 1	a 1	b 2	c 3	d 4	e 5	6	7	Left 8
	%	%	%	%	%	%	%	%	%	%	%	%	%	%	%	%
Deciduous																
Sound				53	57	95	93	73	73	94	95	57	51			
Filled				9	8	–	–	–	–	–	–	7	11			
Decayed				28	27	5	2	1	1	2	5	27	28			
Unerupted	100	100	78	10	8	–	3	2	3	2	–	9	10	77	100	100
Permanent																
Sound	–	–	21	–	–	–	2	24	23	2	–	–	–	22	–	–
Filled	–	–	–	–	–	–	–	–	–	–	–	–	–	–	–	–
Decayed	–	–	1	–	–	–	–	–	–	–	–	–	–	1	–	–
Missing, decayed	–	–	–	–	–	–	–	–	–	–	–	–	–	–	–	–
" trauma	–	–	–	–	–	–	–	–	–	–	–	–	–	–	–	–
" ortho	–	–	–	–	–	–	–	–	–	–	–	–	–	–	–	–
Decay categories																
Deciduous																
Decayed				15	13	4	2	1	1	2	4	14	16			
Unrestorable				10	13	1	–	–	–	–	1	12	9			
Filled & decayed				3	1	–	–	–	–	–	–	1	3			
Permanent																
Decayed	–	–	1	–	–	–	–	–	–	–	–	–	–	1	–	–
Unrestorable	–	–	–	–	–	–	–	–	–	–	–	–	–	–	–	–
Filled & decayed	–	–	–	–	–	–	–	–	–	–	–	–	–	–	–	–

Table 64
Known disease experience of individual teeth for children aged six

(a) Upper jaw

Condition of teeth	Left 8	7	6	e 5	d 4	c 3	b 2	a 1	a 1	b 2	c 3	d 4	e 5	6	7	Right 8
Deciduous	%	%	%	%	%	%	%	%	%	%	%	%	%	%	%	%
Sound				52	65	93	80	52	52	80	94	66	52			
Filled				15	7	1	-	-	-	-	1	8	16			
Decayed				27	21	6	7	9	10	6	5	18	25			
Unerupted	100	100	33	6	7	-	10	11	10	10	-	8	7	32	100	100
Permanent																
Sound	-	-	60	-	-	-	3	28	28	4	-	-	-	61	-	-
Filled	-	-	2	-	-	-	-	-	-	-	-	-	-	2	-	-
Decayed	-	-	5	-	-	-	-	-	-	-	-	-	-	5	-	-
Missing, decayed	-	-	-	-	-	-	-	-	-	-	-	-	-	-	-	-
" trauma	-	-	-	-	-	-	-	-	-	-	-	-	-	-	-	-
" ortho	-	-	-	-	-	-	-	-	-	-	-	-	-	-	-	-
Decay Categories																
Deciduous																
Decayed				16	13	4	5	7	8	4	3	10	15			
Unrestorable				8	7	2	2	2	2	2	1	7	7			
Filled & decayed				3	1	-	-	-	-	-	1	1	3			
Permanent																
Decayed	-	-	4	-	-	-	-	-	-	-	-	-	-	4	-	-
Unrestorable	-	-	}1	-	-	-	-	-	-	-	-	-	-	}1	-	-
Filled & decayed	-	-		-	-	-	-	-	-	-	-	-	-		-	-

(b) Lower jaw

Condition of teeth	Right 8	7	6	e 5	d 4	c 3	b 2	a 1	a 1	b 2	c 3	d 4	e 5	6	7	Left 8
Deciduous	%	%	%	%	%	%	%	%	%	%	%	%	%	%	%	%
Sound				43	46	93	68	23	24	70	93	46	41			
Filled				16	12	1	-	-	-	-	1	12	16			
Decayed				27	26	5	2	-	-	2	5	26	27			
Unerupted	100	100	31	14	16	1	8	3	3	7	1	16	16	30	100	100
Permanent																
Sound	-	-	62	-	-	-	22	74	73	21	-	-	-	62	-	-
Filled	-	-	2	-	-	-	-	-	-	-	-	-	-	2	-	-
Decayed	-	-	5	-	-	-	-	-	-	-	-	-	-	6	-	-
Missing, decayed	-	-	-	-	-	-	-	-	-	-	-	-	-	-	-	-
" trauma	-	-	-	-	-	-	-	-	-	-	-	-	-	-	-	-
" ortho	-	-	-	-	-	-	-	-	-	-	-	-	-	-	-	-
Decay Categories																
Deciduous																
Decayed				13	12	4	1	-	-	1	4	11	13			
Unrestorable				9	12	1	1	-	-	1	1	13	10			
Filled & decayed				5	2	-	-	-	-	-	-	2	4			
Permanent																
Decayed	-	-	5	-	-	-	-	-	-	-	-	-	-	5	-	-
Unrestorable	-	-	-	-	-	-	-	-	-	-	-	-	-	}1	-	-
Filled & decayed	-	-	-	-	-	-	-	-	-	-	-	-	-		-	-

Table 65
Crown disease experience of individual teeth for children aged seven

a) Upper jaw

Condition of teeth	Left 8	7	6	e/5	d/4	c/3	b/2	a/1	a/1	b/2	c/3	d/4	e/5	6	7	Right 8
	%	%	%	%	%	%	%	%	%	%	%	%	%	%	%	%
Deciduous																
Sound				43	55	91	46	14	15	45	91	56	43			
Filled				17	9	1	–	–	–	–	1	7	18			
Decayed				27	22	6	4	3	2	3	5	24	26			
erupted	100	100	6	12	12	2	22	7	7	25	3	11	12	7	100	100
Permanent																
Sound	–	–	72	1	2	–	28	76	76	27	–	2	1	73	–	–
Filled	–	–	9	–	–	–	–	–	–	–	–	–	–	7	–	–
Decayed	–	–	12	–	–	–	–	–	–	–	–	–	–	12	–	–
Missing, decayed	–	–	1	–	–	–	–	–	–	–	–	–	–	1	–	–
" trauma	–	–	–	–	–	–	–	–	–	–	–	–	–	–	–	–
" ortho	–	–	–	–	–	–	–	–	–	–	–	–	–	–	–	–

Decay Categories

Deciduous	8	7	6	e/5	d/4	c/3	b/2	a/1	a/1	b/2	c/3	d/4	e/5	6	7	8
Decayed				14	12	4	3	2	2	2	3	12	13			
Unrestorable				11	8	2	1	1	–	1	2	9	10			
Filled & decayed				2	2	–	–	–	–	–	–	3	3			
Permanent																
Decayed	–	–	11	–	–	–	–	–	–	–	–	–	–	11	–	–
Unrestorable	–	–	1	–	–	–	–	–	–	–	–	–	–	}1	–	–
Filled & decayed	–	–	–	–	–	–	–	–	–	–	–	–	–		–	–

b) Lower jaw

Condition of teeth	Right 8	7	6	e/5	d/4	c/3	b/2	a/1	a/1	b/2	c/3	d/4	e/5	6	7	Left 8
	%	%	%	%	%	%	%	%	%	%	%	%	%	%	%	%
Deciduous																
Sound				35	40	86	24	3	2	24	87	42	36			
Filled				18	11	1	–	–	–	–	1	10	17			
Decayed				24	25	6	1	–	–	1	6	24	23			
erupted	100	100	6	23	23	6	7	1	1	8	5	24	24	6	100	100
Permanent																
Sound	–	–	74	–	1	1	68	96	97	67	1	–	–	72	–	–
Filled	–	–	9	–	–	–	–	–	–	–	–	–	–	8	–	–
Decayed	–	–	10	–	–	–	–	–	–	–	–	–	–	13	–	–
Missing, decayed	–	–	1	–	–	–	–	–	–	–	–	–	–	1	–	–
" trauma	–	–	–	–	–	–	–	–	–	–	–	–	–	–	–	–
" ortho	–	–	–	–	–	–	–	–	–	–	–	–	–	–	–	–

Decay Categories

Deciduous	8	7	6	e/5	d/4	c/3	b/2	a/1	a/1	b/2	c/3	d/4	e/5	6	7	8
Decayed				10	9	4	1	–	–	}1	5	9	9			
Unrestorable				11	15	2	–	–	–		1	13	11			
Filled & decayed				3	1	–	–	–	–	–	–	2	3			
Permanent																
Decayed	–	–	9	–	–	–	–	–	–	–	–	–	–	11	–	–
Unrestorable	–	–	1	–	–	–	–	–	–	–	–	–	–	1	–	–
Filled & decayed	–	–	–	–	–	–	–	–	–	–	–	–	–	1	–	–

Table 66
Known disease experience of individual teeth for children aged eight

(a) Upper jaw

Condition of teeth	Left 8	7	6	e 5	d 4	c 3	b 2	a 1	a 1	b 2	c 3	d 4	e 5	6	7	Right 8
	%	%	%	%	%	%	%	%	%	%	%	%	%	%	%	%
Deciduous																
Sound				34	45	82	16	2	3	14	82	46	32			
Filled				20	9	1	–	–	–	–	2	10	21			
Decayed				26	20	7	1	1	1	1	7	19	26			
Unerupted	100	100	1	16	15	8	14	2	1	16	8	14	16	1	100	100
Permanent																
Sound	–	–	58	4	11	2	69	95	95	69	1	11	5	57	–	–
Filled	–	–	21	–	–	–	–	–	–	–	–	–	–	22	–	–
Decayed	–	–	19	–	–	–	–	–	–	–	–	–	–	19	–	–
Missing, decayed	–	–	1	–	–	–	–	–	–	–	–	–	–	1	–	–
" trauma	–	–	–	–	–	–	–	–	–	–	–	–	–	–	–	–
" ortho	–	–	–	–	–	–	–	–	–	–	–	–	–	–	–	–
Decay Categories																
Deciduous																
Decayed				11	10	5	1	}1	}1	1	6	9	12			
Unrestorable				10	8	2	–			–	1	8	10			
Filled & decayed				5	2	–	–	–	–	–	2	4				
Permanent																
Decayed	–	–	15	–	–	–	–	–	–	–	–	–	–	16	–	–
Unrestorable	–	–	1	–	–	–	–	–	–	–	–	–	–	1	–	–
Filled & decayed	–	–	3	–	–	–	–	–	–	–	–	–	–	2	–	–

(b) Lower jaw

Condition of teeth	Right 8	7	6	e 5	d 4	c 3	b 2	a 1	a 1	b 2	c 3	d 4	e 5	6	7	Left 8
	%	%	%	%	%	%	%	%	%	%	%	%	%	%	%	%
Deciduous																
Sound				29	31	74	7	–	–	5	75	33	28			
Filled				19	12	–	–	–	–	–	1	10	18			
Decayed				21	22	5	–	–	–	–	5	22	21			
Unerupted	100	100	1	30	30	11	2	–	–	3	9	29	31	1	100	100
Permanent																
Sound	–	–	56	1	5	10	91	99	99	92	10	6	2	57	–	–
Filled	–	–	22	–	–	–	–	–	–	–	–	–	–	23	–	–
Decayed	–	–	19	–	–	–	–	1	1	–	–	–	–	17	–	–
Missing, decayed	–	–	2	–	–	–	–	–	–	–	–	–	–	2	–	–
" trauma	–	–	–	–	–	–	–	–	–	–	–	–	–	–	–	–
" ortho	–	–	–	–	–	–	–	–	–	–	–	–	–	–	–	–
Decay Categories																
Deciduous																
Decayed				7	8	4	–	–	–	–	4	9	7			
Unrestorable				10	13	1	–	–	–	–	1	11	9			
Filled & decayed				4	1	–	–	–	–	–	–	2	5			
Permanent																
Decayed	–	–	15	–	–	–	–	1	1	–	–	–	–	13	–	–
Unrestorable	–	–	2	–	–	–	–	–	–	–	–	–	–	2	–	–
Filled & decayed	–	–	2	–	–	–	–	–	–	–	–	–	–	2	–	–

Table 67
Known disease experience of individual teeth for children aged nine

(a) Upper jaw

Condition of teeth	Left 8	7	6	e 5	d 4	c 3	b 2	a 1	a 1	b 2	c 3	d 4	e 5	6	7	8 Right
	%	%	%	%	%	%	%	%	%	%	%	%	%	%	%	%
Deciduous																
Sound				31	34	69	3	–	–	4	69	34	29			
Filled				21	8	1	–	–	–	–	1	9	20			
Decayed				20	17	6	–	–	–	–	6	17	23			
Unerupted	100	99	–	14	12	12	5	–	–	4	13	11	14	–	99	100
Permanent																
Sound	–	1	46	14	29	12	91	99	99	90	11	28	14	48	1	–
Filled	–	–	33	–	–	–	–	–	–	1	–	1	–	31	–	–
Decayed	–	–	19	–	–	–	1	1	1	1	–	–	–	18	–	–
Missing, decayed	–	–	2	–	–	–	–	–	–	–	–	–	–	3	–	–
" trauma	–	–	–	–	–	–	–	–	–	–	–	–	–	–	–	–
" ortho	–	–	–	–	–	–	–	–	–	–	–	–	–	–	–	–

Decay Categories

Deciduous																
Decayed				9	10	5	–	–	–	–	4	7	10			
Unrestorable				8	6	1	–	–	–	–	2	8	10			
Filled & decayed				3	1	–	–	–	–	–	–	2	3			
Permanent																
Decayed	–	–	14	–	–	–	1	1	1	1	–	–	–	14	–	–
Unrestorable	–	–	2	–	–	–	–	–	–	–	–	–	–	1	–	–
Filled & decayed	–	–	3	–	–	–	–	–	–	–	–	–	–	3	–	–

(b) Lower jaw

Condition of teeth	Right 8	7	6	e 5	d 4	c 3	b 2	a 1	a 1	b 2	c 3	d 4	e 5	6	7	8 Left
	%	%	%	%	%	%	%	%	%	%	%	%	%	%	%	%
Deciduous																
Sound				26	24	50	1	–	–	1	51	25	24			
Filled				16	8	–	–	–	–	–	1	9	18			
Decayed				19	16	4	–	–	–	–	3	13	19			
Unerupted	100	97	–	28	26	11	–	–	–	1	11	28	29	–	96	100
Permanent																
Sound	–	3	47	11	26	35	99	99	99	98	34	25	9	47	4	–
Filled	–	–	29	–	–	–	–	–	–	–	–	–	–	28	–	–
Decayed	–	–	19	–	–	–	–	1	1	–	–	–	1	20	–	–
Missing, decayed	–	–	5	–	–	–	–	–	–	–	–	–	–	5	–	–
" trauma	–	–	–	–	–	–	–	–	–	–	–	–	–	–	–	–
" ortho	–	–	–	–	–	–	–	–	–	–	–	–	–	–	–	–

Decay Categories

Deciduous																
Decayed				5	6	3	–	–	–	–	}3		5	6		
Unrestorable				9	8	1	–	–	–	–			7	9		
Filled & decayed				5	2	–	–	–	–	–			1	4		
Permanent																
Decayed	–	–	12	–	–	–	–	1	1	–	–	–	}1	13	–	–
Unrestorable	–	–	3	–	–	–	–	–	–	–	–	–		2	–	–
Filled & decayed	–	–	4	–	–	–	–	–	–	–	–	–		5	–	–

Table 68
Known disease experience of individual teeth for children aged ten

(a) Upper jaw

Condition of teeth	Left 8	7	6	e 5	d 4	c 3	b 2	a 1	a 1	b 2	c 3	d 4	e 5	6	7	Right 8
	%	%	%	%	%	%	%	%	%	%	%	%	%	%	%	%
Deciduous																
Sound				25	21	47	1	–	–	1	48	22	23			
Filled				15	5	1	–	–	–	–	1	5	12			
Decayed				14	10	7	–	–	–	–	6	11	17			
Unerupted	100	90	–	13	8	13	1	–	–	1	13	8	15	–	91	100
Permanent																
Sound	–	9	32	32	54	32	94	97	96	93	32	51	32	36	9	–
Filled	–	–	41	1	1	–	1	1	1	1	–	1	1	40	–	–
Decayed	–	1	21	–	–	–	3	2	3	4	–	1	–	18	–	–
Missing, decayed	–	–	6	–	–	–	–	–	–	–	–	–	–	6	–	–
" trauma	–	–	–	–	–	–	–	–	–	–	–	–	–	–	–	–
" ortho	–	–	–	–	1	–	–	–	–	–	–	1	–	–	–	–
Decay Categories																
Deciduous																
Decayed				6	5	5	–	–	–	–	5	5	7			
Unrestorable				6	4	2	–	–	–	–	1	5	7			
Filled & decayed				2	1	–	–	–	–	–	–	1	3			
Permanent																
Decayed	–	1	14	–	–	–	3	2	3	4	–	}1	–	12	–	–
Unrestorable	–	–	2	–	–	–	–	–	–	–	–	–	–	1	–	–
Filled & decayed	–	–	5	–	–	–	–	–	–	–	–	–	–	5	–	–

(b) Lower jaw

Condition of teeth	Right 8	7	6	e 5	d 4	c 3	b 2	a 1	a 1	b 2	c 3	d 4	e 5	6	7	Left 8
	%	%	%	%	%	%	%	%	%	%	%	%	%	%	%	%
Deciduous																
Sound				17	14	28	–	–	–	–	27	14	17			
Filled				12	5	–	–	–	–	–	–	6	12			
Decayed				17	9	1	–	–	–	–	2	8	15			
Unerupted	100	83	–	29	22	6	–	–	–	–	5	24	30	–	81	100
Permanent																
Sound	–	15	34	25	49	65	99	99	99	100	66	47	25	31	17	–
Filled	–	1	39	–	–	–	–	–	–	–	–	–	1	40	1	–
Decayed	–	1	19	–	–	–	1	1	1	–	–	–	–	20	1	–
Missing, decayed	–	–	8	–	–	–	–	–	–	–	–	–	–	9	–	–
" trauma	–	–	–	}1			–	–	–	–	}1			–	–	–
" ortho	–	–	–				–	–	–	–				–	–	–
Decay Categories																
Deciduous																
Decayed				5	4	1	–	–	–	–	}2	2	5			
Unrestorable				8	5	–	–	–	–	–		5	6			
Filled & decayed				4	–	–	–	–	–	–	–	1	4			
Permanent																
Decayed	–	–	12	–	–	–	1	1	1	–	–	–	–	11	1	–
Unrestorable	–	–	2	–	–	–	–	–	–	–	–	–	–	4	–	–
Filled & decayed	–	–	5	–	–	–	–	–	–	–	–	–	–	5	–	–

Table 69
Known disease experience of individual teeth for children aged eleven

(a) Upper jaw

Condition of teeth	Left 8	7	6	e 5	d 4	c 3	b 2	a 1	a 1	b 2	c 3	d 4	e 5	6	7	Right 8
	%	%	%	%	%	%	%	%	%	%	%	%	%	%	%	%
Deciduous																
Sound				12	8	23	-	-	-	-	24	9	10			
Filled				8	2	1	-	-	-	-	-	2	9			
Decayed				11	5	3	-	-	-	-	3	4	9			
Unerupted	100	60	-	8	5	9	1	-	-	2	10	4	10	-	63	100
Permanent																
Sound	-	34	27	56	70	64	90	92	92	90	63	72	58	26	31	-
Filled	-	4	45	3	3	-	4	3	3	3	-	3	3	46	3	-
Decayed	-	2	21	1	2	-	5	4	4	5	-	1	1	21	3	-
Missing, decayed	-	-	7	-	-	-	-	-	-	-	-	-	-	7	-	-
" trauma	-	-	-	-	-	-	-	1	1	-	-	-	-	-	-	-
" ortho	-	-	-	1	5	-	-	-	-	-	-	5	-	-	-	-

Decay Categories

Condition of teeth	8	7	6	e 5	d 4	c 3	b 2	a 1	a 1	b 2	c 3	d 4	e 5	6	7	8
Deciduous																
Decayed				3	2	2	-	-	-	-	2	2	3			
Unrestorable				6	2	1	-	-	-	-	1	1	4			
Filled & decayed				2	1	-	-	-	-	-	-	1	2			
Permanent																
Decayed	-	2	12	1	2	-	}5	4	}4	5	-	1	1	13	3	-
Unrestorable	-	-	3	-	-	-	(}5)	-	(}4)	-	-	-	-	3	-	-
Filled & decayed	-	-	6	-	-	-	-	-	-	-	-	-	-	5	-	-

(b) Lower jaw

Condition of teeth	Right 8	7	6	e 5	d 4	c 3	b 2	a 1	a 1	b 2	c 3	d 4	e 5	6	7	Left 8
	%	%	%	%	%	%	%	%	%	%	%	%	%	%	%	%
Deciduous																
Sound				10	5	8	-	-	-	-	7	5	10			
Filled				8	2	-	-	-	-	-	-	2	7			
Decayed				10	3	-	-	-	-	-	1	4	9			
Unerupted	100	50	-	20	14	3	-	-	-	-	4	14	22	-	48	100
Permanent																
Sound	-	41	27	50	72	89	98	97	98	98	88	71	49	23	42	-
Filled	-	6	39	1	1	-	1	1	1	1	-	1	1	43	6	-
Decayed	-	3	22	1	-	-	1	2	1	1	-	-	1	23	4	-
Missing, decayed	-	-	12	-	-	-	-	-	-	-	-	-	-	11	-	-
" trauma	-	-	-	-	-	-	-	-	-	-	-	-	}1	-	-	-
" ortho	-	-	-	-	3	-	-	-	-	-	-	3	-	-	-	-

Decay Categories

Condition of teeth	8	7	6	e 5	d 4	c 3	b 2	a 1	a 1	b 2	c 3	d 4	e 5	6	7	8
Deciduous																
Decayed				3	1	-	-	-	-	-	}1	2	3			
Unrestorable				5	2	-	-	-	-	-	(}1)	1	4			
Filled & decayed				2	-	-	-	-	-	-	-	1	2			
Permanent																
Decayed	-	3	10	1	-	-	1	}2	1	1	-	-	1	12	4	-
Unrestorable	-	-	4	-	-	-	-	(}2)	-	-	-	-	-	4	-	-
Filled & decayed	-	-	8	-	-	-	-	-	-	-	-	-	-	7	-	-

Table 70
Known disease experience of individual teeth for children aged twelve

(a) Upper jaw

Teeth are shown from Left (8 7 6 …) to Right (… 6 7 8).

Condition of teeth	8	7	6	e/5	d/4	c/3	b/2	a/1	a/1	b/2	c/3	d/4	e/5	6	7	8
Deciduous (%)																
Sound				6	2	7	–	–	–	–	9	2	6			
Filled				4	1	–	–	–	–	–	–	1	4			
Decayed				5	1	1	–	–	–	–	1	2	4			
Unerupted	100	32	–	4	2	5	2	–	–	2	5	1	4	–	33	100
Permanent																
Sound	–	53	21	71	76	87	86	90	90	88	85	77	72	21	51	–
Filled	–	9	51	6	6	–	6	4	4	5	–	5	5	49	9	–
Decayed	–	6	18	3	3	–	5	5	5	5	–	3	3	20	7	–
Missing, decayed	–	–	10	–	–	–	1	}1	}1	–	–	–	10	–	–	
" trauma	–	–	–	–	–	–	–		}2		–	–	–	–	–	
" ortho	–	–	–	1	9	–	–	–	–	–	–	9	–	–	–	–

Decay Categories

Condition of teeth	8	7	6	e/5	d/4	c/3	b/2	a/1	a/1	b/2	c/3	d/4	e/5	6	7	8
Deciduous																
Decayed				2	}1	}1	–	–	–	–	}1	1	2			
Unrestorable				2	}1	}1	–	–	–	–	}1	1	2			
Filled & decayed				1	–	–	–	–	–	–	–	–	–			
Permanent																
Decayed	–	6	9	3	}3	–	4	4	4	5	–	2	}3	9	6	–
Unrestorable	–	–	2	–	}3	–	}1	}1	–	–	–	}1	}3	3	–	–
Filled & decayed	–	–	7	–	–	–	}1	}1	1	–	–	}1	8	1	–	–

(b) Lower jaw

Teeth are shown from Right (8 7 6 …) to Left (… 6 7 8).

Condition of teeth	8	7	6	e/5	d/4	c/3	b/2	a/1	a/1	b/2	c/3	d/4	e/5	6	7	8
Deciduous (%)																
Sound				5	1	2	–	–	–	–	2	2	4			
Filled				3	–	–	–	–	–	–	–	–	3			
Decayed				4	1	–	–	–	–	–	–	1	4			
Unerupted	100	25	–	12	5	1	–	–	–	–	1	5	12	–	22	100
Permanent																
Sound	–	56	23	70	84	97	98	97	97	98	97	84	69	23	56	–
Filled	–	11	44	3	2	–	1	1	2	1	–	2	3	46	12	–
Decayed	–	8	18	2	1	–	1	2	1	1	–	1	2	16	10	–
Missing, decayed	–	–	15	–	–	–	–	–	–	–	–	–	15	–	–	
" trauma	–	–	–	–	–	–	–	–	–	–	–	}3		–	–	–
" ortho	–	–	–	1	6	–	–	–	–	–	–	5	–	–	–	–

Decay categories

Condition of teeth	8	7	6	e/5	d/4	c/3	b/2	a/1	a/1	b/2	c/3	d/4	e/5	6	7	8
Deciduous																
Decayed				1	1	–	–	–	–	–	–	}1	1			
Unrestorable				2	–	–	–	–	–	–	–	}1	2			
Filled & decayed				1	–	–	–	–	–	–	–	}1	1			
Permanent																
Decayed	–	6	8	2	1	–	1	}2	1	1	–	1	2	5	8	–
Unrestorable	–	1	3	–	–	–	–	–	–	–	–	–	–	4	1	–
Filled & decayed	–	1	7	–	–	–	–	–	–	–	–	–	–	7	1	–

Table 71
Known disease experience of individual teeth for children aged thirteen

(a) Upper jaw

Condition of teeth	Left 8	7	6	e 5	d 4	c 3	b 2	a 1	a 1	b 2	c 3	d 4	e 5	6	7	Right 8
	%	%	%	%	%	%	%	%	%	%	%	%	%	%	%	%
Deciduous																
Sound				3	–	3	–	–	–	–	3	1	3			
Filled				1	–	–	–	–	–	–	–	–	1			
Decayed				2	1	1	–	–	–	–	1	1	2			
Unerupted	100	12	–	3	1	2	1	–	–	1	3	–	3	–	13	100
Permanent																
Sound	–	59	21	74	73	92	84	88	88	85	91	74	75	19	58	–
Filled	–	18	52	12	10	–	8	6	5	7	–	9	10	51	19	–
Decayed	–	11	16	4	3	1	7	5	6	6	1	3	4	16	10	–
Missing, decayed	–	–	11	–	–	–	–	–	–	–	–	–	–	14	–	–
" trauma	–	–	–	–	–	–	–	1	1	}1	–	–	–	–	–	–
" ortho	–	–	–	1	12	1	–	–	–	–	1	12	2	–	–	–

Decay Categories

	Left 8	7	6	e 5	d 4	c 3	b 2	a 1	a 1	b 2	c 3	d 4	e 5	6	7	Right 8
Deciduous																
Decayed				1	}1	1	–	–	–	–	1	}1	1			
Unrestorable				1	}	–	–	–	–	–	–	}	1			
Filled & decayed				–	}	–	–	–	–	–	–	}	–			
Permanent																
Decayed	–	9	8	3	3	1	5	4	–	5	1	2	2	8	8	–
Unrestorable	–	}2	3	–	–	–	1	–	1	–	–	1	1	2	1	–
Filled & decayed	–	}	5	1	–	–	1	1	5	1	–	–	1	6	1	–

(b) Lower jaw

Condition of teeth	Right 8	7	6	e 5	d 4	c 3	b 2	a 1	a 1	b 2	c 3	d 4	e 5	6	7	Left 8
	%	%	%	%	%	%	%	%	%	%	%	%	%	%	%	%
Deciduous																
Sound				3	–	1	–	–	–	–	1	–	3			
Filled				1	–	–	–	–	–	–	–	–	1			
Decayed				2	–	–	–	–	–	–	–	–	1			
Unerupted	100	9	–	7	2	–	–	–	–	–	1	2	9	–	8	100
Permanent																
Sound	–	54	17	74	86	99	98	97	97	98	98	86	72	18	53	–
Filled	–	25	48	8	4	–	1	2	1	1	–	4	8	48	27	–
Decayed	–	11	18	3	2	–	1	1	2	1	–	1	3	17	11	–
Missing, decayed	–	1	17	1	–	–	–	–	–	–	–	1	1	17	}1	–
" trauma	–	–	–	–	–	–	–	–	–	–	–	–	–	–	}	–
" ortho	–	–	–	1	6	–	–	–	–	–	–	6	2	–	–	–

Decay Categories

	Right 8	7	6	e 5	d 4	c 3	b 2	a 1	a 1	b 2	c 3	d 4	e 5	6	7	Left 8
Deciduous																
Decayed				1	–	–	–	–	–	–	–	–	}1			
Unrestorable				1	–	–	–	–	–	–	–	–	}			
Filled & decayed				–	–	–	–	–	–	–	–	–	}			
Permanent																
Decayed	–	9	8	2	}2	–	}1	1	}2	1	–	1	2	7	9	–
Unrestorable	–	1	3	1	}	–	}	–	}	–	–	–	1	3	1	–
Filled & decayed	–	1	7	–	}	–	}	–	}	–	–	–	–	7	1	–

Table 72
Known disease experience of individual teeth for children aged fourteen

(a) Upper jaw

Condition of teeth	Left 8	7	6	e 5	d 4	c 3	b 2	a 1	a 1	b 2	c 3	d 4	e 5	6	7	Right 8
	%	%	%	%	%	%	%	%	%	%	%	%	%	%	%	%
Deciduous																
Sound				1	-	2	-	-	-	-	-	1	-			
Filled				-	-	-	-	-	-	-	-	-	-			
Decayed				-	-	-	-	-	-	-	-	-	1			
Unerupted	99	3	-	3	1	1	1	-	-	1	1	1	2	-	3	99
Permanent																
Sound	1	53	17	73	70	93	80	86	85	80	94	69	73	17	51	1
Filled	-	30	53	16	12	1	11	8	8	11	1	12	15	53	32	-
Decayed	-	14	17	4	4	2	8	6	7	7	2	5	5	16	13	-
Missing, decayed	-	-	13	1	1	-	-	-	-	1	-	-	1	14	1	-
" trauma	-	-	-	-	-	-	-	-	-	-	-	-	-	-	-	-
" ortho	-	-	-	2	12	1	-	-	-	-	1	13	3	-	-	-

Decay Categories

	8	7	6	e 5	d 4	c 3	b 2	a 1	a 1	b 2	c 3	d 4	e 5	6	7	8
Deciduous																
Decayed				-	-	-	-	-	-	-	-	-				
Unrestorable				-	-	-	-	-	-	-	-	-	} 1			
Filled & decayed				-	-	-	-	-	-	-	-	-				
Permanent																
Decayed	-	10	9	2	3	2	5	3	5	5		4	3	9	10	-
Unrestorable	-	1	3	1	-	-	1	1	1	1	} 2	-	1	3	1	-
Filled & decayed	-	3	5	1	1	-	2	2	1	1		1	1	4	2	-

(b) Lower jaw

Condition of teeth	Right 8	7	6	e 5	d 4	c 3	b 2	a 1	a 1	b 2	c 3	d 4	e 5	6	7	Left 8
	%	%	%	%	%	%	%	%	%	%	%	%	%	%	%	%
Deciduous																
Sound				1	-	-	-	-	-	-	-	-	1			
Filled				-	-	-	-	-	-	-	-	-	-			
Decayed				1	-	-	-	-	-	-	-	-	-			
Unerupted	100	2	-	3	1	-	-	-	-	-	-	1	5	-	2	100
Permanent																
Sound	-	45	16	76	84	99	98	97	97	97	99	84	76	14	45	-
Filled	-	35	48	12	5	-	1	2	2	1	-	6	12	50	37	-
Decayed	-	16	17	4	1	1	1	1	1	1	1	1	3	15	14	-
Missing, decayed	-	1	19	2	1	-	-	-			-	-	1	21	1	-
" trauma	-	-	-	-	-	-	-	-	} 1		-	-	-	-	-	-
" ortho	-	1	-	1	8	-	-	-			-	8	2	-	1	-

Decay Categories

	8	7	6	e 5	d 4	c 3	b 2	a 1	a 1	b 2	c 3	d 4	e 5	6	7	8
Deciduous																
Decayed				-	-	-	-	-	-	-	-	-				
Unrestorable				1	-	-	-	-	-	-	-	-				
Filled & decayed				-	-	-	-	-	-	-	-	-				
Permanent																
Decayed	-	11	6	3	1	1	1	1	1	1	1	1	2	6	11	-
Unrestorable	-	2	4	1	-	-	-	-	-	-	-	-	-	4	1	-
Filled & decayed	-	3	7	-	-	-	-	-	-	-	-	-	1	5	2	-

Table 73
Known disease experience of individual teeth for children aged fifteen

(a) Upper jaw

Condition of teeth	Left 8	7	6	e 5	d 4	c 3	b 2	a 1	a 1	b 2	c 3	d 4	e 5	6	7	8 Right
	%	%	%	%	%	%	%	%	%	%	%	%	%	%	%	%
Deciduous																
Sound				–	–	I	–	–	–	–	I	–	–			
Filled				–	–	–	–	–	–	–	–	–	–			
Decayed				–	–	–	–	–	–	–	I	–	–			
Unerupted	99	2	–	I	I	I	I	–	–	I	–	–	I	–	2	99
Permanent																
Sound	I	41	12	67	65	95	80	85	84	82	94	67	69	12	41	I
Filled	–	43	63	23	17	I	12	8	10	11	I	16	22	61	42	–
Decayed	–	13	11	6	4	I	6	6	5	5	2	4	5	11	14	–
Missing, decayed	–	I	14	I	I	–	–	I	} 1	I	–	I	I	16	I	–
" trauma	–	–	–	–	–	–	–	–	} (1)	–	–	–	–	–	–	–
" ortho	–	–	–	2	12	I	I	–	}	–	I	12	2	–	–	–
Decay Categories																
Deciduous																
Decayed				–	–	–	–	–	–	–	} 1	–	–			
Unrestorable				–	–	–	–	–	–	–	}	–	–			
Filled & decayed				–	–	–	–	–	–	–	}	–	–			
Permanent																
Decayed	–	9	5	4	3	I	5	4	4	4	2	3	4	5	9	–
Unrestorable	–	I	2	I	–	–	–	–	–	–	–	–	–	I	I	–
Filled & decayed	–	3	4	I	I	–	I	2	I	I	–	I	I	5	4	–

(b) Lower jaw

Condition of teeth	Right 8	7	6	e 5	d 4	c 3	b 2	a 1	a 1	b 2	c 3	d 4	e 5	6	7	8 Left
	%	%	%	%	%	%	%	%	%	%	%	%	%	%	%	%
Deciduous																
Sound				–	–	–	–	–	–	–	–	–	–			
Filled				–	–	–	–	–	–	–	–	–	–			
Decayed				–	–	–	–	–	–	–	–	–	–			
Unerupted	99	2	–	2	–	–	–	–	–	–	–	–	2	–	2	99
Permanent																
Sound	I	34	13	74	84	98	97	96	96	97	99	85	69	12	35	I
Filled	–	47	56	17	6	I	2	3	2	2	I	8	19	56	48	–
Decayed	–	15	13	4	2	I	I	I	I	I	–	–	4	13	13	–
Missing, decayed	–	2	18	I	–	–	–	–	} 1	–	–	–	3	19	2	–
" trauma	–	–	–	–	–	–	–	–	}	–	–	–	–	–	–	–
" ortho	–	–	–	2	8	–	–	–	}	–	–	7	3	–	–	–
Decay Categories																
Deciduous																
Decayed				–	–	–	–	–	–	–	–	–	–			
Unrestorable				–	–	–	–	–	–	–	–	–	–			
Filled & decayed				–	–	–	–	–	–	–	–	–	–			
Permanent																
Decayed	–	10	4	3	} 2	I	I	I	I	I	–	–	3	5	9	–
Unrestorable	–	I	2	–	}	–	–	–	–	–	–	–	–	2	–	–
Filled & decayed	–	4	7	I	}	–	–	–	–	–	–	–	I	6	4	–

Table 74   Distribution of the number of segments
                with some gum inflammation for children   *All children,*
                of different ages   *sex and racial origin*

Number of segments with gum inflammation	Age at 31 December 1972										
	5+	6+	7+	8+	9+	10+	11+	12+	13+	14+	15+
All children	%	%	%	%	%	%	%	%	%	%	%
0	74	65	50	44	44	44	41	43	45	45	49
1	14	16	24	23	23	20	21	21	19	18	19
2	7	10	13	17	15	17	16	14	14	14	12
3	2	5	7	6	8	7	8	9	7	7	7
4	2	2	3	4	6	6	7	6	7	7	6
5	1	2	1	3	2	2	3	3	3	3	2
6	-	-	2	3	2	4	4	4	5	6	5
	100	100	100	100	100	100	100	100	100	100	100
Male	%	%	%	%	%	%	%	%	%	%	%
0	72	67	50	41	41	41	38	38	37	36	39
1	15	14	26	25	24	20	20	21	22	19	20
2	7	10	12	19	16	18	19	15	14	15	13
3	3	4	6	5	8	8	7	9	9	8	10
4	2	3	4	5	6	7	8	9	8	10	8
5	1	2	1	2	3	2	2	3	3	3	3
6	-	-	1	3	2	4	6	5	7	9	7
	100	100	100	100	100	100	100	100	100	100	100
Female	%	%	%	%	%	%	%	%	%	%	%
0	76	63	50	47	47	47	44	49	53	55	57
1	13	18	22	21	23	20	22	20	16	17	17
2	7	11	15	15	14	17	14	13	14	13	12
3	2	4	7	7	7	6	9	8	6	6	5
4	1	1	3	4	5	5	5	4	5	3	4
5	-	2	1	3	1	2	3	2	2	2	2
6	1	1	2	3	3	3	3	4	4	4	3
	100	100	100	100	100	100	100	100	100	100	100
White	%	%	%	%	%	%	%	%	%	%	%
0	74	65	49	43	43	43	40	43	45	45	48
1	14	16	25	24	24	20	21	20	19	18	18
2	7	11	13	17	15	18	17	15	13	14	12
3	2	4	7	6	8	7	8	9	7	7	8
4	2	2	3	4	5	6	7	6	7	7	6
5	1	2	1	3	2	2	3	3	3	3	3
6	-	-	2	3	3	4	4	4	6	6	5
	100	100	100	100	100	100	100	100	100	100	100
Non-White	%	%	%	%	%	%	%	%	%	%	%
0	72	73	65	55	62	60	52	55	36	57	51
1	16	12	14	19	14	19	26	24	24	11	22
2	3	7	16	14	10	7	10	5	15	9	16
3	5	4	5	2	2	4	3	6	17	6	5
4	2	-	-	7	7	6	3	8	4	11	2
5	2	3	-	-	2	2	3	-	2	6	-
6	-	1	-	3	3	2	3	2	2	-	4
	100	100	100	100	100	100	100	100	100	100	100

For bases see Tables 1, 39, 45, 51, 57

Table 75   Distribution of the number of segments
            with some gum inflammation for children
            of different ages

Number of segments with gum inflammation	Age at 31 December 1972										
	5+	6+	7+	8+	9+	10+	11+	12+	13+	14+	15+
North	%	%	%	%	%	%	%	%	%	%	%
0	72	63	50	40	46	41	36	40	45	42	51
1	13	13	22	24	23	19	20	20	16	17	18
2	8	12	13	17	13	21	20	13	15	16	10
3	3	6	8	7	8	7	10	10	8	8	7
4	2	3	4	6	6	6	5	6	8	7	6
5	2	3	1	4	2	2	5	6	2	4	4
6	-	-	2	2	2	4	4	5	6	6	4
	100	100	100	100	100	100	100	100	100	100	100
M&EA	%	%	%	%	%	%	%	%	%	%	%
0	68	67	52	46	46	45	49	42	43	47	51
1	16	16	22	22	20	22	17	22	23	20	17
2	8	10	14	18	18	16	15	16	13	9	12
3	4	3	6	6	6	7	5	6	6	5	5
4	2	1	2	1	5	6	6	9	6	5	8
5	1	2	1	2	1	-	1	1	2	4	1
6	1	1	3	5	4	4	7	4	7	10	6
	100	100	100	100	100	100	100	100	100	100	100
W&SW	%	%	%	%	%	%	%	%	%	%	%
0	75	66	47	46	45	47	40	37	41	51	47
1	15	14	23	18	21	14	20	22	23	15	21
2	8	9	15	16	15	17	13	16	10	14	14
3	1	5	8	6	9	9	9	11	9	5	6
4	1	3	3	6	6	6	11	7	7	8	5
5	-	2	3	2	1	2	3	2	2	2	3
6	-	1	1	6	3	5	4	5	8	5	4
	100	100	100	100	100	100	100	100	100	100	100
L&SE	%	%	%	%	%	%	%	%	%	%	%
0	79	65	50	46	40	45	41	50	47	45	46
1	13	18	28	26	26	23	26	19	19	18	19
2	5	10	12	17	15	16	16	14	15	16	13
3	2	4	6	4	7	5	6	8	7	8	9
4	1	2	2	4	6	6	6	5	5	6	5
5	-	1	1	2	3	2	2	1	4	2	2
6	-	-	1	1	3	3	3	3	3	5	6
	100	100	100	100	100	100	100	100	100	100	100
Wales	%	%	%	%	%	%	%	%	%	%	%
0	78	72	60	54	50	48	40	38	42	49	45
1	13	11	16	18	21	19	25	26	19	17	22
2	5	8	12	10	13	14	15	15	15	18	15
3	1	4	6	4	6	6	5	8	11	4	8
4	1	3	3	7	6	6	7	6	4	7	5
5	1	-	3	2	2	2	5	3	4	2	3
6	1	2	-	5	2	5	3	4	5	3	2
	100	100	100	100	100	100	100	100	100	100	100

For bases see Tables 9, 15, 21, 27, 33

Table 76　　Distribution of the number of segments
　　　　　　with some debris for children of　　　　　　*All children,*
　　　　　　different ages　　　　　　　　　　　　　　*sex and racial origin*

Number of segments with debris	Age at 31 December 1972										
	5+	6+	7+	8+	9+	10+	11+	12+	13+	14+	15+
All children	%	%	%	%	%	%	%	%	%	%	%
0	61	52	38	33	33	35	35	36	41	44	49
1	13	16	20	20	20	19	18	16	14	13	13
2	10	13	15	16	15	15	15	15	14	12	11
3	5	6	9	10	10	10	9	8	7	7	7
4	4	5	7	8	9	8	8	9	9	8	7
5	3	4	5	5	4	5	5	5	4	4	5
6	4	4	6	8	9	8	10	11	11	12	8
	100	100	100	100	100	100	100	100	100	100	100
Male	%	%	%	%	%	%	%	%	%	%	%
0	57	53	39	31	26	28	29	27	32	32	37
1	15	14	18	20	20	19	15	16	15	12	15
2	11	13	16	16	16	17	18	18	15	15	11
3	6	6	9	8	11	11	10	7	8	9	10
4	5	5	8	10	11	9	9	11	10	10	8
5	2	5	4	6	5	5	7	6	5	5	5
6	4	4	6	9	11	11	12	15	15	17	14
	100	100	100	100	100	100	100	100	100	100	100
Female	%	%	%	%	%	%	%	%	%	%	%
0	65	50	38	36	40	42	41	46	50	55	60
1	11	19	22	20	19	18	20	16	14	14	12
2	10	13	15	15	14	14	12	12	13	9	11
3	4	6	8	11	9	8	8	8	6	6	4
4	3	5	6	7	6	7	7	6	8	6	6
5	3	4	6	4	4	5	4	5	3	3	4
6	4	3	5	7	8	6	8	7	6	7	3
	100	100	100	100	100	100	100	100	100	100	100
White	%	%	%	%	%	%	%	%	%	%	%
0	61	52	39	34	33	35	35	36	42	43	49
1	13	16	20	20	20	18	17	16	14	13	13
2	10	13	15	15	15	15	15	15	14	12	11
3	5	6	8	10	10	10	9	8	7	8	7
4	4	5	7	8	9	9	8	9	8	8	7
5	3	4	5	5	4	5	6	5	4	4	5
6	4	4	6	8	9	8	10	11	11	12	8
	100	100	100	100	100	100	100	100	100	100	100
Non-White	%	%	%	%	%	%	%	%	%	%	%
0	53	46	31	27	41	26	32	42	24	57	56
1	16	19	16	18	9	23	22	18	24	14	11
2	14	9	19	17	10	19	10	8	19	12	16
3	3	4	14	5	8	7	5	5	5	-	7
4	5	8	9	14	5	7	11	5	16	3	4
5	2	7	4	7	7	5	7	9	7	6	2
6	7	7	7	12	20	13	13	13	5	8	4
	100	100	100	100	100	100	100	100	100	100	100

For bases see Tables 1, 39, 45, 51, 57

Table 77   Distribution of the number of segments
            with some debris for children of
            different ages

Region

Number of segments with debris	Age at 31 December 1972										
	5+	6+	7+	8+	9+	10+	11+	12+	13+	14+	15+
North	%	%	%	%	%	%	%	%	%	%	%
0	60	51	38	29	34	32	32	36	37	42	48
1	11	17	20	18	19	19	19	15	13	16	13
2	10	11	13	15	15	15	16	15	13	8	10
3	7	5	9	14	10	9	8	6	10	7	7
4	5	6	7	8	8	9	9	9	8	10	7
5	3	7	5	6	4	7	5	9	6	5	7
6	4	3	8	10	10	9	11	10	13	12	8
	100	100	100	100	100	100	100	100	100	100	100
M&EA	%	%	%	%	%	%	%	%	%	%	%
0	63	56	43	34	31	37	30	30	41	44	51
1	13	15	19	22	23	16	17	22	18	8	9
2	9	15	14	14	14	16	14	14	10	13	11
3	4	5	7	9	9	10	10	8	6	9	12
4	4	3	7	9	12	9	11	10	10	9	6
5	5	3	4	5	4	7	7	4	3	2	4
6	2	3	6	7	7	5	11	12	12	15	7
	100	100	100	100	100	100	100	100	100	100	100
W&SW	%	%	%	%	%	%	%	%	%	%	%
0	59	47	29	31	28	35	34	33	36	37	50
1	15	20	20	19	17	14	17	17	15	13	15
2	12	12	15	20	16	15	18	17	16	16	10
3	6	7	14	8	14	15	9	8	7	9	5
4	4	4	10	8	12	8	7	8	10	9	10
5	1	5	6	4	4	5	7	6	7	6	5
6	3	5	6	10	9	8	8	11	9	10	5
	100	100	100	100	100	100	100	100	100	100	100
L&SE	%	%	%	%	%	%	%	%	%	%	%
0	62	51	41	39	35	36	41	42	48	49	49
1	13	15	21	22	20	21	17	14	13	13	14
2	11	15	19	16	15	15	13	13	15	14	12
3	3	6	6	5	10	9	9	9	6	6	6
4	3	5	6	8	5	7	6	8	7	5	7
5	2	3	4	4	4	2	4	3	2	3	2
6	6	5	3	6	11	10	10	11	9	10	10
	100	100	100	100	100	100	100	100	100	100	100
Wales	%	%	%	%	%	%	%	%	%	%	%
0	66	55	38	39	39	34	33	32	39	46	48
1	10	16	26	20	20	18	20	24	16	16	18
2	11	9	11	15	16	20	20	17	14	14	11
3	4	6	9	5	8	9	6	6	8	6	8
4	3	5	5	8	7	7	8	6	7	5	8
5	2	6	4	5	4	3	5	6	6	4	2
6	4	3	7	8	6	9	8	9	10	9	5
	100	100	100	100	100	100	100	100	100	100	100

For bases see Tables 9, 15, 21, 27, 33

Table 78   Distribution of the number of segments with some calculus for children of different ages   *All children, sex and racial origin*

Number of segments with calculus	Age at 31 December 1972										
	5+	6+	7+	8+	9+	10+	11+	12+	13+	14+	15+
All children	%	%	%	%	%	%	%	%	%	%	%
0	96	95	91	85	83	79	75	72	69	67	66
1	4	4	8	13	14	18	20	22	24	23	22
2	-	-	-	1	1	2	3	2	3	5	5
3	-	1	-	1	1	1	2	3	3	4	4
4	-	-	-	-	-	-	-	1	1	1	2
5	-	-	-	-	-	-	-	-	-	-	1
6	-	-	-	-	-	-	-	-	-	-	-
	100	100	100	100	100	100	100	100	100	100	100
Male	%	%	%	%	%	%	%	%	%	%	%
0	96	95	91	84	83	77	72	70	63	65	63
1	4	4	8	15	15	19	23	22	29	24	23
2	-	-	1	1	2	3	3	3	3	5	6
3	-	1	-	-	-	1	2	4	3	5	5
4	-	-	-	-	-	-	-	1	2	1	2
5	-	-	-	-	-	-	-	-	-	-	1
6	-	-	-	-	-	-	-	-	-	-	-
	100	100	100	100	100	100	100	100	100	100	100
Female	%	%	%	%	%	%	%	%	%	%	%
0	96	96	91	86	84	81	77	74	75	70	70
1	4	4	8	12	14	17	17	22	19	21	21
2	-	-	1	-	1	1	3	2	2	4	4
3	-	-	-	1	1	1	2	2	2	3	3
4	-	-	-	1	-	-	1	-	1	1	1
5	-	-	-	-	-	-	-	-	1	1	1
6	-	-	-	-	-	-	-	-	-	-	-
	100	100	100	100	100	100	100	100	100	100	100
White	%	%	%	%	%	%	%	%	%	%	%
0	96	96	92	86	85	79	76	73	70	68	68
1	4	4	7	13	14	18	21	22	24	23	22
2	-	-	1	1	1	2	2	2	2	4	5
3	-	-	-	-	-	1	1	3	3	4	3
4	-	-	-	-	-	-	-	-	1	1	1
5	-	-	-	-	-	-	-	-	-	-	1
6	-	-	-	-	-	-	-	-	-	-	-
	100	100	100	100	100	100	100	100	100	100	100
Non-White	%	%	%	%	%	%	%	%	%	%	%
0	90	84	77	74	60	73	58	56	48	52	49
1	10	11	21	20	27	22	20	23	29	20	27
2	-	1	-	2	5	2	8	3	7	8	7
3	-	3	2	-	6	2	8	10	9	14	9
4	-	-	-	2	2	-	3	3	5	-	4
5	-	1	-	2	-	1	3	5	2	6	2
6	-	-	-	-	-	-	-	-	-	-	2
	100	100	100	100	100	100	100	100	100	100	100

For bases see Tables 1, 39, 45, 51, 57

Table 79   Distribution of the number of segments with some calculus for children of different ages

Region

Number of segments with calculus	5+	6+	7+	8+	9+	10+	11+	12+	13+	14+	15+
North	%	%	%	%	%	%	%	%	%	%	%
0	98	94	92	85	85	82	77	77	74	73	71
1	2	6	7	14	13	15	19	15	21	21	17
2	-	-	1	1	1	2	2	2	2	3	6
3	-	-	-	-	1	1	1	5	1	3	4
4	-	-	-	-	-	-	-	1	1	-	2
5	-	-	-	-	-	-	1	-	1	-	-
6	-	-	-	-	-	-	-	-	-	-	-
	100	100	100	100	100	100	100	100	100	100	100
M&EA	%	%	%	%	%	%	%	%	%	%	%
0	94	95	88	83	81	77	68	66	67	66	64
1	4	3	10	14	16	20	22	25	23	19	22
2	1	1	1	1	1	1	4	2	2	6	4
3	1	1	1	1	2	2	5	6	5	7	4
4	-	-	-	1	-	-	1	-	3	1	5
5	-	-	-	-	-	-	-	1	-	1	1
6	-	-	-	-	-	-	-	-	-	-	-
	100	100	100	100	100	100	100	100	100	100	100
W&SW	%	%	%	%	%	%	%	%	%	%	%
0	94	96	93	86	84	72	74	71	59	64	65
1	5	4	7	13	14	24	24	24	33	27	28
2	-	-	-	1	2	3	2	3	4	6	5
3	-	-	-	-	-	1	-	1	3	1	1
4	-	-	-	-	-	-	-	1	-	2	-
5	-	-	-	-	-	-	-	-	1	-	1
6	1	-	-	-	-	-	-	-	-	-	-
	100	100	100	100	100	100	100	100	100	100	100
L&SE	%	%	%	%	%	%	%	%	%	%	%
0	94	96	92	86	83	80	76	71	71	64	65
1	6	4	8	13	15	18	20	25	23	26	24
2	-	-	-	1	2	2	3	3	2	5	5
3	-	-	-	-	-	-	1	1	3	5	4
4	-	-	-	-	-	-	-	-	1	-	-
5	-	-	-	-	-	-	-	-	-	-	1
6	-	-	-	-	-	-	-	-	-	-	1
Wales	%	%	%	%	%	%	%	%	%	%	%
0	95	95	93	88	80	77	73	70	59	61	53
1	5	3	6	12	16	21	22	24	32	30	35
2	-	1	-	-	3	2	3	3	4	4	6
3	-	1	1	-	1	-	1	1	2	3	3
4	-	-	-	-	-	-	1	1	1	2	1
5	-	-	-	-	-	-	-	1	2	-	2
6	-	-	-	-	-	-	-	-	-	-	-
	100	100	100	100	100	100	100	100	100	100	100

Age at 31 December 1972

For bases see Tables 9, 15, 21, 27, 33

Table 80   Distribution of the number of segments with some crowding for children of different ages   *All children, sex and racial origin*

Number of segments with crowding	Age at 31 December 1972										
	5+	6+	7+	8+	9+	10+	11+	12+	13+	14+	15+
All children	%	%	%	%	%	%	%	%	%	%	%
0	82	60	40	35	37	38	42	45	48	50	47
1	13	26	30	26	26	27	25	27	28	25	28
2	4	11	21	25	23	21	20	18	16	17	18
3	1	2	5	8	8	8	7	6	5	5	5
4	–	1	2	4	5	4	4	2	2	2	2
5	–	–	1	1	1	1	1	1	–	1	–
6	–	–	1	1	–	1	1	1	1	–	–
	100	100	100	100	100	100	100	100	100	100	100
Male	%	%	%	%	%	%	%	%	%	%	%
0	85	65	44	36	39	40	41	46	49	49	47
1	12	22	29	27	28	27	25	28	28	27	30
2	3	11	17	25	22	21	20	17	17	16	17
3	–	1	6	7	5	7	8	5	5	5	5
4	–	1	3	4	4	4	5	2	1	2	1
5	–	–	1	1	2	1	1	2	–	1	–
6	–	–	–	–	–	–	–	–	–	–	–
	100	100	100	100	100	100	100	100	100	100	100
Female	%	%	%	%	%	%	%	%	%	%	%
0	79	56	36	33	34	36	42	45	47	51	48
1	15	30	31	25	24	26	24	25	28	23	27
2	5	11	24	26	25	22	20	19	15	17	19
3	1	2	5	9	10	9	7	7	5	5	4
4	–	1	2	5	6	4	4	2	3	3	1
5	–	–	1	1	1	2	1	1	1	1	1
6	–	–	1	1	–	1	2	1	1	–	–
	100	100	100	100	100	100	100	100	100	100	100
White	%	%	%	%	%	%	%	%	%	%	%
0	82	60	39	34	36	37	41	45	48	49	46
1	14	26	31	26	26	27	25	27	28	26	29
2	4	11	21	26	24	22	20	18	16	17	18
3	–	2	5	8	8	8	8	6	5	5	5
4	–	1	2	4	5	4	4	2	2	2	1
5	–	–	1	1	1	1	1	1	–	1	1
6	–	–	1	1	–	1	1	1	1	–	–
	100	100	100	100	100	100	100	100	100	100	100
Non-White	%	%	%	%	%	%	%	%	%	%	%
0	87	64	57	44	53	56	49	59	53	74	62
1	11	29	18	32	25	23	26	15	31	15	22
2	2	7	20	19	14	14	10	18	14	11	16
3	–	–	5	2	6	7	7	8	2	–	–
4	–	–	–	3	2	–	5	–	–	–	–
5	–	–	–	–	–	–	–	–	–	–	–
6	–	–	–	–	–	–	3	–	–	–	–
	100	100	100	100	100	100	100	100	100	100	100

For bases see Tables 1, 39, 45, 51, 57

Table 81 — Distribution of the number of segments with some crowding for children of different ages

Age at 31 December 1972

North

Number of segments with crowding	5+	6+	7+	8+	9+	10+	11+	12+	13+	14+	15+
	%	%	%	%	%	%	%	%	%	%	%
0	85	62	43	34	41	39	44	50	50	52	49
1	12	29	30	28	27	27	27	23	30	24	29
2	3	8	20	24	18	20	18	19	14	17	16
3	-	1	4	9	7	8	6	5	4	5	4
4	-	-	2	4	6	4	3	2	2	1	1
5	-	-	-	1	1	1	-	1	-	1	1
6	-	-	1	-	-	1	2	-	-	-	-
	100	100	100	100	100	100	100	100	100	100	100

M&EA

	5+	6+	7+	8+	9+	10+	11+	12+	13+	14+	15+
	%	%	%	%	%	%	%	%	%	%	%
0	81	65	39	35	33	38	37	45	47	51	49
1	15	20	32	27	25	24	23	26	23	26	29
2	3	12	19	21	27	23	22	14	21	14	15
3	1	1	7	10	8	8	9	9	5	3	6
4	-	2	2	5	4	5	5	3	3	5	1
5	-	-	1	1	3	1	3	2	-	1	-
6	-	-	-	1	-	1	1	1	1	-	-
	100	100	100	100	100	100	100	100	100	100	100

W&SW

	5+	6+	7+	8+	9+	10+	11+	12+	13+	14+	15+
	%	%	%	%	%	%	%	%	%	%	%
0	83	58	35	31	34	32	41	42	43	48	43
1	10	23	29	28	23	34	29	28	33	26	32
2	6	15	25	30	28	19	19	21	18	18	17
3	1	2	7	6	8	8	5	6	3	5	4
4	-	2	3	4	5	3	5	1	1	2	3
5	-	-	-	-	1	3	1	1	1	1	1
6	-	-	1	1	1	1	-	1	1	-	-
	100	100	100	100	100	100	100	100	100	100	100

L&SE

	5+	6+	7+	8+	9+	10+	11+	12+	13+	14+	15+
	%	%	%	%	%	%	%	%	%	%	%
0	78	56	41	38	36	40	42	43	50	47	47
1	15	29	30	22	27	25	22	30	27	27	26
2	6	12	19	28	24	23	21	17	14	18	21
3	1	2	5	6	8	8	8	6	6	6	5
4	-	1	2	5	4	3	5	3	2	2	1
5	-	-	2	1	1	1	1	1	-	-	-
6	-	-	1	-	-	-	1	-	1	-	-
	100	100	100	100	100	100	100	100	100	100	100

Wales

	5+	6+	7+	8+	9+	10+	11+	12+	13+	14+	15+
	%	%	%	%	%	%	%	%	%	%	%
0	83	61	44	38	40	43	44	49	46	50	48
1	14	26	29	25	30	30	29	23	29	28	24
2	3	10	20	28	20	18	17	18	18	15	18
3	-	1	7	4	6	6	6	6	4	5	8
4	-	1	-	4	3	2	3	2	1	2	2
5	-	-	-	1	1	1	-	1	1	-	-
6	-	1	-	-	-	-	1	1	1	-	-
	100	100	100	100	100	100	100	100	100	100	100

For bases see Tables 9, 15, 21, 27, 33

Table 82   Occlusion and overbite, for
children of different ages

England and Wales

Occlusion and overbite	Age at 31 December 1972										
	5+	6+	7+	8+	9+	10+	11+	12+	13+	14+	15+
Occlusion	%	%	%	%	%	%	%	%	%	%	%
Class 1	73	73	65	61	64	64	62	64	65	67	68
Class 2, division 1	9	8	16	18	17	17	19	18	14	13	12
Class 2, division 2	–	1	3	6	5	4	5	4	5	5	5
Class 2*, unknown	13	13	12	11	10	11	10	11	11	10	8
Class 3	4	4	3	3	3	3	3	3	4	5	6
Not classified	1	1	1	1	1	1	1	–	1	–	1
	100	100	100	100	100	100	100	100	100	100	100
Overbite	%	%	%	%	%	%	%	%	%	%	%
Anterior open bite	11	18	10	6	3	3	2	2	2	2	2
Zero overbite	10	9	7	4	2	2	2	2	3	4	3
Up to a third	30	32	33	33	33	30	26	30	32	35	37
Over a third, up to two-thirds	24	18	29	38	44	46	49	48	46	42	42
Over two-thirds	17	11	12	17	17	18	19	16	16	15	14
Not measured	8	12	9	2	1	1	2	2	1	2	2
	100	100	100	100	100	100	100	100	100	100	100
Base	*952*	*1080*	*1137*	*1091*	*1129*	*1092*	*986*	*956*	*915*	*923*	*696*

Table 83   Overjet as measured for the upper left and right central incisors, for children of different ages

England and Wales

Overjet measurement for upper central incisors in mm	Age at 31 December 1972										
	5+	6+	7+	8+	9+	10+	11+	12+	13+	14+	15+
Right	%	%	%	%	%	%	%	%	%	%	%
-1 or less	1	1	2	1	1	1	1	1	1	1	1
Zero	7	6	4	3	1	2	2	2	2	3	3
+1	29	27	21	17	16	15	13	17	18	20	24
+2	30	28	26	25	29	28	26	24	28	29	28
+3	16	18	20	21	21	23	24	23	22	13	20
+4	8	10	11	13	13	14	14	14	15	7	9
+5	4	6	6	9	7	7	8	8	8	4	7
+6	3	2	4	4	5	5	5	5	2	2	3
+7	1	1	2	3	3	2	2	2	1	1	2
+8	1	1	2	2	3	2	2	2	1	1	1
+9	-	-	2	1	1	-	1	1	-	-	1
+10	-	-	-	1	-	1	1	1	1	-	1
+11 or more	-	-	-	-	-	-	1	-	1	-	-
	100	100	100	100	100	100	100	100	100	100	100
Not measured	19%	26%	17%	6%	4%	3%	4%	3%	4%	4%	4%
Left	%	%	%	%	%	%	%	%	%	%	%
-1 or less	1	1	2	1	1	1	1	1	1	1	1
Zero	7	5	3	3	1	2	2	2	2	3	4
+1	33	30	20	16	15	14	14	16	18	19	20
+2	29	27	25	24	27	30	24	24	29	28	29
+3	13	18	21	22	21	23	23	23	22	22	23
+4	8	9	13	15	15	13	14	16	13	11	9
+5	5	6	6	9	8	8	10	6	8	8	7
+6	2	2	4	3	5	4	5	5	4	3	4
+7	1	1	2	3	3	2	2	3	1	2	2
+8	1	1	2	2	1	1	2	2	1	1	1
+9	-	-	2	1	2	1	1	1	1	1	-
+10	-	-	-	1	1	1	1	1	-	1	-
+11 or more	-	-	-	-	-	-	1	-	-	-	-
	100	100	100	100	100	100	100	100	100	100	100
Not measured	20%	27%	17%	6%	4%	3%	3%	3%	5%	4%	5%
Base	*952*	*1080*	*1137*	*1091*	*1129*	*1092*	*986*	*956*	*915*	*923*	*696*

Table 84   Orthodontic assessments for children
of different ages

Assessments of edge to edge or instanding incisors, buccal crossbite and mucosal trauma	Age at 31 December 1972										
	5+	6+	7+	8+	9+	10+	11+	12+	13+	14+	15+
Proportion of children with											
Edge to edge or instanding incisors	13%	14%	13%	12%	11%	11%	10%	9%	9%	10%	9%
Buccal crossbite or cusp to cusp occlusion	2%	9%	16%	15%	14%	14%	11%	11%	13%	10%	9%
Mucosal trauma	2%	2%	4%	4%	4%	4%	3%	2%	2%	2%	2%
Edge to edge or instanding incisors	Rate per thousand										
Upper left lateral incisor											
Edge to edge	26	23	21	33	43	36	33	27	35	39	16
Instanding	66	69	33	22	22	28	26	25	33	31	33
Upper left central incisor											
Edge to edge	12	13	26	20	19	14	15	16	7	11	4
Instanding	56	34	22	12	6	14	11	8	16	20	26
Upper right central incisor											
Edge to edge	11	13	24	16	12	18	11	16	8	12	6
Instanding	51	33	26	20	6	11	18	9	15	17	29
Upper right lateral incisor											
Edge to edge	26	21	23	28	43	41	41	38	33	33	29
Instanding	67	63	41	32	19	24	23	24	25	29	30
Buccal crossbite or cusp to cusp occlusion	Rate per thousand										
Left side											
Cusp to cusp	4	34	55	49	40	33	20	21	39	31	29
Buccal crossbite	4	23	35	48	38	44	35	38	45	36	33
Right side											
Cusp to cusp	5	35	68	59	50	51	35	32	36	24	30
Buccal crossbite	6	25	48	39	42	47	40	44	43	36	50
Base	*952*	*1080*	*1137*	*1091*	*1129*	*1092*	*986*	*956*	*915*	*923*	*696*

Table 85   Other conditions for children
            of different ages

England and Wales

Proportion of children with some other conditions	Age at 31 December 1972										
	5+	6+	7+	8+	9+	10+	11+	12+	13+	14+	15+
Ulceration of soft tissues	1%	1%	1%	1%	1%	1%	–	1%	1%	1%	1%
Abscess	6%	5%	5%	4%	4%	3%	1%	–	–	1%	–
Acquired conditions	3%	3%	2%	1%	1%	1%	1%	1%	–	1%	–
Developmental conditions											
Enamel, dentine	2%	3%	4%	3%	5%	4%	5%	4%	3%	3%	2%
Teeth	1%	2%	2%	3%	3%	5%	4%	4%	4%	5%	3%
Face and jaws	1%	2%	2%	2%	1%	1%	1%	–	1%	1%	1%
Base	952	1080	1137	1091	1129	1092	986	956	915	923	696

Part V

Appendices

A   Glossary of general dental terms

Deciduous teeth (dentition)   - also called "primary" or "milk" teeth

Permanent teeth (dentition)   - also called "secondary" teeth

Mixed dentition   - a situation where a child has some deciduous and some permanent teeth present

Exfoliation   - the natural shedding of deciduous teeth

Eruption   - the process by which teeth break through the gum and establish their position in the mouth

Quadrant   - one quarter of the mouth (half of one jaw). The teeth in each quadrant are classified from front to back eg UR6 = "upper right permanent first molar"; LLb = "lower left deciduous lateral incisor".

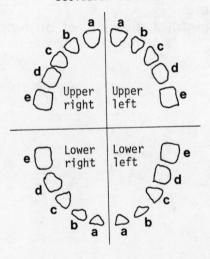

Deciduous dentition

a - central incisor
b - lateral incisor
c - canine
d - first molar
e - second molar

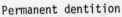
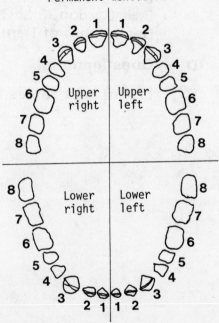

Permanent dentition

1 - central incisor
2 - lateral incisor
3 - canine
4 - first premolar
5 - second premolar
6 - first molar
7 - second molar
8 - third molar (wisdom)

Segment	- part of the mouth - in this survey the six segments referred to are those involving the teeth: 8-4; 3-3; and 4-8 in each jaw.
Anterior teeth	- 'c' - 'c' deciduous teeth and 3-3 permanent teeth
Posterior teeth	- 'd' - 'e' deciduous teeth and 4-8 permanent teeth
Caries	- decay
Filled, otherwise sound	- denotes a tooth which has been decayed but is currently soundly restored, thus distinguishing it from a tooth which has been filled but is currently decayed, the latter being included in the catagory of decayed teeth.
Trauma	- injury
Periodontal disease	- disease of the gums and supporting tissues of the teeth, in this survey measured in terms of gum inflammation
Plaque	- bacterial substance adhering to teeth
Debris	- food material, materia alba, plaque
Calculus	- hard deposit sometimes found on teeth, also known as "tartar".
Orthodontic	- pertaining to the position and development of the teeth and jaws.
Occlusion	- the relationship between contact points of the upper and lower teeth
Potential crowding	- current evidence that in the future there will be insufficient space for all the teeth to erupt without crowding

The above definitions are of a very general nature. Readers interested in the more specialised dental terminology used in the examination should refer to Annexe C.1 where the definitions of the criteria provide a description of the measurements which the dentists undertook.

B Calculating the estimated total deciduous decay experience among children over the age of five

We began by using the estimated decay experience of each tooth type among five year olds as our base line. The assumptions of Estimate III meant that at the age of five all missing deciduous teeth other than incisors were assumed to have been extracted due to caries. But we felt that even among five year olds natural exfoliation was already playing too great a part in deciduous tooth loss to assume that all missing deciduous incisors had been extracted for decay reasons. We therefore estimated the decay experience of the missing deciduous incisors from the state of health of the other anterior teeth, (see Section 4.1).

When proceeding to the older age groups we immediately had to define at what ages deciduous canines and molars become involved with natural exfoliation, and thus over what age range a missing deciduous tooth was likely to have been extracted for caries and over what age range one can no longer make such a simple assumption.

We examined the proportion of each permanent tooth type erupted for children of different ages, and also the rate at which the proportion was changing from age group to age group. On this evidence we made a decision, albeit arbitrary, about the age at which we could no longer state with any reliability that deciduous loss was due to extraction rather than exfoliation, thus deriving a definition of the age at which natural exfoliation can be expected to begin for a particular tooth type. The ages so defined were as follows:-

Tooth type	Age of child at which natural exfoliation is assumed possible
Upper left 'a' Lower left 'a' Upper left 'b' Lower left 'b'	5 years or more
Upper left 'c' Lower left 'c'	9 years or more 8 years or more
Upper left 'd' Lower left 'd'	8 years or more 9 years or more
Upper left 'e' Lower left 'e'	9 years or more 9 years or more

For each age group and each deciduous tooth type* we wrote down how many deciduous teeth were present but decayed or filled, and how many were absent (either due to exfoliation or extraction). We then had to estimate how many of the absent deciduous teeth had been decayed before they were lost.

In the cases where the children were younger than the age when exfoliation was defined as possible for a particular tooth type then all the absent teeth of that type were assumed to have been extracted because of decay. Where exfoliation was possible a more complicated procedure was followed.

Since the loss of a tooth is irreversible, any count of missing teeth includes all the accumulated loss from the past. Consequently some of the teeth missing among eight year olds (for example) were lost recently and some were lost years earlier. Assuming that no major changes have taken place in dental health and treatment during the lifetime of the children in the survey, it is reasonable to suppose that the rate of loss experienced by the older children in earlier years is approximately equal to the rate of loss currently being experienced by younger children. We therefore apportioned missing teeth to the likely age of loss, using the younger age groups as an estimate.

For example, among eight year olds 97% of the upper left 'a's were missing. Among seven year olds 83% were missing, among six year olds 39% were missing and among five five year olds 8% were missing. We therefore assumed that the 97% missing among eight year olds was made up of 8% that had been lost at five, 31% that had been lost at six, 44% that had been lost at seven and 14% that had been lost when they were eight.

Those teeth estimated as being lost at an age when exfoliation was defined to be unlikely were assumed to have all been diseased. For the teeth estimated to have been lost at an age when exfoliation was possible we needed to estimate their probable disease experience. In these cases we assumed that teeth lost at eight, for example, but present at seven had a similar disease experience to the same tooth type currently present in seven year olds.

This procedure is probably more easily explained by a worked example.

B.1 Calculation of estimated total disease experience of the upper left 'e's for children aged ten

We use three basic assumptions in this estimation:-

(i)   The rate of loss experienced by the older children in earlier years is approximately equal to the rate of loss currently being experienced by the younger children.

---

* We tested for symmetry of caries and found the two sides of the mouth so close in decay experience that we carried out the detailed calculations for each tooth on the left and doubled the results to obtain the total decay experience for the whole mouth.

(ii)   The upper left 'e's can be expected to be involved with natural
        exfoliation for children aged nine years or more, thus, any missing
        before the age of nine can be assumed to have been extracted for
        caries.

(iii)   For those upper left 'e's lost at the age of nine or more the
        proportion which were diseased before they were lost is approximately
        equal to the proportion of teeth present and diseased among children
        a year younger.

        Number of children aged ten   1092

        Number of decayed or filled
        upper left 'e's present   312

        Number of missing upper left 'e's   509

We apportioned the missing upper left 'e's in accordance with the proportion of
upper left 'e's lost among the younger age groups, which led to the following
distribution of age at loss:-

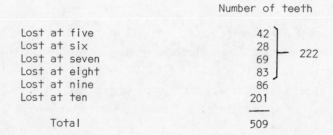

	Number of teeth	
Lost at five	42	
Lost at six	28	222
Lost at seven	69	
Lost at eight	83	
Lost at nine	86	
Lost at ten	201	
Total	509	

All of the 222 teeth estimated to have been lost before the age of nine were assumed
to have been extracted for caries.

Of the 86 teeth estimated to have been lost at nine 57%, i.e. 49 teeth, were
estimated to have been diseased (this was the proportion of upper left 'e's present
and either decayed or filled among eight year olds).

Of the 201 teeth estimated to have been lost at ten 57% i.e. 115 teeth, were
estimated to have been diseased (this was the proportion of upper left 'e's present
and either decayed or filled among nine year olds).

Thus the total number of upper left 'e's estimated as being diseased was:-

Present and diseased		312
Missing but estimated		
diseased	(i)	222
	(ii)	49
	(iii)	115
Total		698

This estimation procedure was used for each of ten tooth types and for each of ten
age groups and the results were then amalgamated to give a whole mouth estimate of
total disease experience.

The criteria for clinical assessments, the conduct of the dental examination and the training of the examiners

C

R.J. Anderson, J.F. Beal, T.D. Foster, P.H. Gordon, P.M.C. James
Department of Dental Health, University of Birmingham.

We wish to acknowledge the University of Birmingham for allowing us to take part
in this study and the Birmingham Dental School and Hospital for the use of their
facilities.

We are indebted to the Health and Education authorities of Birmingham City, Solihull
County Borough and Warwickshire County Councils for permission to visit schools in
their areas during the development, training and calibration programmes. In
particular, we would like to thank the head teachers and staff of the following
schools:- Foundry Junior School, Birmingham; Chapel Fields, Langley and St.
Margarets Church of England Junior Schools, Solihull; and Kineton High School and
Wootton Wawen Church of England Junior and Infants School, Warwickshire. Our thanks
are also due to the children of these schools who cheerfully allowed themselves to
be examined on many occasions. Without their particular help the training of the
large number of dental examiners would have been impossible.

We are also most grateful to the postgraduate students and dentists who took part
in the development programme and the pre-pilot and pilot studies, to Mr. R. Bettles
and Mr. J. Onions who assisted in the training programme, and to the technical and
secretarial staff of the Department of Dental Health, University of Birmingham for
their assistance at every stage.

Finally we wish to thank all the dentists who undertook the examinations for the
good humoured way they approached a most intensive training course. Their names
are given in Annex C.3.

Introduction

A study such as this has certain necessary limitations, one of which is the time that can be allowed for the examination of each child. Early in the planning it was decided that this must be restricted to a period of six minutes, and this had a considerable effect on the extent and conduct of the examination.

There is a second limiting factor - the results and conclusions of epidemiological studies are invalid unless the methods of data collection are standardised and the criteria for identifying the conditions are clearly defined and reproducible. The accomplishment of these essentials presented some difficulty in this large scale study, where it was necessary to employ many examining dentists, most of whom had long-established opinions about the diagnosis and grading of clinical features. It was very important to overcome this difficulty; the examiners were to examine children in their own areas only, so variation between them could easily account for apparent area differences.

When establishing a set of criteria for diagnosis it is necessary to compromise. It must extract as much information as possible while avoiding the grey area of potential massive disagreement. Refinement of detail must often be sacrificed for the achievement of standardisation and reproducibility, with full recognition of the fact that the results will almost certainly be an understatement.

The clinical information required from the survey was agreed with representatives of the Department of Health and Social Security and for a period of approximately twelve months examination methods and diagnostic criteria were discussed, tested, modified and re-tested by members of the Department of Dental Health, University of Birmingham, until there was reasonable certainty that the above compromise had been achieved.

The development programme included initial calibration exercises, a pre-pilot study and a pilot study.

Initial calibration exercises

These were carried out in the Birmingham Dental Hospital in March, 1972, using Hospital patients as examination subjects and members of the Department of Dental Health, with seven postgraduate students, as examiners. Equipment, method and criteria were tested and a provisional protocol and dental examination chart were drawn up.

Pre-pilot study

To test the practicability of the examination and collection document a pre-pilot trial was undertaken in June, 1972, at Kineton High School and Wootton Wawen C of E Infant and Junior School, in Warwickshire. Five examiners spent one day at each school conducting dental examinations on children grouped in appropriate age ranges between 5 and 15 years. Recording of data was carried out by a team from the Office of Population Censuses and Surveys. As a result of this exercise, some modifications of the equipment, techniques, criteria and collection method were proposed and agreed.

Pilot study

The revised protocol was used as a basis for further testing. Six Public Dental Officers from different parts of the country attended a training course at the Birmingham Dental School in October, 1972, during which they conducted dental examinations in the two Warwickshire schools. After a calibration exercise at a third school, they carried out a trial of the whole technique of clinical examinations and interviews in six pilot study areas in England. The degree of standardisation achieved was investigated by the Office of Population Censuses and Surveys' representatives and, again, modifications and improvements to the protocol and techniques were suggested and agreed. A final document was drawn up and this, with the addition of a few minor points of clarification that arose during the training period, was adopted for the study proper. It is shown in Annex C.1 together with some explanatory notes and the dental examination chart.

Main training and calibration programme

This took place during the two weeks beginning 15th and 22nd January, 1973. About 35 examiners attended each week and they brought, or were issued with, the equipment listed in Annex C.2. The instructors in the training courses were four members of staff from the Department of Dental Health, who had developed and become accustomed to the examination techniques in the pre-pilot study and who had carried out the training of observers in the pilot investigation. They were assisted by two of the dentists trained in the pilot study.

At the outset of the training courses the necessity for the standardisation of diagnostic criteria was emphasized to the participants. During the first training period the objective was to achieve this standardisation between each examiner and the group as a whole, and care was taken not to influence individuals towards the personal interpretations of the instructors if these were found to differ from the majority opinion of the group. During the next week the second group of dentists was trained in accordance with the majority views of the first group.

Standardisation exercises were conducted after each course of training so that the residual differences between the examiners could be measured. These were repeated after the national study, to detect possible changes in diagnostic criteria either as the group or as individual members of it.

Training Programme

The observers spent the first three sessions at the Dental School receiving instruction on the conditions to be recorded, their diagnostic criteria and the appropriate codes. Each session followed the same basic pattern: the conditions to be recorded were described in detail with as much visual aid as possible, and this was followed by practical tests using slides, models of the dental arches, or plaster blocks containing extracted teeth. The interchange of study material between individuals permitted a wide range of experience and the material itself was chosen so as to be representative of extensive variation. Demonstrations and practice were given in the methods of recording in conjunction with a member of staff from the Office of Population Censuses and Surveys.

After this initial training period the observers went into the field and examined children in selected schools under the supervision of their instructors. They worked in pairs, one examining the children and the other recording, using the appropriate codes. At set intervals they changed places to ensure equal examination experience. At each of these five clinical sessions staff from the Office of Population Censuses and Surveys were present for checking examination forms and analysing the data as they were collected.

The first clinical session was used to familiarise the dentists with the various criteria and examination techniques, while the Office of Population Censuses and Surveys' representatives merely scrutinised the records for errors and omissions in recording. The next two days were devoted to the standardisation of the examiners. The two schools involved in the pre-pilot and pilot studies were re-visited and the same children examined again. Briefly, two groups of children were established in each of the age ranges 5 to 6, 8 to 9, 12 and 15 years. The dentists were again paired and one of each pair saw the whole of one group in every age range, each child being examined by each dentist in turn. In the afternoon the dentists in each pair exchanged roles as before and the second group of children were examined by the other dentist. All the examiners saw approximately ten children in each age range and their recorded findings could be compared in detail.

As the sessions proceeded, differences between the examiners became apparent. Discussions were held with individual dentists throughout the whole period and on the completion of a batch of children a general conference took place to resolve any problems, with the children available for scrutiny. As the examiners became more confident they needed less guidance with the examination technique. Instructors then followed the same child around all the dentists, taking note of the recorded differences in diagnoses. This was particularly useful for discovering and correcting discrepancies as they arose.

On their last day the dentists returned to the Dental School and spent the first part of the morning discussing problems that had arisen during the clinical sessions. They were then joined by their recorders for the national study and each pair practised their calling and recording techniques, with the dentists dictating from existing examination records and the recorders transcribing onto new sheets. This permitted the two members of each team to work together before the calibration exercise, which took place in the afternoon.

Calibration

Examiners and their recorders were divided into three groups. Each group attended a different junior school in Solihull where every dentist examined between 10 and 13 children. Dental instructors and a member of the Office of Population Censuses and Surveys' field staff were present at the schools to ensure that the examiners and recorders were working well together, but there was no attempt to alter the diagnostic standards in any way.

Re-calibration

After the national study the examiners returned and re-examined the same children that they had seen in the calibration trial. Results from the calibration and re-calibration trials were scrutinised to discover the degree of standardisation and reproducibility of the observers.

Calibration results

There were, in all, 69 dentists who carried out examinations for the survey; of these, two were unable to attend the re-calibration session which took place once all the fieldwork was completed. We have calculated the calibration results for the 67 dentists who were at both calibration sessions so that the data can be compared for the 'before' and 'after' tests. Similarly we included in the tests only those children who had been present at both test sessions. As described earlier the calibration exercise took place in three separate schools on two half days before the fieldwork and two half days after the fieldwork. Although initially it was hoped that the same group of children would be examined on the two half days in each school by two groups of dental examiners, sickness among the children prevented this and on the second half day different children were substituted to maintain the numbers. Therefore instead of being able to reduce the presentation of calibration results to three larger groups of dentists we have to present the results separately for the six groups of dentists. Although the numbers in each group are rather small we have calculated the coefficient of variation for each group, and for each condition tested so that some comparison can be made of the variability of examiners in different groups, and the variability in the measurement of different dental health indicators.

The results show (see Table C.1) that among the measurements of decay experience and its treatment the number of actively decayed teeth was the most variable. There was little variation in the measurement of filled teeth and very few of the children in the calibration study had any missing permanent teeth. Since the number of filled teeth among these groups of children was much higher than the number of actively decayed teeth the total number of decayed, missing or filled teeth was dominated by the last component and, in consequence, the measurement of the variability was low.

The amount of variability in the measurement of active decay was, generally speaking, similar at the calibration and re-calibration sessions. There was more variability between dentists in different groups than between the same group of dentists on different occasions. With the relatively small numbers of children examined it is possible that some groups of dentists examined children for whom the dental assessments involved a greater number of border line decisions.

Table C.1
Calibration and recalibration results for the measurements of decayed, missing and filled teeth.

	Group A	Group B	Group C	Group D	Group E	Group F
Number of children	9	9	11	11	12	13
Number of dentists	9	11	12	10	13	12

Decayed teeth

Calibration

	Group A	Group B	Group C	Group D	Group E	Group F
Mean[†]	10.4	10.4	14.8	13.4	12.3	21.2
Standard deviation	3.5	3.6	2.7	3.1	5.7	6.5
Coeff. of variation*	0.34	0.34	0.18	0.23	0.47	0.31

Recalibration

	Group A	Group B	Group C	Group D	Group E	Group F
Mean[†]	9.0	11.3	13.1	11.9	15.0	17.7
Standard deviation	2.7	2.9	3.9	2.0	6.2	6.1
Coeff. of variation*	0.30	0.26	0.30	0.17	0.41	0.34

Missing teeth

Calibration

	Group A	Group B	Group C	Group D	Group E	Group F
Mean[†]	–	–	–	–	2.1	2.8
Standard deviation	–	–	–	–	0.3	1.7
Coeff. of variation*	–	–	–	–	0.13	0.59

Recalibration

	Group A	Group B	Group C	Group D	Group E	Group F
Mean[†]	–	–	–	–	2.0	1.8
Standard deviation	–	–	–	–	0.0	0.6
Coeff. of variation*	–	–	–	–	0.00	0.31

Filled teeth

Calibration

	Group A	Group B	Group C	Group D	Group E	Group F
Mean[†]	42.3	50.4	26.2	25.9	45.8	51.6
Standard deviation	2.4	2.4	1.6	1.5	3.1	3.5
Coeff. of variation*	0.06	0.05	0.06	0.06	0.07	0.07

Recalibration

	Group A	Group B	Group C	Group D	Group E	Group F
Mean[†]	45.3	50.9	26.7	26.8	44.8	53.7
Standard deviation	1.2	2.4	1.2	1.2	3.0	3.4
Coeff. of variation*	0.03	0.05	0.05	0.04	0.07	0.06

Decayed, missing and filled teeth

Calibration

	Group A	Group B	Group C	Group D	Group E	Group F
Mean[†]	52.8	60.7	41.0	39.3	60.3	75.6
Standard deviation	1.6	2.2	1.7	2.5	2.9	3.8
Coeff. of variation*	0.03	0.04	0.04	0.06	0.05	0.05

Recalibration

	Group A	Group B	Group C	Group D	Group E	Group F
Mean[†]	54.3	62.2	39.8	38.7	61.8	73.2
Standard deviation	1.8	1.6	3.1	2.0	3.8	3.6
Coeff. of variation*	0.03	0.02	0.08	0.05	0.06	0.05

* Coefficient of variation = $\dfrac{\text{Standard deviation}}{\text{Mean}}$

[†] Mean per dentist for all children in group

333

Table C.2
Calibration and recalibration results for the measurements of gum condition, crowding, and orthodontic referral

	Group A	Group B	Group C	Group D	Group E	Group F
Number of children	9	9	11	11	12	13
Number of dentists	9	11	12	10	13	12

Gum inflammation [+]

Calibration

	Group A	Group B	Group C	Group D	Group E	Group F
Mean[+]	17.6	19.3	11.2	8.2	10.5	9.7
Standard deviation	3.7	3.8	11.3	6.1	7.3	5.4
Coeff. of variation*	0.21	0.20	1.01	0.74	0.70	0.56

Recalibration

	Group A	Group B	Group C	Group D	Group E	Group F
Mean[+]	13.4	18.0	10.6	5.7	11.1	13.1
Standard deviation	4.4	3.0	8.8	6.8	8.5	6.8
Coeff. of variation*	0.32	0.17	0.83	1.20	0.77	0.52

Debris [+]

Calibration

	Group A	Group B	Group C	Group D	Group E	Group F
Mean[+]	17.0	20.3	14.2	14.9	15.9	14.1
Standard deviation	10.3	4.8	11.9	3.7	10.9	6.7
Coeff. of variation*	0.61	0.24	0.84	0.25	0.68	0.48

Recalibration

	Group A	Group B	Group C	Group D	Group E	Group F
Mean[+]	19.7	23.6	10.9	9.9	18.5	9.7
Standard deviation	7.4	5.9	5.4	3.7	13.9	6.6
Coeff. of variation*	0.37	0.25	0.49	0.37	0.75	0.68

Calculus [+]

Calibration

	Group A	Group B	Group C	Group D	Group E	Group F
Mean[+]	6.4	14.5	3.1	2.1	2.9	4.2
Standard deviation	0.7	1.8	1.4	1.6	2.7	3.1
Coeff. of variation*	0.11	0.13	0.44	0.78	0.93	0.75

Recalibration

	Group A	Group B	Group C	Group D	Group E	Group F
Mean[+]	7.0	14.2	3.0	1.9	3.5	2.2
Standard deviation	1.2	1.6	2.1	2.2	3.1	1.7
Coeff. of variation*	0.18	0.12	0.71	1.14	0.89	0.77

Crowding [+]

Calibration

	Group A	Group B	Group C	Group D	Group E	Group F
Mean[+]	17.0	23.7	12.6	11.6	18.3	14.3
Standard deviation	2.9	2.1	2.6	2.2	3.8	4.4
Coeff. of variation*	0.17	0.09	0.20	0.19	0.21	0.31

Recalibration

	Group A	Group B	Group C	Group D	Group E	Group F
Mean[+]	17.0	23.7	12.2	13.6	18.5	11.5
Standard deviation	4.0	2.8	3.8	4.5	5.2	5.1
Coeff. of variation*	0.24	0.12	0.31	0.33	0.28	0.44

Orthodontic referral

Calibration

	Group A	Group B	Group C	Group D	Group E	Group F
Mean[+]	5.9	5.4	6.6	6.9	7.2	5.2
Standard deviation	0.9	1.9	1.5	1.3	1.6	1.2
Coeff. of variation*	0.15	0.35	0.23	0.19	0.22	0.23

Recalibration

	Group A	Group B	Group C	Group D	Group E	Group F
Mean[+]	5.3	5.5	6.6	6.6	7.6	5.1
Standard deviation	1.4	1.4	1.7	1.3	1.1	1.3
Coeff. of variation*	0.27	0.25	0.26	0.19	0.14	0.26

* Coefficient of variation = $\dfrac{\text{Standard deviation}}{\text{Mean}}$ [+] Number of segments with ......

[+] Mean per dentist for all children in group

Table C.2 shows the variability in the measurements of the childrens' gum conditions, crowding and whether the dentist considered they needed or would need orthodontic referral or treatment.

The variability in the measurement of gum inflammation was fairly similar at the calibration and recalibration sessions. In groups A and B the variability in the number of segments recorded as having some gum inflammation was much lower than for the other groups.

As far as debris was concerned there was considerable variation in the coefficient of variation both between groups of dentists and in some cases between sessions. It is perhaps unreasonable, however, to expect the debris condition to remain constant over time.

The number of segments found to have calculus was fairly small. The variability in groups A and B was much lower than the other groups, a result similar to that found for the measurement of gum inflammation. The children examined at this school were a little younger than those at the other schools, a fact which may well have contributed to this difference. As with the measurement of gum inflammation variability was, on the whole, greater among the different dentists than between the same group seeing the same children on different occasions.

The variation in the assessment of the number of segments that were crowded and the number of children needing orthodontic referral or treatment was of the same order as the variation in the number of teeth said to be actively decayed. For these measurements the variability was not as large between different groups of dentists as was the case with gum inflammation, debris and calculus.

The numbers of children involved in the calibration exercise were very small and so it is difficult to make precise estimates of examiner variability. The calibration and recalibration results show in general that the measurement of filled teeth, missing teeth and DMF teeth was very reliable. The measurements of decayed teeth, crowded teeth and the need for orthodontic referral showed some examiner variability but, as previous studies have shown, the greatest examiner variability was found in the measurement of gum conditions.

We examined the calibration and recalibration results according to the region in which the dentist carried out his fieldwork and established that there was no domination of any region by either high scoring or low scoring dentists.

Study of child dental health
in England and Wales
1973

The conduct of the dental examination
and criteria for the assessments

*(Notes in italics indicate points of clarification
made during the main training course)*

Racial Origin

The racial origin of the child will be recorded. This may not be the same as the nationality or country of birth. There is considerable variation between individuals of the same race, especially in skin colour. Classification is to be assessed by physical appearance only.

White/Caucasian (Code 1)

Only those of 'white' European origin are recorded in this category. Individuals have a 'white' skin and fair, brown, red or black hair, which may be wavy or straight.

Negro (Code 2)

These individuals have a dark ('black') skin and black woolly hair.

Indian/Pakistani (Code 3)

Features include a light brown skin, black straight hair and a narrow nose.

Oriental/Mongoloid (Code 4)

These have a 'yellow' skin, black coarse straight hair and a low bridge of the nose; the eyes often slant and the cheekbones are prominent.

Other (Code 5)

Specify any individual who can be classified into a racial group other than those above.

Not known (Code 6)

This category is to be used when the examiner is unable to classify the subject into any racial group.

The Teeth

Teeth will be examined in the following order:

Upper left - upper right - lower right - lower left

In the first instance the teeth present will be identified and recorded. In cases where both primary tooth and its permanent successor are present, both will be identified and called but further details will be recorded for the permanent tooth only. Subsequently every tooth will be identified and called, indicating the primary or permanent dentition, as appropriate.

A tooth is deemed to be present if any part of it is visible. Teeth may be absent for a number of reasons, as follows:

Code U	Unerupted
Code M	Extracted due to caries
Code T	Missing due to trauma
Code O	Extracted for orthodontic reasons

In most cases the reason for the absence of a tooth will be obvious and the appropriate code may be called and recorded at once. Sometimes questioning the child will be necessary - "Did you have those teeth taken out to make room for the others?" "Was that front tooth knocked out?"

Tooth Surfaces

If a tooth is present each surface will be examined, coded and called in the following order:

Mesial - occlusal - distal - buccal - lingual
(in the case of anterior teeth "occlusal" is, of course, omitted.)

"Buccal" and "lingual" should be used for all teeth; other descriptive terms such as "labial" and "palatal" must be avoided.

The surface coding is as follows:

Code G   Present and sound
In the case of partly-erupted teeth, where some surfaces may not be visible, these will be considered as sound and called under this category.

Code F   Filled
Surfaces containing a permanent restoration of any material will be coded under this category. Lesions or cavities containing a temporary dressing, or cavities from which a restoration has been lost, will be coded in the appropriate category of 'decayed'.
Petralit fillings are to be regarded as temporary and classified as 'decayed'.

Code 2   Decayed
Surfaces are regarded as decayed if, in the opinion of the examiner, after visual inspection, there is a carious cavity that does not involve the pulp. (The cavity that requires filling). If doubt exists the surface will be investigated with the probe supplied and unless the point enters the lesion the surface will be recorded as sound (G). The catching of the probe in a pit or fissure is not enough to warrant the diagnosis of caries unless there is additional visual evidence of it.
Hard arrested caries is not diagnosed as 'decayed' as no treatment is indicated.

Code 3   Unrestorable
Surfaces are regarded as falling into this category if, in the opinion of the examiner, after scrutiny and testing as above, there

is a carious cavity that involves the pulp. (The cavity that necessitates extraction or pulp treatment).

As a rough guide a primary tooth with a break in the marginal ridge of more than two-thirds its width is usually regarded as 'unrestorable'.

NB WHERE DOUBT EXISTS IN THE DIFFERENTIATION BETWEEN THE CATEGORIES (CODES G, 2 AND 3), THE LESS SEVERE CATEGORY SHOULD ALWAYS BE CALLED.

Code 4   Filled and decayed
            A surface that has a filling and a carious lesion will fall into this category unless the carious lesion would be coded as "unrestorable", in which case the filling will be ignored and the surface classified as Code 3.

Communication of Codes to the Recorder

When calling alphabetic codes the letter alone may be used. When calling numeric codes the number must be preceded by the word "code" - this will avoid confusion between code numbers and tooth numbers.

Trauma of incisors

Upper and lower incisors will be examined for traumatic injury. If none exists in any of these teeth, this is stated and recorded (A). If there is injury to any tooth, every incisor will be identified and allocated to one or more of the following categories:

    1   Discolouration
    2   Fracture involving enamel
    3   Fracture involving enamel and dentine
    4   Fracture involving enamel, dentine and pulp
    5   Missing due to trauma
    6   Temporary crown fitted
    7   Permanent or semi-permanent restoration fitted
        Include Class IV inlays if restoring a fracture.
    8   Displacement
    X   No trauma to this tooth

Multi-coding is possible in this section.

Categories 1-5, 8 and X are self-explanatory.

Temporary crowns

(6) refers to items of immediate treatment, such as foil, steel caps, pinch bands, acetate crowns, etc.

Permanent and semi-permanent restorations

(7) includes basket crowns, veneer crowns, post crowns, pinned inlays, etc.

340

Dentures

If the child wears a denture, the type will be recorded for each jaw involved. The categories are:

1	Partial denture
2	Full denture
X	No denture in this jaw.

If the child does not wear a denture, this should be recorded (A).
Bridges are excluded, these should be written in under 'further conditions'.

Gums, Debris, Calculus

For these assessments each jaw is divided into three segments, as follows:

The middle segment: extending from the distal surface of the canine on one side to the distal surface of the canine on the other side.

The left and right segments: extending from the distal surfaces of the canines to the distal surfaces of the most posterior teeth present.

The examiner will look at each of these segments in the prescribed order (upper left, upper middle, upper right, lower right, lower middle, lower left) three times; once for the assessment of the gum condition, once for estimating the amount of debris on the teeth and, once to determine the presence or absence of calculus.
The average condition of the gums or debris in the segment should be recorded and not the worst area in that segment.

Gums

Each segment will be examined both buccally and lingually and its state recorded according to one of the following categories:

0. The gums appear healthy. No treatment is needed.
1. The gums are not healthy. The condition is reversible; treatment in the form of prophylaxis and the correction of oral hygiene should restore them to health.
2. There is considerable redness and swelling of the gums. The condition is irreversible and the patient cannot be restored to health without the intervention of a dental surgeon.
   Such as surgery, extraction or replacing faulty restorations.
   Abscesses are ignored in assessing the gum condition, these should be recorded under 'dentists comments'.

Debris (food material, materia alba, plaque)
Each segment will be examined visually both buccally and lingually and its state recorded according to one of the following categories:

0. The teeth are clean. No debris is evident.
1. There is a small quantity of debris of recent origin.
   Ignore recent debris such as small pieces of potato crisp found in an otherwise clean mouth immediately following a school breaktime.
2. The teeth are dirty. There is considerable debris of long standing.

Calculus

Each segment will be examined visually and with the probe and the presence of calculus recorded as follows:

0.   No calculus
1.   Calculus is present

> IT MUST BE STRESSED THAT WHEN THERE IS
> DOUBT ABOUT THE CLASSIFICATION OF ANY
> CONDITION, THE LOWER CATEGORY SHOULD
> BE RECORDED.

Occlusal Assessment

The assessment of overbite, overjet, buccal cross-bite, occlusal classification and incisor relationship should be made with the teeth in centric occlusion. The assessment of overbite and overjet should be made with the Frankfort plane horizontal.

Overbite

The amount by which the upper incisor overlaps the lower incisor in the vertical dimension.

The overbite should be assessed at the level of the centre of the incisal edge of the upper left central incisor. If this tooth is missing or instanding, assess the right upper central incisor. If both are missing or instanding, mark "not measurable" (Y).

Assess and record the proportion of the crown of the lower incisor overlapped by the upper incisor in the following categories:

(Y) **Not measurable**	No assessment possible.
(1) **Anterior open bite**	The upper incisor does not overlap the lower incisor and does not fall into category 2 below.
(2) **Zero overbite**	The upper and lower incisal edges are in the same horizontal plane. (Not necessarily in contact.)
(3) **Up to and including** $\frac{1}{3}$	The upper incisor overlaps the lower incisor by not more than one-third of the clinical crown of the lower incisor.
(4) **Over** $\frac{1}{3}$, **up to and including** $\frac{2}{3}$	The upper incisor overlaps the lower incisor by more than one-third but not more than two-thirds of the clinical crown of the lower incisor.
(5) **Over** $\frac{2}{3}$	The upper incisor overlaps the lower incisor by more than two-thirds of the clinical crown of the lower incisor.

This assessment is to be made irrespective of the state of eruption of the tooth.

342

Overjet

The horizontal distance between the labial surfaces of the upper and lower central incisors in occlusion.

Measure, with the gauge supplied, at the centre of the incisal edge of:

    a)   left upper central and,

    b)   right upper central incisor (see diagram)

If the upper and lower central incisor edges are in contact, record 0.

A reversed overjet, ie. with the upper incisor in lingual relation to the lower incisor, should be recorded with a minus sign.

If the measurement falls between marks on the gauge, record the lower mark.

If no assessment is possible, record at (Y).

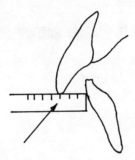

Buccal Crossbite

Record the lateral relationship of the first permanent molars in one of the following categories:

    (Y) **6's not in occlusion** (or missing)

    (0) **None** (normal relationship - see diagram)

    (1) **Cusp-to-cusp** (see diagram)

    (2) **Crossbite** (see diagram)

Record each side separately.

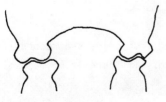 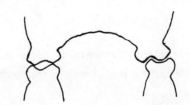

         Normal   Cusp-to-cusp   Crossbite

343

Occlusion

Record the antero-posterior relationship of the dental arches, assessed after allowing for the drifting of individual teeth.

Class 1 Within the limits of the "ideal" dental arch relationship, Code
typified by the intercuspation of the canine teeth with
the tip of the upper canine on the same vertical plane as   4
the distal edge of the lower canine in occlusion and
corresponding intercuspation of the other buccal teeth.

Class 2 A post-normal relationship of the lower dental arch to the
upper dental arch.
Division 1: increased overjet, usually with proclined
upper central incisors.   5
Division 2: retroclined upper central incisors.   6
Indefinite: a Class 2 relationship which does not fall
clearly into Division 1 or 2.   7

Class 3 A pre-normal relationship of the lower dental arch to the
upper dental arch.   8

If it is not possible to classify the occlusion in the
above categories, record "not classified".   9

Incisors

Upper incisors will be examined for instanding or edge-to-edge relationships. If none is instanding or edge-to-edge, this is recorded (A). If any incisor is instanding or edge-to-edge, every incisor will be examined and allocated to one of the following categories:

(1) This incisor is instanding (ie. behind the lower incisor or canine).
(2) This incisor is edge-to-edge (any part of its incisal edge is touching that of the opposing lower tooth).
(X) This incisor is neither instanding nor edge-to-edge.

Mucosal Trauma

Record the contact of teeth on gingival tissue or mucoperiosteum in occlusion, with apparent inflammation or other soft tissue damage.

Assess for middle segments of upper and lower arch only, and record lingual (palatal) and labial sides of the dental arch. If there is no mucosal trauma, record at A.

Crowding

This is defined as insufficient space in the existing dental arch for the teeth to be accommodated without overlap or irregularity. Potential crowding should be included, ie. any teeth which are assumed to be unerupted should be included in the assessment. Teeth which are assumed to be missing should not be included in the assessment.

Record each segment separately, the middle segments to include incisors and canines, and the left and right segments to include premolars and molars.

Record in the following categories:

0.   No crowding. The teeth, erupted and unerupted, can be fitted into that segment of the dental arch without overlapping or irregularity.

1.   There is shortage of space in that segment of not more than one premolar width (left and right segments), or one lower lateral incisor width (lower middle segment), or one upper lateral incisor width (upper middle segment).

2.   There is shortage of space in that segment to a greater extent than in the previous category (1).

Appliances

Record the presence of orthodontic appliances in each arch in one of the following categories:

> (1)   Removable orthodontic appliance.
> (2)   Fixed orthodontic appliance.
> (3)   Other (eg fixed/removable appliance). In this case, specify the type of appliance worn.
> (X)   No appliance in this jaw.

If no appliance is present in either jaw record at (A) and, in this case, if the child was born before 1965 ask whether a 'brace' has ever been worn. If the answer is 'yes', ask whether or not they still have to wear it.

Referral

a)   Record whether or not in your opinion the child needs, or will need, orthodontic assessment or treatment. If the child is undergoing orthodontic appliance treatment, record at (1).

b)   Record your opinion on what form of orthodontic treatment, if any, will be required. Assess the need for treatment on the actual or potential occlusion and position of the teeth, ignoring any consideration of patient co-operation or availability, or other aspects of oral health. The following categories will be used:

0.   No orthodontic treatment will be necessary.

1.   The child is currently undergoing orthodontic appliance treatment.

3.   The child will need extraction of teeth for the relief of potential or actual crowding and/or irregularity, but will not need appliance treatment for the alignment of teeth.

4.   The child will need appliance treatment for alignment of the teeth, either in conjunction with, or without, extraction of teeth.

5.   The form of treatment required is not known.

Dentists' comments

The dentist will be asked if he wishes to make any comments. If so, they will be recorded on the back of the card by the dentist. The check list should be used, where appropriate, to insert the code number alongside the comment. If it is felt that the condition described requires treatment, a tick should be placed in the appropriate column.

Check List

    10   Ulceration of soft tissues
           11   Infective (eg Vincent's, herpetic or other)
           12   Traumatic (eg biting cheek)
           13   Aphthous

    20   Tumour
           21   Hard tissue (eg cyst, odontome)
           22   Soft tissue (eg epulis)

    30   Abscess (eg gingival, apical or inter-radicular)

    40   Gross enlargement of gingival tissue (eg epanutin, blood
                                                  dyscrasias)

    50   Developmental anomalies: enamel and/or dentine
           51   Hypoplasia
           52   Amelogenesis imperfecta
           53   Dentinogenesis imperfecta (hereditary opalescent dentine)
           54   Gross enamel discolouration (intrinsic)
           55   Tetracycline staining

    60   Developmental anomalies: teeth
           61   Supplemental teeth
           62   Supernumerary teeth
           63   Geminated teeth
           64   Teeth of unusual form (e.g. peg-shaped laterals)
           65   Hypodontia
           66   Gross displacement or rotation of incisor teeth

    70   Developmental anomalies: face and jaws
           71   Cleft palate
           72   Cleft lip
           73   Cleft lip and palate
           74   Lingual fraenum
           75   Labial fraenum

    80   Acquired anomalies
           81   Attrition
           82   Abrasion

*This list is not exhaustive, other abnormal conditions should be
recorded by giving a main category code and describing the clinical findings.*

Notes on the oral examination

The objective of the clinical part of this investigation was to indicate treatment needs, so the data to be collected were chosen as indicating clinical necessity. The temptation to enlarge the scope of the examination for other research purposes had to be resisted. Some clinical features, included at the outset of the development programme, were later excluded for various reasons as this programme proceeded; some were too time-consuming to identify and record, while others required diagnostic experience that was impossible to impart and standardise during a short training period. The use of radiographs and models of the dental arches would have contributed considerably to the information gained, but considerations of time and cost made them impracticable. The limitations dictated by necessity were especially relevant to the occlusal assessment and consideration is given to the problem in the comments that follow under that heading.

These notes are intended to clarify the examination protocol and to explain, when appropriate, why a particular technique was adopted.

Racial Origin

The assessment of racial origin was made by the examining dentist, who usually had the advantage of local knowledge. It was done by appearance only; the children were allocated to four easily identifiable categories; white caucasian, negroid, Indian/Pakistani or oriental/mongoloid. When the child could be positively identified as belonging to another group, space was available for this to be entered on the sheet. In cases where the examiner was unsure of the racial origin or considered the child to be of mixed parentage, the 'not known' category was recorded.

The Teeth

The data relating to the state of the dentition were recorded for each tooth surface to gain the maximum possible information from the dental examination. To ensure uniformity between examiners and their recorders, it was necessary to standardise the order in which the teeth and tooth surfaces were examined.

All surfaces of a tooth were assumed to be erupted if any part of it was visible. If a tooth was not present a decision had to be made as to why it was missing. It could have been (1) unerupted, (2) congenitally absent, or (3) extracted. Without radiographs it was impossible to decide with certainty between the first two categories, so these were together classified as 'unerupted'. In most cases it was considered possible, using clinical judgment, to decide whether or not a tooth had been extracted. If there was doubt it was also designated as 'unerupted'. In cases of extraction it was necessary to decide on the reason. Factors taken into account included the particular tooth concerned, the condition of corresponding teeth in other segments of the mouth, the general oral state, etc., and usually the reason for the extraction was obvious. Sometimes it was necessary to question the child. Answers to such questions as: "was that front tooth knocked out?" or "did you have those teeth taken out to make room for the others?", often confirmed suspicions of trauma or extractions for orthodontic reasons, and these were recorded as such. Other extractions were recorded as missing (due to caries).

Dental Caries

Dental caries is a continuous process starting with the minute lesion only visible under a microscope and progressing until most of the tooth is involved. It is necessary in any study to define the stage in this process at which the lesion should be positively diagnosed. It is also essential to make the criteria as objective as possible so that all the examiners can agree on what to diagnose as caries. It has been shown that the greatest inter-examiner variation occurs in the case of the early enamel lesion, especially in the interpretation of the pit or fissure in which a sharp probe sticks and requires a positive effort to withdraw it. To avoid this difficulty it was decided that the examination should be primarily a visual one; a surface on which caries could be seen was recorded as carious using the appropriate code and if no lesion was visible the surface was scored as sound. A sickle probe blunted to a diameter of 0.4 mm at the tip was issued to the examiners. This was only used to investigate surfaces where doubt existed after the visual inspection. If the probe tip could not be inserted into the suspect lesion the surface was recorded as sound. It was thought that this would give an underestimate of the total prevalence of caries, but Downer and O'Mullane (1973)* have shown that the accuracy of diagnosis with initial lesions included, is rather lower than that for the diagnosis of cavities used in this study.

The carious lesion was divided into two categories according to the treatment needed. It was recorded as 'decayed' where in the opinion of the examiner the cavity could be filled, and 'unrestorable' when the cavity was thought to necessitate extraction or pulp treatment of the tooth.

During the pre-pilot and pilot studies each tooth was examined once, the dentist first identifying the tooth and then calling the surface codes in the predetermined order. This was found to cause confusion, especially in the anterior part of the mouth. For example, the tooth designation of 2 or 3 (lateral incisor or canine) could be mistaken for the surface codes 2 or 3 (decayed or unrestorable). For this reason the dentists in the main training programme were asked to examine all the·teeth twice, the first time to identify and record each tooth present in the mouth and the second to diagnose the state of the surfaces. They were also asked to use the word 'code' as a prefix when calling surface conditions.

On the few occasions when both a primary tooth and its permanent successor were present in the mouth, the surface data were recorded for the permanent tooth.

---

*Manchester Dental School, personal communication

Trauma of Incisors

The dentist first observed the upper and lower incisors collectively. If there was an injury to any of these teeth he examined each in turn and recorded the degree of traumatic effect and the presence of crowns as appropriate.

Dentures

These were recorded as present or absent.

Gums and Calculus

Assessments of the gum condition, the amount of debris on the teeth and the presence or absence of calculus followed in sequence. The word 'debris' was used instead of plaque as this was found to be more definitive in the minds of observers. The mouth was divided into six segments for each of these items as indicated earlier. During the development programme two methods of examination were tried.   The first was to examine each segment for the three conditions in turn before passing on to the next, the second was to record each feature in turn for the whole mouth. Although this second method involved going round the mouth three times it was found easier to perform as the dentist was able to concentrate on one aspect of the diagnosis at a time.

The criteria for the assessment of the gum condition were based upon the treatment requirements of that segment. The debris was recorded according to absence or amount present, and the calculus was a straightforward present or absent assessment.

The Occlusal Assessment

The occlusion and position of the teeth are made up by a number of features, each of which is subject to a continuous range of variation. Deviation from the ideal state in any of these features does not necessarily constitute a need for treatment. Any assessment of the occlusion can be divided into three categories:

1. Occlusal features.
2. Aetiological features.
3. The need for orthodontic treatment.

Occlusal features are the end result, which can be observed and assessed on the same basis as any other oral condition.

Aetiological features are the causative mechanisms of the existing occlusion, which may have a profound effect on the possibility or difficulty of corrective treatment. They are, however, more difficult to assess.

The need for orthodontic treatment is recognised as being, to a large extent, a subjective assessment. It is usually accepted that orthodontic treatment is necessary if the occlusion or position of the teeth adversely affects oral function, oral health or personal appearance. No wholly satisfactory objective measure of these conditions has been devised. Assessments of treatment needs have, therefore, always been made on the basis of personal opinion, or by measuring the deviation from the ideal of various occlusal features. The latter method depends on the subjective assumption that deviation from the ideal beyond a certain point constitutes need for treatment.

With these points in mind, and in view of the facts that the dental examination
would be carried out by dentists after only one week's specific training; with no
radiographic examination; and with an average of only 6 minutes for the whole
examination, it was decided to make an assessment of observable occlusal features
only, excluding aetiological factors. In addition the examiner was asked for a
personal opinion regarding the necessity for and type of orthodontic treatment.
It was hoped to choose occlusal features which could be reliably assessed, indicate
the range of occlusal variation in the sample, and provide a basis for an
assessment of the potential treatment load.

After testing the reproducibility of various diagnostic features in the development
programme, and the two pilot studies, the following were selected for assessment:-

    1.   The incisal overbite.
    2.   The incisal overjet.
    3.   Buccal crossbite.
    4.   The antero-posterior relationship of the dental arches.
    5.   The presence of instanding upper incisors.
    6.   The presence of mucosal trauma.
    7.   Actual or potential crowding of the teeth.

Other features which were originally included in the test programme were finally
excluded, either because of the difficulty of assessment or because of the time
limitations. It will be appreciated that, without radiographs, a small proportion
of occlusal problems will not be observed, but it was felt that the main features
of the occlusion were covered and that variation in these features constituted the
main load of orthodontic treatment.

The criteria for the assessments are given earlier.

Other oral conditions

There are many relatively uncommon conditions about which information would be of
value but which would necessitate recording a negative finding in the majority of
children. To save examination time space was left on the back of the recording
sheet in which this information could be written. Each examiner was given a check
list containing a number of such conditions and after the formal part of the
examination the recorder prompted him to mention any additional clinical feature.
When this was on the check list the appropriate code number was recorded. The
list was by no means comprehensive, so many conditions were not included. In these
cases the examiner indicated the code of the group to which that condition belonged,
together with brief details of the clinical finding.

SS1011   # DENTAL EXAMINATION

	Area	School	Child	Int.
Serial number							

Name...

	Day	Mth.	Yr.
Date of birth			

	M	F
Sex	1	2

School..

Interviewer's name................................. No. □

Dentist's name.................................... No. □

Date of examination | | | |

Rac. Orig.		
W. Cauc.	1
Neg.	2
Ind./ Pak.	3
Orien./ Mong.	4
.... Other (specify)	5
Not known	6

IF NO EXAMINATION: WHY NOT?

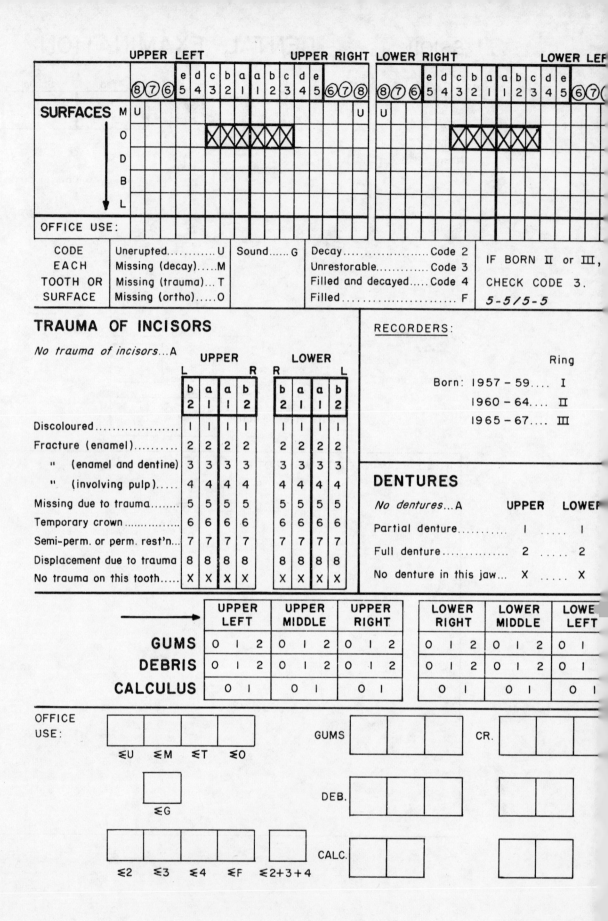

		UPPER LEFT										UPPER RIGHT				LOWER RIGHT									LOWER LEFT	
		⑧⑦⑥	e 5	d 4	c 3	b 2	a 1	a 1	b 2	c 3	d 4	e 5	⑥⑦⑧	⑧⑦⑥	e 5	d 4	c 3	b 2	a 1	a 1	b 2	c 3	d 4	e 5	⑥⑦

SURFACES

M	U												U	U											
O					☒	☒	☒	☒									☒	☒	☒	☒				
D																								
B																								
L																								

OFFICE USE:

CODE EACH TOOTH OR SURFACE	Unerupted............U Missing (decay).....M Missing (trauma)...T Missing (ortho).....O	Sound......G	Decay....................Code 2 Unrestorable............Code 3 Filled and decayed.....Code 4 Filled......................F	IF BORN II or III, CHECK CODE 3. *5-5/5-5*

TRAUMA OF INCISORS

No trauma of incisors...A

	UPPER				LOWER			
	L			R	R			L
	b 2	a 1	a 1	b 2	b 2	a 1	a 1	b 2
Discoloured.....................	1	1	1	1	1	1	1	1
Fracture (enamel)..........	2	2	2	2	2	2	2	2
" (enamel and dentine)	3	3	3	3	3	3	3	3
" (involving pulp).....	4	4	4	4	4	4	4	4
Missing due to trauma........	5	5	5	5	5	5	5	5
Temporary crown...............	6	6	6	6	6	6	6	6
Semi-perm. or perm. rest'n...	7	7	7	7	7	7	7	7
Displacement due to trauma	8	8	8	8	8	8	8	8
No trauma on this tooth.....	X	X	X	X	X	X	X	X

RECORDERS:

Ring

Born: 1957 – 59.... I
1960 – 64.... II
1965 – 67.... III

DENTURES

No dentures...A   UPPER   LOWER

Partial denture.......... 1 1

Full denture.............. 2 2

No denture in this jaw... X X

→	UPPER LEFT			UPPER MIDDLE			UPPER RIGHT			LOWER RIGHT			LOWER MIDDLE			LOWE LEFT	
GUMS	0	1	2	0	1	2	0	1	2	0	1	2	0	1	2	0	1
DEBRIS	0	1	2	0	1	2	0	1	2	0	1	2	0	1	2	0	1
CALCULUS	0	1		0	1		0	1		0	1		0	1		0	1

OFFICE USE:

≤U   ≤M   ≤T   ≤O   GUMS   CR.

≤G

≤2   ≤3   ≤4   ≤F   ≤2+3+4   CALC.

DEB.

OVERBITE (upper left incisor)

Not measurable.................. Y
Anterior open bite............. 1
Zero overbite.................. 2
Up to and including $\frac{1}{3}$ 3
Over $\frac{1}{3}$, up to and including $\frac{2}{3}$ ... 4
Over $\frac{2}{3}$ 5

OVERJET

	+/−	mm
Upper **LEFT** central incisor ......Y.....		

	+/−	mm
Upper **RIGHT** central incisor .....Y.....		

BUCCAL CROSSBITE

	LEFT	RIGHT
'6' not in occlusion	Y	Y
None....................	0	0
Cusp to cusp..........	1	1
Crossbite............	2	2

OCCLUSION

Class I.................. 4
Class 2 Division I....... 5
Class 2 Division 2...... 6
Class 2 Indefinite........ 7
Class 3.................. 8
Not classified........... 9

INCISORS

No incisors instanding or edge to edge...A

UPPER

	L			R
	b 2	a 1	a 1	b 2
This incisor is instanding....	1	1	1	1
This incisor is edge to edge	2	2	2	2
Is neither...................	X	X	X	X

MUCOSAL TRAUMA

No trauma...A

UPPER		LOWER	
Palatal	1	Lingual	1
Labial	2	Labial	2
Neither	X	Neither	X

CROWDING

UPPER LEFT			UPPER MIDDLE			UPPER RIGHT			LOWER RIGHT			LOWER MIDDLE			LOWER LEFT		
0	1	2	0	1	2	0	1	2	0	1	2	0	1	2	0	1	2

APPLIANCES (Ortho)

No appliances...A

	UPPER	LOWER
Removable ortho. appliance	1	1
Fixed ortho. appliance.....	2	2
Other (specify)............	3	3
No appliance in this jaw....	X	X

IF NO APPLIANCES (A) *and* CHILD BORN
I OR II, DENTIST ASK:

*Have you ever had to wear a brace,
or anything like that?*............... Yes 1
                                              No 0

IF YES:
*Do you still have to wear it, or
have you finished with it now?*

Still wears it 2
Not 3

REFERRAL (Ortho)

a) *In your opinion, will orthodontic
treatment or referral
be necessary?*.................... No 0
Under treatment now 1
Treatment needed 2

b) *In your opinion, what form of
treatment will be required?*

No treatment necessary 0
Under treatment now 1
Extractions only 3
Appliance (with or without extractions) 4
Not known 5

ASK DENTIST: *Any more?*   Yes 1
                                      No 2

FURTHER CONDITIONS AND DENTIST'S COMMENTS: P.T.O. ⟶

CHECK LIST NUMBER	TICK IF TREATMENT NEEDED	COMMENT

CHECK LIST NUMBER	TICK IF TREATMENT NEEDED	COMMENT

Each examiner was asked to provide the following equipment:

1) Two towels.

2) A minimum of four mouth mirrors with new No. 4 plane mirrors.

3) Two tumblers or containers to hold mirrors and probes in an antiseptic solution.

4) One chip syringe.

5) One hand sponge (for washing hands when no running water was available).

6) One polythene bag at least 1' square (in which to place the sponge).

7) Anglepoise lamp.

Each examiner was issued with:

1) 4 - Sickle Probes, the points of which had been blunted to a diameter of 0.4 mm.

2) One 60W bulb for lamp.

3) One device for measuring the incisal overjet.

Pilot Study

Mr R H Bettles

Mr P I Christensen

Mr C Howard

Mr J M James

Mr J P Onions

Mrs J M Scarborough

Mr L J Wallace

Main Study

Miss M Armitage

Mrs M Attrill

Mr J M Bain

Mr L W Brockhurst

Mr C L Carmichael

Mr H R Carter

Miss M B Cogan

Mr J W Coombs

Mr A N Crawford

Mr J B C Cuzner

Mr P G Davies

Mr D R Edwards

Col E Ferguson

Mr A D French

Mr J S Furniss

Mr P Gore

Mr G E Griffith

Mrs E M M Hague

Mrs C L Haine

Mr J F Higson

Mr D M Hobbs

Mr I Hopes

Mr J R Humphreys

Mr R J Izon

Mr J M James

Mr C W D Jones

Mr L Jones

Mr N Kipps

Mr J W Lewis

Mrs M A Libbey

Mr J O Lofthouse

Mr T S Longworth

Mr R Lovewell

Mr W McKay

Mr D C McKendrick

Mr G Morgan

Mr J A E Morris

Mrs E A Morse

Mr K J Moss

Mr J I Munro

Mr J Naylor

Miss J Neden

Dr D M O'Mullane

Mr J D Palmer

Miss A M Paterson

Mr D R Pearse

Mr A R Peck

Mr J P S Pengelly

Mr P C Perkins

Mr J H Pitman

Mrs M B Redfern

Mr S J Redding

Mr L Richardson

Mr H R Rippon

Mr B K Robinson

Mr W L Rothwell

Mrs J A D Saunders

Mr R F Sawle

Miss D E Smith

Mr A C Sorrell

Miss D A Stockel

Miss J Stocks

Mr G O Taylor

Mr W E Titley

Mr G H Tucker

Mr N H Whitehouse

Mr T A Williams

Mrs G M Yates

Appendix D

Questionnaire

CHILDREN'S DENTAL HEALTH

SS 1011

Area	School	Child	Int

Child's Name ....

Date
of
Birth

Day	Month	Year

School ....

Sex   M 1
      F 2

Interviewer's Name .... Date of Interview ....

Auth. No. .... Length of Interview ....

- 1 -

360

(Right section)

INTRODUCE AS NECESSARY
You've told me about all the children in the family, but I would particularly like to talk just about (NAMED CHILD) and not the others for the moment.

2 Has ___ ever been to a dentist's surgery, either for treatment or for any other reason?
EXCLUDE INSPECTION CARRIED OUT AT SCHOOL

Been to dentist's surgery	1	ask (a)-(d)
Not	2	Go to Q41 p19

IF BEEN TO DENTIST'S SURGERY (1)

(a) About how many times, in all, has ___ sat in a dentist's chair?

PROMPT AS NECESSARY

None	0 .... Go to Q5 p5
Once only	1
2 - 4 times	2
5 - 9 times	3
10 - 14 times	4
15 or more times	5
Other (SPECIFY)	6

(b) You say that ___ has sat in the dentist's chair ___ times in all; about how many times would that be in ......

INDIVIDUAL PROMPT

...... the last 6 mths? ....
...... the last year? ....
...... the last 2 years? ....

(c) Has ___ always been seen by the same dentist (same person) or not?

Same dentist	2
Not	3

(d) Has ___ ever had any dental treatment?

Has had treatment	1	ask Q3
Has not	2	Go to Q5 p5

- 3 -

(Left section)

Number ....

1 Can you tell me how many children you have altogether including any not living at home?

STARTING WITH THE ELDEST, ASK FOR EACH CHILD:-

(i) What is his/her name?
(ii) What was his/her age last birthday?
(iii) (May I just check) Does he/she live at home?

ENTER DETAILS IN BOX

Child RING NO.	(i) Name	Br.	Sist.	Named Child	(ii) Age last birth.	(iii) At home Yes	No
1		7	8	9		1	2
2		7	8	9		1	2
3		7	8	9		1	2
4		7	8	9		1	2
5		7	8	9		1	2
6		7	8	9		1	2
7		7	8	9		1	2
8		7	8	9		1	2
9		7	8	9		1	2
10		7	8	9		1	2

- 2 -

I'd like to talk generally about treatment for teeth .....

IF HAS HAD DENTAL TREATMENT (Q2(d) code 1)

3 Has ___ ever had any teeth filled?

   Yes, filled ...... A .... ask (a)
   Not 1

   IF HAD TEETH FILLED (A)

   (a) Has he/she ever had an injection
       to freeze the gum before having
       a filling or not?

   Had injection 2
   Not 3

5 If ___ had a bad back tooth and it was a baby
   (milk) tooth would you rather it was filled, or
   would you rather it was taken out?
   PROMPT AS NEC. "SUPPOSING IT COULD BE FILLED"

   Filled 1
   Taken out 2   } ask (a)
   Other 3
   (SPECIFY)

   (a) Why would you rather ......

4 Has ___ ever had any teeth
   taken out by the dentist?

   Teeth out by dentist ...... B ... ask (a)-(c)
   Not .... 1 ... Go to Q5

   IF HAD TEETH TAKEN OUT (B)

   (a) The teeth ___ had out, were
       these milk (baby) teeth,
       second (permanent) teeth, or
       some of each?

   Milk teeth only 2
   Second teeth only 3
   Some of each 4

   Other (SPECIFY) 5

6 If ___ had a bad back tooth and it was not a
   baby (milk) tooth, but a second (permanent)
   tooth would you rather it was filled, or would
   you rather it was taken out?
   PROMPT AS NEC. "SUPPOSING IT COULD BE FILLED"

   Filled 1
   Taken out 2   } ask (a)
   Other 3
   (SPECIFY)

   (a) Why would you rather ......

   (b) Has ___ ever had gas to
       have a tooth out?

   Had gas 1
   Has not 2

   (c) Has ___ ever had an injection
       to have a tooth out?

   Had injection ...... C ... ask (i)
   Not 1

   IF HAD INJECTION (C)

   (i) Was this injection
       to freeze the gum, or to
       put him to sleep while
       he/she had the tooth out?

   Freeze gum only 2
   Put to sleep 3
   Had both types 4

7 If ___ had a bad front tooth and it was not
   a baby (milk) tooth, but a second (permanent)
   tooth would you rather it was filled, or would
   you rather it was taken out?
   PROMPT AS NEC. "SUPPOSING IT COULD BE FILLED"

   Filled 1
   Taken out 2   } ask (a)
   Other 3
   (SPECIFY)

   (a) Why would you rather ......

8 If ___ went to a dentist tomorrow do you think he/she would need any treatment or not?

Need treatment	1	ask (a)-(b)
Would not	2	
DK	3	Go to Q9

IF WOULD NEED TREATMENT (1)

(a) Do you think ___ would need any fillings?

Need fillings	4
Not	5
DK	6

(b) Do you think ___ would need any teeth taken out?

Need teeth out	7
Not	8
DK	9

9 If ___ had to have any teeth taken out would you prefer this to be done with gas or with injection?

Gas	1	
Injection	2	ask (a)
Other (SPECIFY)	3	
PROBE FULLY		

(a) Why would you prefer that?

10 There are several types of surgeries where a child can have dental treatment. Has ___ ever had dental treatment from ... RUNNING PROMPT ...

INTERVIEWER CHECK:
Was this under the NHS or did you
have to pay?
RECODE IF NEC.

CODE
ALL
THAT
APPLY

... a dentist in the NHS	1	
... a dentist in private practice	2	CHECK
... a school dental clinic	3	
... a (LA) clinic for the under 5's	4	
... or a dental hospital?	5	

see (a) or (b)

IF ONLY ONE TYPE OF DENTIST ATTENDED (Q10 single coded)

(a) Why did ___ go to a .....
(rather than a ..... ?)
PROBE FULLY

(i) 1 or 2 rather than 3(4)
(ii) 3 or 4 rather than 1
(iii) 5

IF MORE THAN ONE TYPE OF DENTIST ATTENDED (Q10 MULTI-CODED)

(b) You say ___ has been to ...
Which type of dentist did
he/she go to first? WRITE IN

1st ....
2nd ....
3rd ....

STARTING WITH THE FIRST:

(i) Why did he/she go to .....(rather than a .....) ?
AS ABOVE at (a)

(ii) Why did he/she change from (1st type) to (2nd type)?

(iii) Why did he/she change from (2nd type) to (3rd type)?

11 Does anyone else in the family go to the same dentist (or group of dentists) as _____ went to last time?

Yes, others go there ..... 1 ... ask (a)
No 2

IF OTHERS IN FAMILY GO THERE (1)

(a) Who else in the family goes to that dentist (or group of dentists)? RELATIONSHIP TO CHILD

All the family 4

12 About how far away from here is the dentist (surgery) _____ went to last time .... RUNNING PROMPT

less than 1 mile 1
1 - 2 miles 2
3 - 4 miles 3
more than that? 4
(SPECIFY)

13 Next time _____ goes to the dentist will he/she go to the same dentist (or group of dentists) as last time or not?

Same dentist 1
Not ..... 2 ... ask (a)
DK 3

IF NOT SAME DENTIST (2)

(a) Why wont _____ be going to the same dentist next time?

14 Beside the special inspection done for this survey has _____ ever had his/her teeth examined at school, by a dentist?

Examined at school ..... 1 ⎱ ask (a)-(b)
Not ..... 2 ⎰ Go to Q15
DK 3

IF EXAMINED AT SCHOOL (1)

(a) Has _____ had his teeth examined while he's/she's been at the school he's/she's at now?

Had teeth examined at this school 4
Not 5
DK 6

(b) About how long ago was the last time he/she had a school dental examination?

.... yrs .... mths
DK 9

15 Has _____ ever brought a note home from school saying that it would be a good idea if he/she went to see a dentist?

Yes ..... 1 ... ask (a)
No 2

IF BROUGHT NOTE HOME (1)

(a) The last time _____ brought a note home did he/she see a dentist within the next month or did you leave it for the time being?

Saw dentist within month 3
Left it for the time being ..... 4 ... ask (i)

IF LEFT IT (4)

(i) Why did you leave it for the time being?

16 Has _____ ever had a fall or some other accident that damaged any of his/her teeth?

Yes .... A ... ask (a)-(g)
No .... O ... Go to Q17

IF YES (A)

	1st time	2nd time	3rd time
(a) How many times has _____ damaged his/her teeth? Number ____			
(b) What was the damage?			
(c) How did it happen?			
(d) Were they (was it) baby (milk) teeth or second teeth?	Baby (milk).. 1 Second 2	1 2	1 2
(e) What was done about the teeth (tooth)?			
(f) May I just check, did _____ go to a dentist to see about the teeth (tooth)?	Yes...3..ask (g) No ...4	3 .. ask (g) 4	3 .. ask (g) 4
IF WENT TO DENTIST (3) (g) Did you have any difficulty at all in getting them treated? (SPECIFY DIFFICULTY)			

- 10 -

17 Has _____ ever had toothache?

Yes .... A ... ask (a)-(f)
No .... O ... Go to Q18

IF YES (A)

	1st time	2nd time	3rd time
(a) How many times has _____ had toothache? Number ____			
(b) How long did the toothache last?			
(c) What did you do about it?			
(d) What happened about the tooth that was aching?			
(e) May I just check, did _____ go to a dentist to see about the tooth (teeth)?	Yes...3..ask (f) No ...4	3 .. ask (f) 4	3 ... ask (f) 4
IF WENT TO DENTIST (3) (f) Did you have any difficulty in getting the toothache treated or not? (SPECIFY DIFFICULTY)			

22 Have any of ____'s teeth ever been ...

INDIVIDUAL PROMPT

	YES	NO
... crossed over	1	...X
... crowded together	2	...X
... sticking out	3	...X
... or anything else like that?	4	...X
(SPECIFY)		
ALL 'NO'	9	Go to Q23

IF YES TO ANY (1 to 4)

(a) Have you asked a dentist if anything should be done about ____'s teeth?

| Asked dentist | 5 | ask (i) |
| Has not | 6 | Go to (b) |

IF ASKED DENTIST (5)

(i) What did the dentist say?

(ii) Has ____ had any dental treatment by the dentist for this?

| Yes, treatment | 7 | ask (iii) |
| Not | 8 | Go to Q23 |

IF TREATMENT (7)

(iii) What kind of treatment did ____ have?

IF HAS NOT ASKED A DENTIST (6)

(b) Why haven't you asked the dentist's advice?

| Corrected itself | 1 | Go to Q23 |

23 Has ____ ever had any other problems with his/her teeth that we haven't talked about?

| Other problems | 1 | ask (a) |
| Not | 2 | |

IF OTHER PROBLEMS (1)

(a) What other problems has he/she had?

- 13 -

Most of the problems that children have with their teeth are because of decay, but sometimes children have other dental problems.

18 Has ____ ever had any trouble with his/her gums?

| Trouble with gums | 1 | ask (a) |
| Not | 2 | |

IF TROUBLE (1)

(a) What kind of trouble?

Another problem that some children have is crooked or protruding teeth.

19 Do you think it is very important, fairly important or not very important that children with crooked or protruding teeth should have them straightened?

Very important	1	
Fairly important	2	ask (a)
Not very important	3	
Other (SPECIFY)	4	

PROBE FULLY

(a) Why do you think it is ____?

20 Do you think that treatment to straighten teeth would be done free for children, or would the parent have to pay?

Free for children	1
Parents have to pay	2
Other (SPECIFY)	3

21 If a child had to wear a brace, about how long would he have to wear it to get his teeth straight?

DO NOT PROMPT

ENTER No. of weeks ....
or months ....
or years ....
or SPECIFY

- 12 -

Could we talk now about the most recent visit or set of visits that ___ has made to the dentist for a check-up, or treatment or any other reason.
EXCLUDE SCHOOL INSPECTION

30 Last time ___ went to the dentist, why did he/she go ... PROMPT AS NECESSARY ... was he/she having trouble with his/her teeth, did you have a note from the school dentist, was it a check-up, or was there some other reason?

CODE ONE ONLY

Trouble 1
Note 2
Check-up 3
Other (SPECIFY) ... 4

31 Did ___ need any treatment?

Treatment needed ...... 1 .... ask (a)
Not 2

IF TREATMENT NEEDED (1)

(a) What kind of treatment was needed?

32 Did you go with ___ last time or not?

With him/her ...... 1 .... ask (a)-(c)
Not .... 2 .... Go to Q33

IF WITH HIM/HER (1)

(a) Did you go into the surgery with ___ when he/she saw the dentist or did you stay in the waiting room?

Went into surgery 3
Stayed in waiting room 4
Other (SPECIFY) 5

(b) Did the dentist say anything to you about ___'s teeth, or not?

Dentist said something ...... 5 .... ask (i)
Did not 6

IF DENTIST SAID SOMETHING (5)

(i) What sort of things did he say?

(c) Would you have liked the dentist to say more (something) or not?

- 15 -

24 Do you usually go with ___ when he/she goes to the dentist or not?

Usually goes ...... 1 .... ask (a)
Does not 2

IF USUALLY GOES (1)

(a) Do you usually go into the surgery with ___ when he/she sees the dentist; or do you stay in the waiting room?

Goes into surgery 3
Stays in waiting room 4
Other (SPECIFY) 5

25 If you can't go, does ___ go by himself/herself or does someone else go with him/her?

By self ...... 1 .... ask (a)
With someone ...... A

IF SOMEONE ELSE (A)

(a) Who goes with him/her if you can't go? (RELATIONSHIP TO CHILD)

26 Can we go back to the first time that ___ ever went to a dentist's surgery.

How old was ___ then, the first time he went to a dentist's surgery?

.... years

27 Why was he/she taken that first time?

28 Did he/she mind going to the dentist that first time?

Did mind 1
Not 2

29 Did he/she need any dental treatment?

Needed treatment ...... 3 .... ask (a)
Did not 4

IF NEEDED TREATMENT (3)

(a) What kind of treatment was needed?

- 14 -

33 Do you think _____ minds going to the dentist or not?

Minds 1
Does not 2

RECORD COMMENTS

34 How do you think he/she feels in the waiting room?

35 How does he/she behave in the dentist's chair?

36 Has _____ ever had an unpleasant experience at the dentist's?

Unpleasant experience ...... 1 .... ask (a)
Not 2

IF UNPLEASANT EXPERIENCE (1)

(a) What was it that made it unpleasant?

37 Has _____ ever been difficult over going to see the dentist?

Difficult ...... 1 ... ask (a)
Not 2

IF DIFFICULT (1)

(a) What did you do about it?

38 Next time _____ goes to the dentist do you think he/she will need any encouragement?

Need encouragement ...... 1 ... ask (a)
Not 2

IF WILL NEED ENCOURAGEMENT (1)

(a) In what ways will you encourage him/her?

39 How will _____ decide when it is time for _____ to go to the dentist again?

Appt. made at last visit 9   Go to Q58 p27

40 How will you make the appointment, will you ......

RUNNING PROMPT

... write 1
will you phone 2
will you call in 3
or will it be some other way? 4
(SPECIFY)

Go to Q58 p27

IF NEVER BEEN TO DENTIST

BEEN TO DENTIST .... Go to Q58 p27

41 Beside the special inspection done for this survey has ___ ever had his/her teeth examined at school?

Examined at school .... 1] ask (a)-(b)
Not .... 2]
DK .... 3] Go to Q42

IF EXAMINED AT SCHOOL (1)

(a) Has ___ had his/her teeth examined while he's/she's been at the school he's/she's at now?

Had teeth examined at this school 4
Not 5
DK 6

(b) About how long ago was the last time he/she had a school dental examination?

.... yrs .... mths

DK 9

42 Has ___ ever brought a note home from school saying that it would be a good idea if he/she went to see a dentist?

Yes ...... 1] ask (a)
No 2

IF BROUGHT NOTE HOME (1)

(a) Why didn't ___ go to see a dentist?

43 There are several types of surgeries where a child can have dental treatment. Where do you think ___ will go if he/she has to ... RUNNING PROMPT ....

... a dentist in the NHS 1
a dentist in private practice .... 2 CHECK
a school dental clinic 3
or a dental hospital? 5

ask (a)

INTERVIEWER CHECK:
Will this be under the NHS or will you expect to pay? RECODE IF NEC.

(a) Why would you take ___ to a ___ (rather than a ___)? PROBE FULLY

(i) 1 or 2 rather than 3
(ii) 3 rather than 1
(iii) 5

- 19 -

- 18 -

I'd like to talk generally about treatment for teeth ......

44 If ___ had a bad back tooth and it was a
baby (milk) tooth would you rather it was
filled, or would you rather it was taken
out?
PROMPT AS NEC. "SUPPOSING IT COULD BE FILLED"

Filled 1	
Taken out 2	} ask (a)
Other 3	
(SPECIFY)	

   (a) Why would you rather ....

45 If ___ had a bad back tooth and it was not
a baby (milk) tooth, but a second (permanent)
tooth would you rather it was filled, or
would you rather it was taken out?
PROMPT AS NEC. "SUPPOSING IT COULD BE FILLED"

Filled 1	
Taken out 2	} ask (a)
Other 3	
(SPECIFY)	

   (a) Why would you rather ....

46 If ___ had a bad front tooth and it was not
a baby (milk) tooth, but a second (permanent)
tooth would you rather it was filled, or
would you rather it was taken out?
PROMPT AS NEC. "SUPPOSING IT COULD BE FILLED"

Filled 1	
Taken out 2	} ask (a)
Other 3	
(SPECIFY)	

   (a) Why would you rather ....

47 If ___ went to a dentist tomorrow do
you think he/she would need any
treatment or not?

Need treatment 1	ask (a)-(b)
Would not 2	
DK 3	Go to Q48

   IF WOULD NEED TREATMENT (1)
   (a) Do you think ___ would need
      any fillings?

Need fillings 4	
Not 5	
DK 6	

   (b) Do you think ___ would need
      any teeth taken out?

Need teeth out 7	ask (a)
Not 8	
DK 9	

48 If ___ had to have any teeth taken
out would you prefer this to be done
with gas or with injection?

Gas 1	
Injection 2	ask (a)
Other (SPECIFY) 3	
PROBE FULLY	

   (a) Why would you prefer that?

370

49 Has ____ ever had a fall or some other accident that damaged any of his/her teeth?

Yes .... A ... ask (a)-(e)
No .... 0 ... Go to Q50

IF YES (A)

(a) How many times has ____ damaged his/her teeth?   Number ...

	1st time	2nd time	3rd time
(b) What was the damage?			
(c) How did it happen?			
(d) Were they (was it) baby (milk) teeth or second teeth?	Baby (milk).. 1 Second 2	Baby (milk).. 1 Second 2	Baby (milk).. 1 Second 2
(e) What was done about the teeth (tooth)?			

50 Has ____ ever had toothache?

Yes .... A ... ask (a)-(d)
No .... 0 ... Go to Q51

IF YES (A)

(a) How many times has ____ had toothache?   Number ____

	1st time	2nd time	3rd time
(b) How long did the toothache last?			
(c) What did you do about it?			
(d) What happened about the tooth that was aching?			

Most of the problems that children have with
their teeth are because of decay, but sometimes
children have other dental problems.

51 Has ___ ever had any trouble
with his/her gums?

Trouble with gums ...... 1 .... ask (a)
Not 2

IF TROUBLE (1)
(a) What kind of trouble?

52 Another problem that some children have is
crooked or protruding teeth.
Do you think it is very important, fairly
important or not very important that
children with crooked or protruding
teeth should have them straightened?

Very important 1
Fairly important 2
Not very important 3
Other (SPECIFY) 4
} ask (a)
PROBE FULLY

(a) Why do you think it is ___ ?

53 Do you think that treatment to
straighten teeth would be done free
for children, or would the parent
have to pay?

Free for children 1
Parents have to pay 2
Other (SPECIFY) 3

54 If a child had to wear a brace,
about how long would he have to
wear it to get his teeth straight?

ENTER No. of weeks ....
or months ....
or years ....
or SPECIFY

DO
NOT
PROMPT

55 Have any of ___ 's teeth ever been ...
INDIVIDUAL PROMPT
... crossed over ......
crowded together ....
sticking out ....
... or anything else like that?
(SPECIFY)

YES NO
1 .. X
2 .. X
3 .. X
4 .. X
} ask (a)

ALL 'NO' .... 9 ..Go to Q56

IF YES TO ANY (1 to 4)
(a) Have you ever thought of asking
a dentist if anything should be
done about ___ 's teeth?
RECORD ALL COMMENTS

Thought of asking 5
Have not 6

56 Has ___ ever had any other dental problems
that we haven't talked about?

Other problems .... 1 ... ask (a)
Not 2

IF OTHER PROBLEMS (1)
(a) What other problems has he/she had?

57 You told me earlier that ___ has not
been to a dentist. Is there any
reason why he/she hasn't been?
(What is the reason?)

None 1

TO ALL

Could we go back to when _____ was very small.

58 When he/she was a baby did you ever take him/her to the baby welfare clinic?

Baby clinic ...... 1 .... ask (a)

Not 2

RECORD COMMENTS

IF BABY CLINIC (1)

(a) How often did you go?

59 When _____ was a baby was he/she breast fed, bottle fed or both?

Breast 1

Bottle ...... 2 } ask (a)

Both 3

....

IF BOTTLE OR BOTH (2,3)

(a) Till what age did he/she have main day-time feeds from the bottle?

60 Once _____ was on solids for main meals did he/she ever have drinks of orange or milk from a bottle?

Yes ...... 1 .... ask (a)

No 2

IF YES (1)

(a) Till what age did he/she sometimes have drinks from a bottle?

61 Did you regularly give _____ any fruit drinks, such as blackcurrant juice or rosehip syrup?

Yes ...... 1 .... ask (a)
No 2

IF YES (1)

(a) What sort of fruit drinks did you give him/her?

62 When _____ was small did he ever have a dummy to suck or not?

Had dummy ...... 3 .... ask (a)
Not 4

IF HAD DUMMY (3)

(a) Till what age did he/she have a dummy?

63 When _____ was small did he/she ever have a dinky or dormel feeder, or not?
SHOW PICTURE AS NECESSARY

Had dinky/dormel ...... 1 .... ask (a)-(b)
Did not ...... 2 .... Go to Q64

IF HAD DINKY/DORMEL FEEDER (1)

(a) Till what age did he/she have a dinky (dormel) feeder?
....

(b) What kinds of things did _____ have in the dinky (dormel) feeder?

64 Some children get into the habit of sucking their thumb. Has _____ ever been in the habit of sucking his/her thumb or fingers?

Sucked thumb or fingers ...... 4 .... ask (a)
Not ...... 5 .... Go to Q65

IF SUCKED (4)

(a) Does _____ suck his/her thumb or fingers now or not?

Yes, now 1
Not now ...... 2 .... ask (i)

IF NOT NOW (2)

(i) At what age did he/she stop?

Now thinking generally about children's teeth.

65 About what age do you think children usually get their first permanent front teeth? .... yrs

66 About what age do you think children usually get their first permanent back teeth? .... yrs

67 About what age do you think children usually lose their last baby back teeth? .... yrs

68 What do you think is the youngest age at which children's teeth can decay (or go bad)? .... yrs

69 What do you think causes teeth to decay (or go bad)?

DK 1

70 What do you think can be done to help prevent decay? (SPECIFY)

DK 1
Nothing 2

71 When do you think children should first be taken to the dentist?

When tooth aches or having trouble with teeth .... 1 .... Go to Q72

FOR ALL EXCEPT "WHEN TOOTH ACHES"

(a) Why do you think children should first be taken to the dentist when ..... ?

74 During the last 6 months have you ever looked inside ____'s mouth to see if his/her back teeth were clean (properly brushed) or not?

Looked 1
Not 2

75 (May I just check) During the last 6 months have you ever brushed ____'s back teeth for him/her or not?

Brushed 3
Not 4

76 During the last 6 months have you ever looked inside ____'s mouth to see if his/her teeth were going bad (decayed) or not?

Looked for bad teeth ...... 5 .... ask (a)
Not 6

IF LOOKED FOR BAD TEETH (5)
(a) How would you tell they were going bad?

72 Do you think children should be encouraged to brush their teeth, or not?

Yes ...... 1 ... ask (a)-(c)
No .... 2 ... ask (a), then go to Q73

(a) Why do you say that?

(b) About what age do you think children should first be encouraged to brush their teeth? .... yrs

(c) About what age do you think children should be able to brush their teeth properly by themselves? .... yrs

73 Does ____ brush his/her teeth at all?

Yes ...... 8 ... ask (a)-(c)
No .... 9 ... Go to Q74

IF YES (8)
(a) How often does ____ brush his/her teeth? .... times per ....

(b) At what times of day does ____ brush his/her teeth?

(c) Do you check in any way whether ____ has brushed his/her teeth or not?

Mother checks ...... 1 ... ask (i) & (ii)
Does not .... 2 ... Go to Q74

IF MOTHER CHECKS (1)
(i) How do you check?

(ii) About how often do you check?

77 Have you ever heard of fluoride?

Yes ...... 1 ... ask (a)-(d)
No ...... 2 ... Go to Q78

IF YES (1)

(a) What effect do you think fluoride has on teeth?

(b) In different parts of the country the water supply has different amounts of fluoride in it.
Some areas have water which naturally contains sufficient fluoride for teeth; do you think your water naturally has sufficient fluoride, or not?

Naturally sufficient ...... 1 ... Go to (c)
Not 2
DK ...... 3 } ask (i)

IF NOT OR DK (2,3)

(i) Has fluoride been added to your water supply or not?

Added ...... 4 ... ask (ii)
Not 5
DK ...... 6 } ask (iii)

IF ADDED (4)

(ii) How long ago was fluoride first introduced in your area?

....

IF NOT OR DK (5,6)

(iii) Would you like fluoride to be added to your water supply or not?

Would like 1
Not 2
RECORD COMMENTS

(c) Besides fluoride in the water do you know of any other ways of getting fluoride? (SPECIFY)

No 1

(d) Have you ever talked to a dentist about fluoride?

Talked to dentist ...... 1 ... ask (i)
Not 2

IF TALKED TO DENTIST (1)

(i) What did the dentist say?

We are interested in the sorts of meals that children have. Could you tell me about ___'s meals for an ordinary weekday (Mon-Fri)?

78 What does ___ usually eat for breakfast?
DO NOT PROMPT LIST

CODE ALL THAT APPLY

Cereal/porridge 1
Cooked breakfast 2
Toast 3
Bread and butter 4
Other (SPECIFY) 5

79 What does he/she usually drink at breakfast?

Water 1
Milk 2
Tea/coffee 3
Other (SPECIFY) 4

80 Does ___ usually have anything to eat in the school break times, or not?

Yes ...... 1 ... ask (a)
No 2
DK 3

IF YES (1)

(a) What sort of things does he/she have?

81 Where does ___ have his/her midday meal during term time?

At home 4
At school 5
Other (SPECIFY) 6

82 What kind of thing does ___ usually eat at midday during term time?

School dinner 1
Other cooked dinner (ie meat & 2 veg plus sweet) 2
Sandwiches 3
Other (SPECIFY) 4

83 When ___ gets home from school in the afternoon does he/she have anything to eat straight away, say within half an hour of getting home, or not?

Eats straight away ...... 1 ... ask (a)
Not 2

IF EATS STRAIGHT AWAY (1)

(a) What kind of thing would he/she usually eat then?

84 If he/she is thirsty, what would he/she be likely to drink when he/she got home from school?

Water 1
Milk 2
Tea/coffee 3
Other (SPECIFY) 4

85 On an ordinary weekday, would ___ usually have any other meals, snacks, and drinks that day, or not?

Yes .... 1 ... ask (a)
No 2

IF YES (1)

(a) What other meals, snacks and drinks would he/she usually have?
COMPLETE EACH COLUMN

Name of meal/snack	What ___ would eat	What ___ would drink

86 Most children are fond of sweet things such as sweets, chocolates and biscuits.

Would you say that ___ is particularly fond of sweet things or about average?

Particularly fond 1
Average 2
Less than average 3

87 Do you usually keep some sweets in the house or not?

Keeps sweets ...... 1 ... ask (a)
Not 2

IF KEEPS SWEETS (1)

(a) If ___ wanted a sweet could he/she help himself/herself or would he/she have to ask you first?

Help self 3
Ask first 4

88 Is there any particular day of the week when ___ usually has more sweets than on other days?
CODE WHICH DAY

No particular day 8
Monday 1
Tuesday 2
Wednesday 3
Thursday 4
Friday 5
Saturday 6
Sunday 7

89 On an average (___) day, what sorts of sweets and about how many would ___ have?

90 Do you usually keep some biscuits or cakes in the house or not?

Keep some biscuits ...... 1 ... ask (a)
Not 2

IF KEEPS BISCUITS (1)

(a) If ___ wanted a biscuit or cake could he/she help himself/herself or would he/she have to ask you first?

Help self 3
Ask first 4

91 Would you say that in a week ___ eats ..... RUNNING PROMPT

a lot of cakes and biscuits 1
a fair number of cakes and biscuits 2
or not many cakes and biscuits 3

RECORD COMMENTS

377

92 Earlier I asked about ____'s brothers and sisters. Now I'd like to ask who else lives here.

CLASSIFICATION

(a) HOUSEHOLD BOX: Standard def. EXCLUDING CHILDREN

	Mother	Father
Ring No.	RELATIONSHIP TO CHILD	
1		
2		
3		
4		
5		
6		

(b) Age last birthday

(c) At what age did you finish your full-time education? (RQ for husband)

	Mother	Father
under 15	1	1
15	2	2
16	3	3
17	4	4
18	5	5
19 or more	6	6

(d) Employment ...

	Mother	Father
full-time	1	1
part-time	2	2
not working	3	3

93 Have you ever worked in any part of the Health Service, or with children?

Yes 1
No 2

94 What is/was your usual job?

Never worked X

95 (Could you tell me) what is/was your husband's occupation?

OCCUPATION

INDUSTRY

We've been talking mostly about ____'s teeth. I'd like to talk now about your own teeth, (and your husband's teeth).

	Mother	Father

96 Have you still got some of your natural teeth or have you lost them all? (Could I ask about your husband?)

	Mother	Father
Some/all natural teeth	1 ask (a)-(c)	1 ask (a)-(c)
None	2 ask (d)	2 ask (d)

FOR PARENTS WITH SOME/ALL NATURAL TEETH (CODE 1)

(a) If you went to the dentist with an aching back tooth would you prefer the dentist to fill it or take it out? (Could I ask about your husband?)

	Mother	Father
Fill it	3	3
Take it out	4	4

(b) In general do you go to the dentist for a regular check-up, an occasional check-up or only when you are having trouble with your teeth? (Could I ask about your husband?)

	Mother	Father
Regular	1	1
Occasional	2	2
Trouble	3	3

(c) Have you ever been fitted with partial dentures (that is false teeth on a plate)? (Could I ask about your husband?)

	Mother	Father
Yes	1	1
No	2	2

FOR PARENTS WITH NO NATURAL TEETH (CODE 2)

(d) How old were you when you lost the last of your natural teeth? (Could I ask about your husband?)

	Mother	Father
	.... yrs	.... yrs

101 (Although it's very difficult to imagine things so far ahead) At some time may need to have a complete set of false teeth.

When would you guess that might be .....

When he/she is in his/her ..... 20's 2
30's 3
40's 4
50's 5
60's or more 6
or Never? 7

DK 9

RECORD COMMENTS

102 Are there any (other) comments that you would like to make about dental health and dentistry?

No 1

97 How long ago did you yourself go to the dentist's, for treatment or a check-up?

.... yrs .... mths

GIVE MONTHS AS WELL IF LESS THAN 2 YRS AGO

98 Some people dislike going to the dentist very much while others don't mind at all. Do you dislike going or don't you mind?

Dislike 1
Don't mind 2

99 What do you yourself find most unpleasant about going to the dentist, if anything?

Nothing 1

100 What do you think children find most unpleasant about going to the dentist, if anything?

Nothing 1

Printed in England for Her Majesty's Stationery Office by Hobbs the Printers Ltd So'ton
(2191) Dd506571 K18 1/75 G1107/2

WEST HERTS & WATFORD
POSTGRADUATE MEDICAL
                CENTRE,
WATFORD GENERAL HOSPITAL,
SHRODELLS WING,
VICARAGE ROAD,
WATFORD, WD1 8HB